Thinking Strategies for Nursing Practice

Thinking Strategies for Nursing Practice

Marsha E. Fonteyn, PhD, RN, CCRN, CS

Associate Professor
School of Nursing
University of San Francisco
San Francisco, California

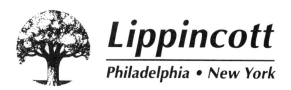

Lippincott
Philadelphia • New York

Acquisitions Editor: Mary P. Gyetvan, RN, MSN
Assistant Editor: Susan M. Keneally
Production Editor: Virginia Barishek
Production Manager: Helen Ewan
Production Service: P.M. Gordon Associates, Inc.

Compositor: Maryland Composition
Printer/Binder: R.R. Donnelley & Sons
   Company/Crawfordsville
Cover Designer: Jerry Cable
Cover Printer: Lehigh Press

9 8 7 6 5 4 3 2 1

Library of Congress Cataloging-in-Publication Data
Fonteyn, Marsha E.
    Thinking strategies for nursing practice / Marsha E. Fonteyn.
       p.   cm.
    Includes bibliographical references and index.
    ISBN 0–397–55274–2
    1. Nursing—Decision making   2. Thought and thinking. I. Title.
    [DNLM: 1. Nursing Process. 2. Mental Processes. WY 100 F683t
    1998
    RT42.F65 1998
    610.73—dc21
    DNLM/DLC   97–17478
    for Library of Congress   CIP

To *the nurses* whose thinking strategies and practice wisdom are the essence of this book.

To *the students* in my course Learning Clinical Reasoning who created the clinical dilemmas presented in this book.

To *my husband, Paul,* whose love and support sustained me throughout this project.

To *my children, John and Mieke,* who keep me humble, and make life fun.

REVIEWERS

Joyce Young Johnson, PhD, RN, CCRN
Assistant Professor, School of Nursing
College of Health Science
Georgia State University
Atlanta, Georgia

Barbara A. Jones, DNSc, RN
Associate Professor, Division of Nursing
Gwynedd-Mercy College
Gwynedd Valley, Pennsylvania

PREFACE

From ancient times, scholars have proposed that the ability to reflect on one's thoughts represents the core of being human. Aristotle told us: "To be conscious that we are perceiving or thinking is to be conscious of our own existence." "Cogito, ergo sum," declared Descartes, "I think, therefore I am." More recently, James Fulbright challenged us to "Dare to think. . . . We must learn to explore all the options and possibilities that confront us in a complex and rapidly changing world." Sound critical thinking is becoming an increasingly vital component for human survival in our complicated modern world. Skill in thinking is particularly important in nursing practice where wise judgments and correct clinical decisions can often mean the difference between life and death.

Although skill in thinking is intrinsic to effective nursing practice, it may not be something that nurses are consciously aware of during their care provision. Nurses may not often give much consideration to the thinking strategies that they use when reasoning and making decisions in clinical practice. As client care becomes increasingly more complex and less predictable and as care is provided in less structured environments, such as the home, busy nurses might wonder how they could find the time or energy to think about their thinking. Indeed, they might even wonder what difference it would make if they were to become more aware of their thinking in practice. A growing body of research suggests that such cognitive awareness is important, and that taking the time and energy to think about one's thinking provides an important means for individuals to improve their thinking strategies and problem-solving skills. The term *metacognition* has been used by cognitive scientists to describe the knowledge and understanding that individuals develop about how they think. Studies in cognitive science support the value of this type of self-reflection for developing and improving thinking skills in any domain, including nursing practice. *Thinking Strategies for Nursing Practice* is intended to help nurses to think better in their practice.

Unit One of this book gives information about what is known about how nurses think in practice, and provides details about the Thinking in Practice (TIP) study on which this book is based. This descriptive study used the think aloud method to identify and describe the thinking strategies that nurses use in practice. The subjects in the study were 15 registered nurses with extensive experience in a specific area of nursing practice, including: critical care, cardiovascular, emergency, home health, obstetric, oncology, pediatric, and psychiatric nursing. In addition, one subject in the TIP study had extensive knowledge and skill in interpreting laboratory data, and one was highly experienced in psychiatric case management. Subjects in the TIP study had been identified by their colleagues as nurses who were particularly skilled in thinking about and caring for clients in their specific area of practice; they were distinguished for their excellence in clinical reasoning and for consistently having positive client outcomes.

Findings from the TIP study revealed 12 predominant thinking strategies that were consistently used by the nurse-subjects regardless of their area of clinical practice. The 12 predominant thinking strategies are:

- Recognizing a pattern
- Setting priorities
- Searching for information
- Generating hypotheses
- Making predictions
- Forming relationships
- Stating a proposition
- Asserting a practice rule
- Making choices
- Judging the value
- Drawing conclusions
- Providing explanations.

Unit Two of the book provides an elaboration of these thinking strategies, with numerous examples from the thoughts of the highly experienced nurses who took part in the TIP study.

Unit Three contains a collection of clinical dilemmas representing a variety of areas of nursing practice. All of the clinical dilemmas contain three important characteristics: data about the dilemma, an inherent goal, and obstacles. The data about the dilemma are revealed in a series of sequential descriptions that are intended to mimic the reality of clinical practice, in which not all information about a dilemma is available upon first encountering the situation; additional information becomes available only as time passes and more data are obtained. Embedded in each dilemma is an inherent goal that represents the desired outcome of the dilemma. The obstacles are the characteristics of the situation that make it difficult for the nurse to resolve the dilemma.

Unit Three allows the reader to closely examine how nurses think when resolving dilemmas that are familiar to them because of their domain (practice) expertise. This part of the book reveals nurses' thinking in action. The same pattern is followed with each chapter in Unit Three: (1) the clinical dilemmas are discussed by experienced nurse clinicians who think aloud as they consider how to resolve each dilemma; (2) each nurse's thoughts about a dilemma are followed by the author's comments about the thinking strategies that the nurse used while thinking and about how those strategies assisted the nurse to resolve the dilemma; (3) the author's comments are then followed by a variety of thinking activities that encourage the individual reader to reflect on his or her thinking in practice. Completion of these thinking activities will assist the reader to develop a repertoire of effective thinking strategies to use in practice, and will help the reader to improve his or her metacognition.

The body of clinical knowledge and information needed for nursing practice is increasing too rapidly for nurses to remember it all. Moreover, possessing an encyclopedic memory of facts and concepts will not ensure effective thinking in practice. An understanding of the thinking strategies that experienced nurses use in their practice coupled with an appreciation of one's own thinking strategies will assist readers to improve their thinking in their practice.

Marsha E. Fonteyn, PhD, RN, CCRN, CS

ACKNOWLEDGMENTS

I am particularly grateful to Dr. Anastasia Fisher, whose contribution to the substance of this book was substantial and who shared a magical time of discovery with me ("Don't let it be forgot that once there was a spot for one brief shining moment that was known as Camelot"). I am also grateful to the many special individuals who provided material for the clinical dilemmas, served as discussants of the dilemmas, or reviewed the manuscript.

I have been incredibly impressed with everyone associated with Lippincott–Raven Publishers; what a class act! I am especially indebted to Susan Keneally, Assistant Editor; Mary Gyetvan, Acquisitions Editor; and Donna Hilton, Vice President and Publisher.

I am also grateful for special friends whose faith in my ability to complete this project was a constant source of strength and encouragement: Mary, Missy, Suzie, Joan, Ellen, Gayle, Jane, and Norma.

CONTENTS

UNIT THREE

Thinking about Clinical Dilemmas

ONE

Introduction

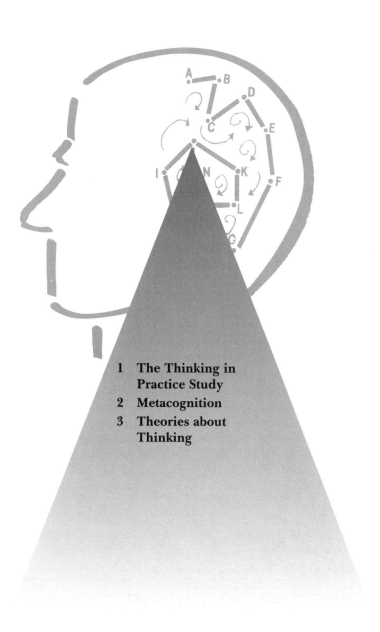

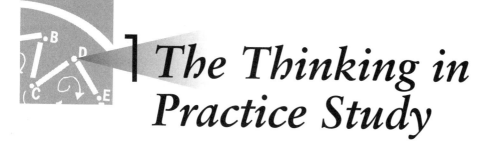

The Thinking in Practice Study

The purpose of this book is twofold: (1) to describe the thinking strategies that nurses use in clinical practice and (2) to assist nurses to develop and improve their own thinking in practice.

This book is based on a descriptive study of nurses' thinking in practice (the Thinking in Practice [TIP] Study), which was conducted between 1994 and 1995. The study was conceived by Dr. Marsha Fonteyn; the coinvestigator of the study was Dr. Anastasia Fisher. The project was funded by the Faculty Development Fund of the University of San Francisco, School of Nursing, and by a grant from Lippincott-Raven Publishing Company. The aims of the study were

1. To identify the predominant thinking strategies that nurses use in practice.
2. To describe the nature of each of these thinking strategies in detail.
3. To identify and describe the other (less dominant) thinking strategies that nurses use in practice.
4. To identify methods to assist nurses to improve their thinking in practice.

The study extended the investigators' earlier work examining nurses' thinking using the think aloud (TA) method and protocol analysis (Grobe, Drew, & Fonteyn, 1991; Fonteyn, 1991; Fonteyn & Grobe, 1993; Fonteyn & Fisher, 1994; Fisher & Fonteyn, 1994; Fonteyn & Fisher, 1995).

The subjects in this study were 15 registered nurses with extensive experience in a specific area of nursing practice, which included critical care, cardiovascular, case management, emergency, trauma, HIV/AIDS, home health, obstetric, oncology, pediatric, and psychiatric nursing. Nurses were chosen for their domain expertise; each had a great deal of knowledge about and experience with client cases within a distinct area of practice. Additionally, one subject was chosen for her extensive knowledge and skill in interpreting laboratory data, and one subject was chosen for her knowledge and skill in psychiatric case management. Subjects were also chosen because they had been identified by their colleagues as nurses who were particularly skilled in thinking about and caring for clients in their specific area of clinical practice; they were distinguished for their excellence in clinical reasoning and for consistently having positive client outcomes.

The findings that are included in this book are from 10 of the 15 study subjects; these 10 represented the greatest diversity of areas of practice.

Clinical dilemmas were constructed to represent each subject's specific area of practice. The dilemmas were designed to represent the typical client situations that the subjects encountered in their particular area of practice. The written descriptions of the dilemmas were presented as scenes, depicting situations that unfolded over time during a nursing shift; additional data about each dilemma were revealed in each subsequent scene, as naturally occurs in real-life situations. The dilemmas included contextual information, such as the time of day that the situation was occurring, and sensory information, such as descriptions of colors, textures, sounds, and temperatures. Each nurse-subject was given an average of three separate dilemmas to think about; each dilemma was made up of an average of three scenes. These clinical dilemmas are displayed in Unit Three.

Each nurse-subject was studied separately on one or two different occasions. Subjects were asked to review and think about the dilemmas that represented client situations from their area of expertise in practice. They were given a written description of the dilemma, one scene at a time, and were instructed to read the information aloud and then think aloud as they considered how to resolve the problems described in the dilemma, so as to continue to reveal their thoughts as consistently and thoroughly as possible. When subjects stated that they were finished with reasoning about a particular scene, they were then given the next scene of the dilemma and were told to read it aloud and then think aloud about the information presented in that scene.

TA studies have commonly used simulation as a stimulus for thinking. Previous investigators have found that clinical simulations, if carefully constructed, are approximately equivalent to real-life situations. The advantages of simulation include predetermination and preselection of the reasoning task, standardization, and compression of real time. Fonteyn, Kuipers, and Grobe (1993, p. 433) propose, "If a case study is presented in segments that provide additional client data and a description of changes in the client's condition that have occurred as time progressed, it will more closely simulate an actual client situation."

The TA method is designed to reveal a subject's thinking at the moment that it is occurring, unhampered by questions or other forms of intrusion into one's thoughts. Until sometime after the turn of the century, the human mind was generally seen as beyond understanding from a scientific perspective. The TA method was first used to study human thinking and problem solving in the 1920s and has been a popular method for studying thinking since the 1950s (Midanik & Hines, 1991). More recently, reports of research using the TA method to study nurses' thinking have begun to appear in the literature (Corcoran, Narayan, & Moreland, 1988; Fonteyn, 1991; Grobe, Drew, & Fonteyn, 1991).

In the TIP Study, as is customary with this method, the TA data were audiotaped and subsequently transcribed before analysis. The total amount of data collected from the 15 nurse-subjects was over 1500 pages of transcribed text from approximately 45 clinical dilemmas with an average of three scenes each. The verbal (qualitative) data were analyzed in a series of steps, as follows:

1.   Transcripts were reviewed generally for initial impressions and to obtain a broad sense of meaning.

2.   Transcripts were imported into a computer program designed to assist investigators in handling qualitative data by supporting the processes of indexing, searching, and theorizing. This program is called NUD·IST, which stands for Nonnumerical Unstructured Data Indexing Searching and Theorizing. The program helps users to "manage, explore and search the text of documents; manage and explore ideas about the data; link ideas and construct theories about the data; test theories about the data; and generate reports including statistical summaries" (NUD·IST program manual, p. 1-1).

3.   A document database was created by importing all of the transcripts of TA data into the NUD·IST program. Each clinical dilemma became a separate document in the database, which was divided into text units, each unit consisting of a sentence within the subject's thoughts. Each document in the database contained 300 to 400 text units. Content method of analysis was used to analyze the text units within each document. The text units were initially examined on-screen and tentatively coded according to the thinking strategies believed to be depicted in that text unit or in several sequential text units. The codes (thinking strategies) were tentatively defined, and the codes and definitions were refined as analysis progressed. Once the initial analysis of a document was completed, a hard copy of the coded text units was closely examined to refine the analysis. All the text units that were given the same code were carefully examined to determine if, indeed, they each fit the code's (thinking strategy's) definition. Those that did not seem to fit the definition were reexamined and recoded.

4.   A feature of NUD·IST that was particularly useful for the purposes of this study is the ability to generate an electronic search of a particular code (thinking strategy) in all the units within all the documents. A printed report of this type of search revealed all text units that were coded as a particular thinking strategy. These reports were then analyzed to identify and define the various features (subcodes) of each thinking strategy. For example, the thinking strategy coded as **recognizing a pattern** was defined as "identifying characteristic pieces of data that fit together." These patterns were found to consist of four distinct types, which were identified and defined as subcodes: **patterns** of case type, **patterns** of standard treatment, **patterns** of familiar circumstances, and **patterns** of lack of fit.

As Hutchinson and Webb (1987, p. 317) so aptly state, "Naming categories of data is tricky and requires close attention to detail." The rich amount of data produced by a qualitative study must be systematically analyzed in a logical fashion. The verbal protocol (TA data) produced in this study revealed the overlapping of certain text units (sentences of the subjects' thoughts) whereby several sequential text units sometimes depicted a single thinking strategy and at other times a single text unit represented more than one thinking strategy. For example, the following sequential text units were both coded as the thinking strategy **asserting a practice rule**: *I mean, his CO_2 is probably a hundred, and you hate to intubate these patients [with chronic obstructive pulmonary disease]. You do everything that you can not to, because you never get them off the ventilator.* Additionally, the first of these text units was also coded as **generating a hypothesis**, and the second text unit was also coded as **providing an explanation**.

External validity of findings from the TIP study is demonstrated by the fit of the thinking strategies identified with what has been previously described in the literature. Each chapter in Unit Two that describes a specific thinking strategy and its varied use in practice is substantiated by a breadth of literature from theory, research, practice, and education. The consistent use of the dominant thinking strategies by each of the subjects, regardless of their area of domain expertise, supports the reliability of study findings. The consistency, repeatability, and stability of the dominant thinking strategies attest to this reliability.

The findings from the TIP Study form the basis for this book. The findings revealed 12 dominant thinking strategies that are used by nurses when thinking about their practice. Also identified were several other less dominant thinking strategies. Each of the dominant thinking strategies is described in detail in separate chapters in Unit Two; those of lesser importance are described in general in the final chapter of Unit Two. The clinical dilemmas and the nurses' "think aloud" responses to them are presented in Unit Three, along with commentary from the investigator (the author of this book). The thinking activities included in each chapter in Unit Three have been designed to give nurses an opportunity to reflect on and practice using the variety of thinking strategies that were demonstrated by the nurse responding to the clinical dilemmas depicted in that chapter.

This book is intended to help nurses improve their metacognitive abilities, that is, their capability to think about their thinking while they are thinking, which makes their thinking better. Increased metacognitive awareness assists nurses to reason more soundly in their practice and to make better and more effective decisions about client care. The next chapter provides further information about metacognition.

References

Corcoran, S., Narayan, S., & Moreland, H. (1998). "Thinking aloud" as a strategy to improve clinical decision-making. *Heart and Lung, 17,* 463–468.

Fisher, A., & Fonteyn, M. (1994). The nature of nursing expertise. In S. Grobe & E. Plutyer-Wenting (Eds.), *Nursing informatics: An international overview for nursing in a technological era* (pp. 331–335). Holland: Elsevier Science B. V.

Fonteyn, M. (1991). *A descriptive analysis of expert critical care nurses' clinical reasoning.* Unpublished doctoral dissertation, University of Texas, Austin.

Fonteyn, M., & Fisher, A. (1994). Critical care nurses' reasoning in practice and associated indicators of patient outcomes. In S. Grobe & E. Plutyer-Wenting (Eds.), *Nursing informatics: An international overview for nursing in a technological era* (pp. 481–485). Holland: Elsevier Science B. V.

Fonteyn, M., & Fisher, A. (1995). Use of think aloud method to study nurses' reasoning and decision making in clinical practice settings. *Journal of Neuroscience Nursing, 27*(2), 121–125.

Fonteyn, M., & Grobe, S. (1993). Expert nurses' clinical reasoning under uncertainty: Representation, structure, and process. *Proceedings of the Sixteenth Annual Symposium on Computer Application in Medical Care.* Los Alimitos, CA: IEEE, Computer Society Press.

Fonteyn, M., Kuipers, B., & Grobe, S. (1993). A description of think aloud methods and protocol analysis. *Qualitative Health Research, 3*(4), 430–441.

Grobe, S., Drew, J., & Fonteyn, M. (1991). A descriptive analysis of experienced nurses' clinical reasoning during a planning task. *Research in Nursing and Health, 14,* 304–314.

Hutchinson, S., & Webb, R. (1987). Teaching qualitative research: Perennial problems and possible solutions. In J. Morse (Ed.), *Qualitative nursing research: A contemporary dialogue* (pp. 301–321). Newbury Park, CA: Sage.

Midanik, L., & Hines, A. (1991). Unstandard ways of answering standard questions: Protocol analysis in alcohol research. *Drug and Alcohol Dependence, 27,* 245–252.

NUD·IST [Computer software]. (1994). Qualitative Solutions and Research Pty, LTD, Melbourne, Australia.

2 Metacognition

A primary goal of this book is to help you develop your metacognitive awareness. Understanding and using metacognition in your practice would be beneficial for several reasons: (1) it would help you to reason more effectively in clinical situations—indeed, in all situations that require critical thinking and problem solving; (2) it would help you to learn and remember new knowledge more easily; and (3) it would allow you to begin to cultivate the habit of continuously developing and refining the important thinking strategies required for sound clinical judgment.

Metacognition is often equated with critical thinking. For example, Paul (1993, p. 91) defines critical thinking as "thinking about your thinking while you're thinking in order to make your thinking better," which is how others define metacognition. Metacognition has been defined as "that body of knowledge and understanding that reflects on cognition itself. That mental activity for which other mental states or processes become the object of reflection." (Yussen, 1985, p. 253). Metacognition consists of both knowledge (about one's ability to think and learn about specific problem tasks as they are encountered) and skill (in thinking and problem solving).

Pesut and Herman (1992, p. 151) propose that "metacognitive skills have always been an implicit part of the nursing process." They contend that the metacognitive skills of monitoring and analyzing are used during the assessment phase of the nursing process, the metacognitive skill of predicting is used during problem identification, the metacognitive skill of planning is useful to the intervention phase of the nursing process, and the metacognitive skills of evaluating and revising are helpful during the evaluative phase of the nursing process.

Paris and Winograd (1990) describe two essential features of metacognition: self-appraisal and self-management. Self-appraisal consists of personal reflections regarding one's knowledge state and abilities. Self-appraisal seeks answers regarding the extent of one's knowledge, the way that one thinks, and the situations and problems in which one uses certain knowledge and thinking skills. As Barrows and Pickell (1991) point out, developing a habit of self-appraisal assists individuals to become more aware of their performance and skills in problem solving and of their need for improving their thinking strategies and for acquiring additional knowledge in specific areas. Likewise, Carnevali and Thomas (1993) stress the importance of self-knowledge for maintaining and increasing one's reasoning and expertise in practice. Higgs and Titchen (1995) propose that the development of metacognitive skills not only enhances problem solving but also assists in the acquisition of new knowledge and thinking strategies. In the text *Critical Thinking in Nursing*, Alfaro-LeFevre (1995) provides guidelines and practice exercises for specific thinking strategies useful in clinical situations. These strategies include checking the accuracy and reliability of data, distinguishing normal from abnormal, identifying patterns, recognizing inconsistencies, identifying missing information, setting priorities, and evaluating and correcting one's thinking. Such practice exercises provide individuals with insightful information about their ability to identify, understand, and use certain thinking strategies, which is foundational to the self-appraisal aspect of metacognition.

Unit Three provides examples of nurses' thinking in practice, followed by thinking activities that will help you learn how to use specific ways of thinking in your nursing practice. These activities are designed to help you improve your ability both to exercise self-appraisal and to execute the second feature of metacognition, self-management.

Self-management is that aspect of metacognition that helps one use thinking strategies for problem solving. It consists of the ability to form good plans, use a variety of thinking strategies, and monitor and revise ongoing reasoning and decision making. Self-management refers to thinking in action; it represents the thinking that one uses to troubleshoot to resolve problems and to avoid worsening of problems or the development of additional problems by regulating one's thinking while the thinking is taking place. Barrows and Pickell (1991) encourage practicing strategies in metacognition until they become a habit and are used automatically as an intrinsic part of the problem-solving process. Rubenfeld and Scheffer (1995) stress the importance of "knowing how you think" to nurture a growing awareness of your thinking styles and abilities.

In his classic work *The Reflective Practitioner*, Schön (1982, p. 50) describes thinking in action as a process that is "central to the art by which practitioners deal well with situations of uncertainty, instability, uniqueness, and value conflict." Schön (p. 337) depicts the practitioner who thinks in action as someone who is inquisitive, reflective, and flexible. It is someone who questions each problem or task to understand its meaning and to identify all of its nuances and subtleties. Schön (p. ix) proposes that it is this ability of practitioners to reflect on their thinking in the midst of action that provides them with "the capacity to cope with the unique, uncertain, and conflicted situations of practice."

As you develop a greater awareness of your thinking (metacognition), you will also become a more active learner, you will learn how to manage your own thinking, and you will begin to take the initiative to discover the solutions to the problems that you encounter, rather than looking for other sources that will provide you with the solutions to these problems. In addition, as you struggle to improve your metacognition, you will find that not only are you becoming better at resolving problems, but also you are learning to develop and refine the thinking strategies important to clinical judgment and are gradually becoming more skillful in your thinking and better and more efficient in resolving the problems and dilemmas that you encounter in your practice.

Paris and Winograd (1990) explain metacognition by using the metaphor of cognitive tools. They propose that just as a good craftsman learns to use a variety of tools wisely and independently for specific tasks and purposes, so too can individuals learn to use a variety of thinking strategies that will both enhance their ability to solve problems and dilemmas as well as increase their inquisitiveness and motivation to acquire new knowledge and cognitive skills.

Interest in metacognition among cognitive psychologists and educators evolved from theoretical inquiry into how thinking strategies are developed and how they can be modified (Ward & Traweek, 1993). Theoretical knowledge about metacognition was acquired through research conducted in the late 1970s and early 1980s by psychologists such as Flavell (1979, 1982) and Brown, Bransford, Ferrara, and Campione (1983). This early work described four general thinking strategies that individuals use when problem solving: planning, predicting, guessing, and monitoring. *Planning* consists of thinking intended to determine how to proceed with a task. *Predicting* involves thinking designed to anticipate outcomes. *Guessing* is thinking that results in the formulation of hunches or hypotheses prior to determining the solution to a problem. And *monitoring* involves thinking designed to assess one's progress toward problem resolution.

Cognitive psychologists have long advocated for further research to identify and describe other thinking strategies that individuals use in problem solving. As explained in Chapter 1, the ways of thinking described in this book were identified through a research study using the think aloud method. The content in Unit Three has been designed to help you learn more about how highly experienced nurses think in their practice and to allow you to practice using specific thinking strategies to improve your metacognitive awareness. Ridley, Schultz, Glanz, and Weinstein (1991, p. 294) describe this as "the process of using reflective thinking to develop awareness about one's own person, task, and strategy knowledge in a given context." Improved metacognitive awareness will help you to reason better in your nursing practice and will enhance your ability to make the type of sound clinical decisions that result in more positive outcomes for your clients.

References

Alfaro-LeFevre, R. (1995). *Critical thinking in nursing: A practical approach*. Philadelphia: Saunders.

Barrows, H. S., & Pickell, G. C. (1991). *Developing clinical problem-solving skills*. New York: Norton.

Brown, A. L., Bransford, J. D., Ferrara, R. A., & Campione, J. (1983). Learning, understanding, and remembering. In P. H. Mussen (Ed.), *Handbook of child psychology* (Vol. 3). New York: Wiley.

Carnevali, D., & Thomas, M. (1993). *Diagnostic reasoning and treatment decision making in nursing*. Philadelphia: Lippincott.

Flavell, J. H. (1979). Metacognition and cognitive monitoring: A new area of psychological inquiry. *American Psychologist, 34*, 906–911.

Flavell, J. H. (1982). On cognitive development. *Child Development, 53*(1), 1–10.

Higgs, J., & Titchen, A. (1995). Propositional, professional, and personal knowledge in clinical reasoning. In J. Higgs & M. Jones (Eds.), *Clinical reasoning in the health professions* (pp. 129–146). Oxford, England: Butterworth-Heinemann.

Paris, W., & Winograd, T. (1990). How metacognition can promote academic learning and instruction. In B. James and L. Idol (Eds.), *Dimensions of thinking and cognition instruction* (pp. 15–51). Hillsdale, NJ: Lawrence Erlbaum.

Paul, R. (1993). *Critical thinking: How to prepare students for a rapidly changing world.* Santa Rosa, CA: Foundation for Critical Thinking.

Pesut, D., & Herman, J. (1992). Metacognitive skills in diagnostic reasoning: Making the implicit explicit. *Nursing Diagnosis, 3*(4), 148–154.

Ridley, D. S., Schultz, P., Glanz, R., & Weinstein, C. (1991). Self-regulated learning: The interactive influence of metacognitive awareness and goal-setting. *Journal of Experimental Education, 60*(4), 293–306.

Rubenfeld, M. G., & Scheffer, B. K. (1995). *Critical thinking in nursing: An interactive approach.* Philadelphia: Lippincott.

Schön, D. (1982). *The reflective practitioner: How professionals think in action.* New York: Basic Books.

Ward, L., & Traweek, D. (1993). Application of a metacognitive strategy to assessment, intervention, and consultation: A think-aloud technique. *Journal of School Psychology, 31,* 469–485.

Yussen, S. (1985). The role of metacognition in contemporary theories of cognitive development. In D. L. Forest-Pressley, G. E. Mackinnon, and T. G. Walker (Eds.), *Metacognition, cognition, and human performance: Vol. I. Theoretical perspectives* (pp. 253–283). Cambridge, MA: MIT Press.

3 Theories about Thinking

Sound critical thinking in professional domains is essential to problem solving, clinical reasoning, clinical judgment, and decision making. The ability to combine one's knowledge and experience with skill in thinking and with consideration of the context in which thinking is occurring is essential for resolving the complex problems and complicated clinical dilemmas that are becoming more and more commonplace in today's nursing practice.

The Influence of Knowledge and Experience on Thinking

Cognitive scientists Glaser and Chi (1988, pp. xvii–xx) identify the following characteristics of experts' thinking: (1) experts excel mainly in their own domains; (2) experts perceive large meaningful patterns in their domains; (3) experts are fast, and they quickly solve problems with little error; (4) experts have superior short-term and long-term memory; (5) experts see and represent a problem in their domain at a deeper (more principled) level; (6) experts spend a great deal of time analyzing a problem qualitatively; and (7) experts have strong self-monitoring skills. Research in cognitive science has consistently demonstrated a strong positive relationship between knowledge and experience and skill in reasoning and problem solving.

Benner's (1984, p. 215) classic work demonstrates this positive relationship in nursing practice: "The expert rapidly grasps the problem by seeing it in relation to past similar and dissimilar situations and rapidly hones in on the correct region of the problem." Benner's subsequent work with Tanner and Chesla (1996) reveals the centrality of experimental learning to the development of expert practice and the practical reasoning and skilled know-how that are characteristic of the expert nurse.

Fonteyn and her co-investigators' (1991, 1993, 1995) research examining the reasoning of nurses with notable knowledge and experience supports the premise that clinical reasoning is significantly enhanced by knowledge and experience, as does the work by Crandall and Gretchell-Reiter (1993) and Jacavone and Dostal (1992).

The Influence of Context on Thinking

Higgs and Jones (1995, p. 4) identify the variety of contextual factors that influence clinical reasoning: "the immediate personal context of the individual client; the unique multifaceted context of the client's clinical problem within the actual clinical setting, the personal and professional framework of the clinician; the broad context of health care delivery; and the complex context of professional decision making." Sound thinking in practice requires consideration of how all of these contextual variables influence one's reasoning and decision making.

Kassirer and Kopelman (1991, p. 75) contend that attention to context assists clinicians in framing the problem that they are attempting to solve. "This cognitive representation has been called the problem space . . . the [problem solver's] representation of the task environment that permits the consideration of different problem situations and sets limitations on possible operations that can be applied to a given problem."

The propensity to spend considerable time analyzing a problem qualitatively was identified earlier in this chapter as characteristic of experts' thinking. Indeed, research has demonstrated that experts typically try to understand a problem, including its associated contextual variables, before attempting to solve it. Novices, in contrast, will try to solve a problem immediately, without taking the time to understand it fully. Research examining expert clinicians' reasoning has shown that it is notably sensitive to contextual clues. Thus, consideration of the influence of context would be important to sound critical thinking in nursing practice.

The Conceptualization of Critical Thinking

Theorists and philosophers provide a conceptual understanding of critical thinking. Scriven and Fisher (forthcoming) offer a concise yet comprehensive definition: "Critical thinking is skilled, active interpretation and evaluation of observations, communications, information, and argumentation as a guide to thought and action." The notion that critical thinking is *skilled* suggests that it is thinking that adheres to standards and that it is contextually dependent on the situation. The idea that critical thinking is *active* assumes that it involves cognition and processing. *Interpretation* and *evaluation* seem to be essential skills associated with critical thinking, and *thought* and *action* are appropriate outcomes of critical thinking. Indeed, the value of critical thinking lies in its ability to result in better plans and actions.

In describing critical thinking, Scriven and Fisher (forthcoming) contrast it with unreflective thinking, which results in jumping to conclusions. According to Scriven and Fisher, the critical thinker adheres to intellectual standards, identifies assumptions, asks pertinent questions, draws out implications, and uses reasoned and reflective thinking. Fisher has assisted the University of Cambridge in the development of an instrument to measure six distinct thinking skills: critical thinking, problem solving, communication, understanding argument, numerical and spatial operations, and literacy. The instrument is an essay test, which is part of the

MENO test, produced by the University of Cambridge; there are also some multiple-choice questions. The test is fairly new and thus is still being evaluated for validity and reliability (Scriven & Fisher, forthcoming).

Paul (1993, p. 526) defines critical thinking in the following manner: "1) disciplined, self-directed thinking which exemplifies the perfections of thinking appropriate to a particular mode or domain of thinking; 2) thinking that displays mastery of intellectual skills and abilities; and 3) the art of thinking about your thinking while you are thinking in order to make your thinking better, more clear, more accurate, more defensible." Paul (p. 131) proposes that intellectual standards are inherent to critical thinking. These intellectual standards include clarity, specificity, relevance, logic, significance, breadth, depth, precision, fairness, accuracy, consistency, and completeness. Paul's understanding of critical thinking is "thinking that deliberately supports the development of *intellectual traits* in the thinker, such as intellectual humility, intellectual integrity, intellectual perseverance, intellectual empathy, and intellectual self-discipline, among others" (p. 22). Additionally, Paul (p. 22) proposes that the critical thinker "can identify the *elements of thought* that are present in all thinking," including purpose, question at issue/problem to be solved, concepts, information, assumptions, inferences and interpretations, points of view, and consequences and implications.

Ennis (1996, p. xvii) defines critical thinking as "a process, the goal of which is to make reasonable decisions about what to believe and what to do." This definition suggests that critical thinking is characterized by sound reasoning rather than by thinking resulting from whim or impulse. Ennis also proposes that critical thinking is reflective, in that it is characterized by thinking that is overt and conscious. Additionally, this definition suggests that critical thinking is thinking that is consciously directed toward a purpose or goal. Finally, this definition says that critical thinking is intended to result in a decision that will guide beliefs and actions.

Ennis has completed extensive work on the development of comprehensive critical thinking tests, including the Cornell Critical Thinking Test, Level X and Level Z, which are multiple-choice tests that focus primarily on the evaluative components of critical thinking, such as identifying assumptions, assessing credibility of sources, assessing the appropriateness of generalizations, and evaluating the relevance of reasons. The Ennis-Weir Critical Thinking Essay Test, which is no longer available commercially, was for a long time the only essay test of critical thinking.

The text by Ennis (1996), entitled *Critical Thinking*, provides a guide to critical thinking, using the acronym FRISCO, "which stands for focus, reasons, inference, situation, clarity and overview" (p. xx). Many of the examples provided in this text come from the author's experience as a juror in a murder trial. The text also provides numerous opportunities for review of the information that is presented in extensive discussions throughout the book, as well as opportunities to assess one's learning of the material presented in individual chapters.

Facione's (1993) definition of critical thinking has resulted from a research study that was conducted from 1988 to 1990 using the Delphi method to obtain a consensus definition of critical thinking from a panel of 46 critical thinking experts. The following definition of critical thinking resulted from this Delphi study: Critical thinking is "purposeful, self-regulatory judgment that results in interpretation, analysis, evaluation, and inference, as well as explanation of the evidential, conceptual, methodological, criteriological, or contextual considerations upon which that judgment is based" (Facione, 1993).

Inherent in this definition of critical thinking are six cognitive skills: (1) *interpretation*, comprehending and expressing meaning and significance; (2) *analysis*, identifying inferential relationships among concepts intended, examining ideas, and detecting and analyzing arguments; (3) *evaluation*, assessing claims and arguments for credibility; (4) *inference*, identifying and securing information needed to draw conclusions, querying evidence, conjecturing alternatives, and drawing conclusions; (5) *explanation*, stating and justifying the results of one's reasoning, including contextual considerations; and (6) *self-regulation*, monitoring and reflecting on one's reasoning and correcting one's reasoning when necessary. Findings from the Delphi study also provided a description of the dispositions toward critical thinking, including inquisitiveness, analyticity, systematicity, truth seeking, cognitive maturity, self-confidence, and open-mindedness.

Facione and several of his colleagues, most notably his wife Noreen, have continued to pursue theoretical development and assessment of the critical skills and dispositions identified by the American Philosophical Association in the Delphi study.

Critical Thinking in Nursing Practice

There is increasing evidence in the literature that critical thinking is an essential component of nursing practice. Through its accreditation process, the National League for Nursing has stipulated that student nurses be taught to think critically and that nursing programs show evidence that students have developed critical thinking skills on completion of their program (National League for Nursing, 1989).

Kataoka-Yahiro and Saylor (1994, p. 351) contend that "nurses need critical thinking in order to be safe, competent, skillful practitioners in their profession. The pace of knowledge development demands that nurses be critical thinkers." Paul and Heaslip (1995, p. 40) concur: "Sound nursing practice, therefore, requires that the nurse be a sound thinker; one who is able to reason things through, to direct her own mind in a way that is disciplined and effective. . . . Practice expertise develops when client experiences are examined through the process of reflective, critical thought so that the nurse gains a clear sense of the elements of the experience and how these elements fit together to form knowledgeable, intuitive practice."

References

Benner, P. (1984). *From novice to expert: Excellence and power in clinical nursing practice*. Menlo Park, CA: Addison Wesley.

Benner, P., Tanner, C., & Chesla, C. (1996). *Expertise in nursing practice: Caring, clinical judgment, and ethics*. New York: Springer.

Crandall, B., & Getchell-Reiter, K. (1993). Critical decision method: A technique for eliciting concrete assessment indicators from the intuition of NICU nurses. *Advances in Nursing Science*, 16(1), 42–51.

Ennis, R. (1996). *Critical thinking*. Upper Saddle River, NJ: Prentice Hall.

Facione, P. (1993). *Critical thinking: A statement of expert consensus for purposes of educational assessment and instruction*. Milbrae, CA: California Academic Press.

Fonteyn, M. (1991). *A descriptive analysis of expert nurses' clinical reasoning*. Unpublished doctoral dissertation, University of Texas, Austin.

Fonteyn, M., & Fisher, A. (1995). Use of think aloud method to study nurses' reasoning and decision making in clinical practice settings. *Journal of Neuroscience Nursing, 27*(2), 121–125.

Fonteyn, M., & Grobe, S. (1993). Expert nurses' clinical reasoning under uncertainty: Representation, structure, and process. In M. Frisse (Ed.), *Sixteenth Annual Symposium on Computer Applications in Medical Care* (pp. 405–409). New York: McGraw-Hill.

Glasser, R., and Chi, M. (1988). Overview. In M. Chi, R. Chi, & M. Farr (Eds.), *The nature of expertise* (pp. xv–xxxvi). Hillsdale, NJ: Lawrence Erlbaum.

Higgs, J., & Jones, M. (1995). *Critical reasoning in the health professions*. London: Butterworth-Heinemann.

Jacavone, J., & Dostal, M. (1992). A descriptive study of nursing judgment in the assessment and management of cardiac pain. *Advances in Nursing Science, 15*(1), 54–63.

Kassirer, J., & Kopelman, R. (1991). *Learning clinical reasoning*. Baltimore: Williams & Wilkins.

Kataoka-Yahiro, M., & Saylor, C. (1994). A critical thinking model for nursing judgment. *Journal of Nursing Education, 33*(8), 351–356.

National League for Nursing (1989). *Criterion for the evaluation of baccalaureate and higher degree programs in nursing* (6th ed.). New York: National League for Nursing.

Paul, R. (1993). *Critical thinking: How to prepare students for a rapidly changing world*. Santa Rosa, CA: Foundation for Critical Thinking.

Paul, R., & Heaslip, P. (1995). Critical thinking and intuitive nursing practice. *Journal of Advanced Nursing, 22*, 40–47.

Scriven, M., & Fisher, A. (forthcoming). *Critical thinking: Defining and assessing it*.

TWO

Thinking Strategies

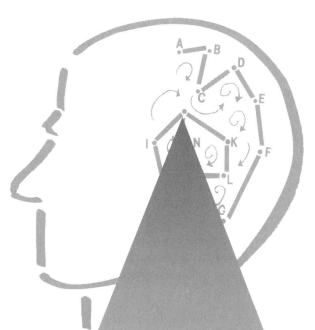

4 Recognizing a Pattern

For the purposes of this book, the thinking strategy **recognizing a pattern** is defined as identifying characteristic pieces of data that fit together. This thinking strategy has also been described as pattern matching (Fisher & Fonteyn, 1995), pattern recognition (Benner & Tanner, 1987; Fonteyn, 1995), feature recognition (Norman, Brooks, Regehr, Marriott, & Shali, 1996), prototype categorization (Murphy & Freidman, 1996), and identifying mental models (Perkins, 1986).

Recognizing a pattern is a very common thinking strategy that people use in ordinary thinking, as well as in skilled thinking (thinking about problems within an area of expertise). In everyday thinking, for example, you are using this thinking strategy when you identify characteristic pieces of data that fit together to alert you to the fact that it is going to rain: the sky is dark and cloudy, the wind is starting to pick up, the air feels damp and heavy, and you hear the distant sounds of thunder. Similarly, if your friend has a scowl on his or her face, a wrinkled brow, and dark and narrowed eyes and is using a sharp tone of voice, you recognize a pattern that indicates anger. These examples should help you to see how commonly you use **recognizing a pattern** in your everyday thinking. Most of the time that you use this skill, you probably are not even aware of it because it has become such an automatic part of the way that you think.

Findings from the Thinking in Practice (TIP) Study, which forms the basis for this book, provide a description of several different varieties of patterns that experienced nurses recognize when thinking: (1) patterns of case type, (2) patterns of standard treatment, (3) patterns of familiar circumstances, and (4) patterns of lack of fit. The following section provides examples of these varieties of patterns taken from the think aloud responses of the nurses who took part in this research study.

Recognizing a Pattern Representing a Case Type

One category of patterns that nurses recognize in practice is patterns depicting a case type. These case types may be of several different varieties: case types repre-

19

senting specific disease conditions, case types representing the most likely explanation of findings (hypotheses), and case types representing the seriousness of a client's condition or the seriousness of a clinical situation.

The following are examples (from the thoughts of nurses who were in the TIP Study) of **recognizing a pattern** that depicts a case type representing a specific medical diagnosis or disease condition:

Case type—heart failure: *She could be in failure. If she's getting a lot of [IV] fluid and getting blood [transfusions], and she has crackles [in her lungs], she is in failure.*

Case type—psychiatric problems: *Lots of times, I can tell that a patient has psychiatric problems by what I see when I walk into their house. They seem perfectly normal until I walk in and see a lot of things: pans with the bottoms burnt out, filthy conditions, and the patient is dirty and denies being dirty.*

Case type—hypoglycemia: *I always think that someone who is unresponsive might be hypoglycemic.*

Case type—cirrhosis: *Looking at his dehydration and his osmolality, it looks like he probably has cirrhosis.*

This skill of **recognizing a pattern** representing a specific type of case, a nursing or medical diagnosis or a disease condition, is very important in nursing practice. Carnevali and Thomas (1993, p. 4) remind us, "Not only is it important that nurses diagnose prior to treatment, but the accuracy and quality of those diagnoses need to be good or the treatment may be ineffective and even harmful."

The following are examples of **recognizing a pattern** of a case type that gives meaning to assessment findings:

Case type—diabetic with an infection: *A fasting blood sugar can sometimes be high if they [diabetic patients] have an infection.*

Case type—anemia related to a bleeding problem: *That degree of anemia would be expected for him [a patient who has a bleeding problem] and would be sort of normal.*

Case type—blood pressure related to size and ethnicity: *Given her size, and considering her ethnic background, I'd expect to see a blood pressure like this.*

Case type—severe fluid overload: *Sometimes, you don't even have to listen to their lungs—you can hear it when you're standing over their bed. I imagine that if he's breathing at 44 breaths per minute and has edema, then this might be one of those times. He's in fluid overload.*

Recognizing a Pattern

Identifying characteristic pieces of data that fit together

Case type—pale conjunctiva related to low hematocrit: *The first hematocrit might come back 26 or 27%, but we'll give the patient a liter of fluids in an hour and the second hematocrit will go down to 18%. The intern will say, "How did you know it would be so low?" And I'd say, "Because I looked at the patient's conjunctiva and it looked like she should be in a wax museum, so I knew that she would have a hematocrit of less than 20%."*

For many conditions, assessment findings can provide valuable clues to the nature of the client's problem. These clues may be explicit and highly diagnostic (such as neck vein distention, rales, and peripheral edema for congestive heart failure), or they may be more conditional (such as age and gender as a condition for pregnancy). **Recognizing a pattern** in assessment findings greatly facilitates interpreting the meaning of the assessment findings.

The following are examples of **recognizing a pattern** of case type depicting the seriousness of a client's condition:

Case type—sick admission: *It sounds like any sick admission.*

Case type—dialysis client with very high serum creatinine levels: *His creatinine is sky-high for somebody who is on dialysis.*

Case type—complicated due to the patient being unarousable: *Anybody who is unarousable is complicated.*

Case type—diabetic getting an infection: *Okay, right then, [when I hear that the client is] complaining of feeling feverish, and they have an incision that is red and sore, that's a big red flag [telling me that] this is somebody who is a diabetic and is getting an infection.*

The skill of recognizing the severity of a client's condition is an essential component of effective nursing practice. Benner (1984, p. 503) refers to this skill as "an essential component of nursing experience. The genius of all successful early warnings based on pattern recognition . . . the most important step is heeding the early warning so that the search for the undetected source of a client's response begins in earnest." Earlier research on nurses' intuition by Pyles and Stern (1983, p. 54) supports the importance of this skill: "All the nurses [highly experienced critical care nurses] reported that they had sensed when a patient had taken a turn for the worse." The nurses in this study described subtle cues as being the basis for their feeling that a client's condition was deteriorating. The subtle cues fit together to form a pattern that indicated deterioration.

Recognizing a Pattern of a Standard Treatment Protocol

The second type of pattern that nurses recognize when thinking is patterns of standard treatment protocols. Some examples from the TIP Study follow:

Recognizing a pattern of the standard treatment protocol for acute respiratory failure: *And they'll give him treatments, and morphine, and steroids, and whatever they need to try to get him past this without having to be intubated.*

Recognizing a pattern of the standard treatment protocol for cerebral vascular accident: *When clients have cerebral vascular accidents (CVAs), they are kept in the hospital for a fairly long time, compared with someone with a heart attack. They usually get a bit of therapy in the hospital before they're sent home.*

Recognizing a pattern of the standard treatment protocol for an unarousable client in the emergency department: *I assume that they would have given him Narcan, and they probably would have given him glucose also.*

Recognizing a pattern of the standard treatment protocol for a client in the emergency department with acute blood loss: *A good nurse would put an IV line in this patient right away. I could tell from looking at this patient that the nurse should put an 18-gauge IV in this patient and at the same time draw blood for an initial hematocrit.*

Recognizing a pattern of the standard treatment protocol for a client in the emergency department with bad skin signs and a drop in blood pressure: *If her blood pressure drops in the face of bad skin signs, she would end up in a trauma room and we would then take her from there to the ICU.*

Recognizing a pattern of the standard treatment protocol for a homeless person found unarousable out on the street: *This guy would be brought in by the paramedics, he'd spend the night in the emergency department with an IV with multivitamins added, and in the morning he'd get a shower, a bag lunch, a full set of clothes, a bus token, and a referral to rehabilitation.*

As nurses gain experience in an area of practice, they learn about a variety of standard treatment protocols that are used to treat the client problems and disease conditions that are encountered in their particular area of practice. Their familiarity with these protocols allows them to recognize the patterns of the conditions that are associated with these protocols and to anticipate, prepare for, and initiate the treatment that is an intrinsic component of these protocols.

Recognizing a Pattern Representing a Familiar Situation

Another category of patterns that nurses recognize in practice represents familiar situations, sometimes even accompanied by a feeling of déjà vu. Some examples of this category of patterns follow:

The familiar situation of a hectic night on the obstetric unit: *Yes, I've been in these situations a lot in my younger days.*

The familiar situation of high client acuity on a unit: *It looks like the acuity is high today.*

The familiar situation of a typical night in the emergency department: *This sounds like a typical night in the emergency department.*

Being able to recognize a familiar situation in practice assists nurses to recall their past actions in similar situations, what strategies worked and what ones didn't work in those situations, how much energy such situations demanded, what resources were needed, and so on. These recollections help nurses to deal more effectively with a current similar situation.

Recognizing a Pattern Representing a Lack of Fit, or Nonpattern

Sometimes, the information that nurses identify in practice (whether signs and symptoms, assessment findings, aspects of treatment, or contextual variables associated with a given situation) does not seem to fit with a typical pattern. This recognition of a lack of fit with an anticipated or customary pattern can also be helpful to nurses' thinking.

Lack of fit with the pattern of a blood transfusion reaction: *If she doesn't have an elevated temperature or back pain or shaking chills or something like that, then she's not having a blood transfusion reaction.*

Lack of fit with what is usually seen in an obstetric client at 25 weeks' gestation: *That's not something that I would expect to see at 25 weeks.*

Lack of fit with the pattern of a typical teenage mother in labor: *This is not our typical teenage mom that we see in labor, especially with this type of family.*

Lack of fit with the pattern of a heart attack: *This presents like a heart attack, but it doesn't meet the kind of things [criteria] that I would look for in a heart attack.*

The skill of recognizing the lack of fit of data with the typical (expected) pattern can be useful to one's thinking because it assists in ruling out various hypotheses concerning the existence of a particular problem or diagnosis. Thus, if some of the usual features associated with a particular health problem or diagnosis are missing from a set of features, such as assessment findings or signs and symptoms, then that particular health problem or diagnosis might more easily be ruled out. If, on the other hand, a set of anticipated features is present, the hypotheses regarding the existence of the problem or diagnosis associated with those features cannot be ruled out (Hammond, Frederick, Robillard, & Victor, 1989).

Recognizing a pattern of lack of fit compares with a skill that has been described in the literature as pattern discrimination: "the ability to correctly discriminate between two or more similar patterns" (Flemming, 1991). In separate studies, Bordage and Zacks (1984) and Grant and Marsden (1987) found that the way in which knowledge is organized in one's mind has a significant influence on one's ability to make decisions. Facility in pattern discrimination seemed to be closely associated with the cognitive organization of one's knowledge. Additionally, Flemming (1991) found that pattern discrimination was a central focus of experienced therapists' early evaluations of client performance and of their subsequent progress in therapy.

Woolery (1990) describes expert nurses' ability to "see familiar situations," and determine when a pattern or rule doesn't fit. Pyles and Stern (1983, p. 54) describe "gut feelings," the sensory or visceral feelings that experienced critical care nurses used to identify that their clients were "falling out of the pattern." The discrepancy between "what is" and "what should be" provided the nurses in this study with the necessary data to determine whether a client's condition is improving or deteriorating.

Improving the Thinking Strategy Recognizing a Pattern

As individuals develop expertise in a certain area, including an area of nursing practice, they accumulate a repertoire of patterns from the experiences that they encounter. In nursing, this collection of patterns includes patterns of case types, patterns of standard treatment protocols, and patterns of familiar situations. Research studies of individuals with expertise from a variety of different disciplines have shown that skill in thinking and problem solving depends in part on a collection of patterns that assists people with expertise to quickly and efficiently understand the problems that they encounter by seeing them as one or more familiar patterns (Perkins, 1986).

Jones (1993) proposes that the ability of experienced practitioners to identify meaningful patterns is related to the way that they have mentally organized the knowledge that they have gained through their experience. Earlier work by cognitive theorists Newell and Simon (1972) supports this premise. Their research indicates that as individuals gain experience resolving problems in a particular area, their knowledge becomes organized in their minds in a manner that permits easy and rapid retrieval of that knowledge the next time a problem is encountered. Once the pattern that a problem represents is recognized, the associated knowledge is readily accessed in one's mind, facilitating rapid problem identification and resolution. Jones (1993, p. 878) explains, "When confronting a familiar presentation, experts utilize rules of action found reliable in their own clinical experience to reach a diagnosis based on pure pattern recognition." Jones's research of experienced physical therapists' reasoning reveals that the therapists examined the features with which each client presented to see if they fit with a recognizable pattern. When a client didn't fit a familiar pattern, the therapists then identified and (mentally) labeled a new and different pattern, which thus extended their knowledge base.

Miller and Babcock (1996) describe how experienced nurses form patterns through recognition of similarities and differences among a repertoire of clinical situations that they encounter in their practice. These patterns become an essential component of the accumulated knowledge that experienced nurses bring to each client interaction and clinical observation.

Kassirer and Kopelman (1991) explain that one way physicians reason is by remembering and indexing specific client cases that they later use to help themselves interpret new cases. This type of thinking is called case-based reasoning, which is reasoning that assists physicians to make routine diagnoses by searching their memory for similar cases that would fit with the pattern they seem to be recognizing. Although this is not the only way that physicians reason and make diagnoses, **recognizing a pattern** is assumed to be a dominant thinking strategy for identifying case types, one used by nurses as well.

Benner and Tanner (1987) suggest that sharing stories of clinical cases with colleagues is a way that nurses could improve and refine their skill in **recognizing patterns**. Pyles and Stern (1983) study of critical care nurses reinforces the importance of this collegial sharing. They recommend that inexperienced nurses work with experienced nurses (described by Pyles and Stern as "Gray Gorillas") who could coach and guide them and help them to gain skill in problem solving and decision making, including skill in **recognizing patterns**. According to Pyles and Stern (1983, p. 56), "In such situations, the Gray Gorilla can mean the difference between the neophytes' success and failure in their professional development and, just as important, in the outcome for their clients."

Developing the habit of reflecting on your practice can also help you to improve your skill in **recognizing patterns**. After a clinical experience, spend some time thinking about the client cases that you encountered. Ask yourself questions such as "What type of cases did I care for today? What problems were associated with each case? What were the features of each problem? What patterns of treatment were associated with each problem? What previous experiences have I had with cases similar to the ones that I encountered today? What was the same and different in the presentation of these similar cases?"

This type of reflection has been described by Donald Schön (1982), in his classic work *The Reflective Practitioner*, as "reflecting-on-action," which he distinguishes from another type of reflection that he calls "reflecting-in-action," both of which can be useful for improving your thinking in practice. Schön (p. 54) compares reflecting-in-action to "thinking on your feet," such as when you collect your thoughts while puzzling about a client problem. Schön (p. 60) explains how reflecting-in-action improves a practitioner's skill in **recognizing patterns**: "As a practitioner experiences many variations of a small number of types of cases, he is able to practice his practice. He develops a repertoire of expectations, images, and techniques. He learns what to look for and how to respond to what he finds."

Wilkinson (1996) describes the process of identifying significant cues as an integral component of diagnostic reasoning. Each cue should be interpreted in the context of the other cues. "Look for cues that are repeated," Wilkinson (p. 104) suggests, then "begin to group together (cluster) the cues that seem related." Wilkinson suggests that nurses use a framework such as Gordon's (1994) functional health patterns to help them cluster cues to identify patterns. For example, client data such as an elevated temperature, decreased skin turgor, skin hot to touch, and dry mucous membranes would cluster under Gordon's nutritional/metabolic functional health patterns, and client data such as decreased urine output and diaphoresis would cluster under the functional health pattern elimination. Clustering data in this manner assists the nurse to interpret the meaning of related data as possible explanations (hypotheses) for each cue cluster (problem identification). After each problem is identified, Wilkinson further advises, a final decision should be made about which of Gordon's functional health problems is represented by each problem. Steps subsequent to clustering cues (i.e., **recognizing patterns**) include determining the etiology of each problem and then establishing a plan for problem resolution. Gordon's functional health patterns are just one of many frameworks nurses can use to develop and refine their ability to employ the thinking strategy **recognizing a pattern**.

Jones (1993, p. 882) cautions that excessive attention to clinical patterns may result in errors in judgment where "anything that resembles a standard pattern will be seen as that pattern." To guard against such errors in judgment, Jones advises that clinicians reason through and reflect on each problem that they encounter in their practice, continuously challenging existing patterns while at the same time acquiring new ones. In the same vein, O'Neil (1994) recommends that clinicians focus on acquiring in-depth knowledge of specific health problems to help prevent their overreliance on standard patterns to the neglect of the clinical information that uniquely depicts each individual client case. Additionally, Bok (1983) insisted that medical students could improve their skill in **recognizing a pattern** by learning less about facts and more about principles, that is, expend less effort in the memorization of the features associated with a particular pattern and more effort in understanding the functional relationship among the variables associated with a particular diagnosis.

References

Benner, P. (1984). *From novice to expert*. Menlo Park, CA: Addison Wesley.

Benner, P., & Tanner, C. (1987). Clinical judgment: How expert nurses use intuition. *American Journal of Nursing, 87,* 23–31.

Bok, D. (1983). *The president's report: 1981–1982*. Cambridge, MA: Harvard University Press.

Bordage, G., & Zacks, R. (1984). The structure of medical knowledge in the memories of medical students and general practitioners: Categories and prototypes. *Medical Education, 18,* 406–416.

Carnevali, D., & Thomas, M. (1993). *Diagnostic reasoning and treatment decision making in nursing*. Philadelphia: Lippincott.

Fisher, A., & Fonteyn, M. (1995). An exploration of an innovative methodological approach for examining nurses' heuristic use in clinical practice. *Journal of Scholarly Inquiry, 9*(3), 263–276.

Flemming, M. (1991). Clinical reasoning in medicine compared with clinical reasoning in occupational therapy. *American Journal of Occupational Therapy, 4*(11), 988–996.

Fonteyn, M. (1995). Clinical reasoning in nursing. In J. Higgs & M. Jones (Eds.), *Clinical reasoning in the health professions*. Jordan Hill, Oxford: Butterworth-Heinemann.

Gordon, M. (1994). *Nursing diagnosis: Process and application* (3rd ed.). St. Louis: Mosby.

Grant, J., & Marsden, P. (1987). The structure of memorized knowledge in students and clinicians: An explanation for diagnostic expertise. *Medical Education, 18,* 406–416.

Hammond, K., Frederick, E., Robillard, N., & Victor, D. (1989). Application of cognitive theory to the student-teacher dialogue. In D. Evans & V. Patel (Eds.), *Cognitive science in medicine: Biomedical modeling*. Cambridge, MA: MIT Press.

Jones, M. (1993). Clinical reasoning in manual therapy. *Physical Therapy, 72*, 875–884.

Kassirer, J., & Kopelman, R. (1991). *Learning clinical reasoning*. Baltimore: Williams & Wilkins.

Miller, M., & Babcock, D. (1996). *Critical thinking applied to nursing*. St. Louis: Mosby.

Murphy, G., & Friedman, C. (1996). Differences in knowledge representations of experienced and inexperienced clinicians as captured by repertory grids. *Academic Medicine, 71*(1/January Suppl.), S16–S18.

Newell, A., & Simon, H. (1972). *Human problem solving*. Englewood Cliffs, NJ: Prentice-Hall.

Norman, G., Brooks, L., Regehr, G., Marriott, M., & Shali, V. (1996). Impact of feature interpretation on medical student diagnostic performance. *Academic Medicine, 71* (1/January Suppl.), S108–109.

O'Neil, E. (1994). Home health nurses' use of base rate information in diagnostic reasoning. *Advances in Nursing Science, 17*(2), 77–85.

Perkins, D. (1986). *Knowledge as design*. Hillsdale, NJ: Lawrence Erlbaum.

Pyles, S., & Stern, P. (1983). Discovery of nursing gestalt in critical care: The importance of the gray gorilla syndrome. *Image: The Journal of Nursing Scholarship, 15*, 51–57.

Schön, D. (1982). *The reflective practitioner: How professionals think in action*. New York: Basic Books.

Wilkinson, J. (1996). *Nursing process: A critical thinking approach* (2nd ed.). Menlo Park, CA: Addison Wesley.

Woolery, L. (1990). Expert nurses and expert systems: Research and development issues. *Computers in Nursing, 8*(1), 23–28.

5 *Setting Priorities*

For the purposes of this book, the thinking strategy **setting priorities** is defined as ordering concepts in terms of importance or urgency. Findings from the Thinking in Practice (TIP) Study, which forms the basis for this book, provided a description of two distinct areas of focus when nurses use the thinking strategy **setting priorities**: plan of action and client concerns. This chapter includes examples from the TIP Study of nurses **setting priorities** regarding these two areas of focus.

Wilkinson (1992, p. 147) describes **setting priorities** as an intrinsic part of the nursing process: "Priorities are assigned on the basis of the nurse's judgment and the client's preferences. . . . Prioritizing problems helps to assure that care is given first for the more important problems [concerns]. This does not necessarily mean that one problem must be resolved before you address another." Carnevali and Thomas (1993) describe how **setting priorities** assists nurses in deciding how to proceed in a given client situation (deciding on a plan of action). As mentioned previously, nurses in the TIP Study used the thinking strategy **setting priorities** both to identify client concerns and to decide on a plan of action.

Setting Priorities That Focus on a Plan of Action

In her text *Plans and Situated Actions*, Suchman (1987, p. 28) defines a plan as "a sequence of actions designed to accomplish some preconceived end." Thinking about a plan can involve thoughts about problems, actions or interventions to resolve problems, or the relationship among these variables. Earlier research has demonstrated that our knowledge of the everyday world is organized by a predetermined sequence of actions (or scripts) for well-known situations. For example, there is a classroom script, a ball game script, a birthday party script, and so on. In other words, every situation has a plan consisting of a sequence of actions. It follows then that situations encountered in nursing practice also have a typical plan of action associated with them, as well as a customary hierarchy or priority for the sequence of actions associated with these plans.

One way that nurses use the thinking strategy **setting priorities** is to choose the order (systematic arrangement) in which they will carry out a plan of action. When nurses are confronted with a clinical dilemma, their thinking focuses on finding a way to resolve the dilemma, including deciding on a plan of action. Since they can't do everything at once, they **set priorities** about what to do first. For example, when a critical care nurse (whose thinking is depicted in detail in Chapter 19) reasons about a clinical dilemma depicting a fire on her critical care unit, she uses the thinking strategy **setting priorities** to guide her plan of action for getting the clients and staff out safely. The following are examples from the critical care nurse's thoughts:

The first thing I'd do is see that the nurses are with their patients.

And as far as who we'd take, we'd get the most ambulatory people out first; the two cardiac patients and the Alzheimer's patient would be out.

Then we'd have to deal with the ventilators.

My feeling is that the main thing is just getting them out of the danger of the fire.

The skill of **setting priorities** for a plan of action is particularly useful when a client is destabilizing and the nurse must choose (from among many possible actions) those actions that are essential for stabilizing the client and must also identify those actions that are not essential and thus could be omitted for the time being. Here are examples of this way of **setting priorities** from an obstetric nurse's thoughts (depicted in detail in Chapter 17) about a client who is in labor and is having difficulty breathing:

We need to get some oxygen on her and make sure that the baby's not getting into trouble.

Given all the other urgent things that are going on with her, I'm not sure I would take the time to listen to her bowel sounds.

I would not do another cervical exam to see if she's dilating further. I'd be more worried about her breathing.

Sometimes **setting priorities** for a plan of action helps nurses to identify the important areas on which to focus when conducting an assessment. In the following example, a nurse from the TIP Study **sets priorities** about the important areas of focus in assessing a 75-year-old client with congestive heart failure:

. . . doing an assessment, listening for breath sounds, seeing if she's got fluid in her lungs, seeing if she has a dysrhythmia.

Setting Priorities

Ordering concepts in terms of importance or urgency

Setting Priorities That Focus on Client Concerns

Another way that nurses use the thinking strategy **setting priorities** in their practice is to decide on the urgency or importance of client concerns. A sense of care or concern for clients is intrinsic to nursing practice, but some concerns are more important than others. A study by Jacavone and Dostal (1992) examined how highly experienced cardiovascular nurses assessed and managed cardiac pain in their clients. Striking among their findings was the ability of the nurses to zero in on the most significant symptoms, without having to examine each clinical finding separately. The following are examples of nurses' using the thinking strategy **setting priorities** to focus on client concerns:

But the immediate problem is this infection. I would always be concerned when anyone post-op got a wound infection.

His pressure is a little high, and his heart rate is a little high, and his respiratory rate is a little high, so that's worrisome.

60 mL of bright red drainage immediately post-op is worrisome. And the fact that her right arm is swollen from a lumpectomy, that would worry me also.

His respirations are at 40, he has decreased blood pressure—I'd be very concerned.

But at this point, I just want the ambulance to get there to evaluate him with a monitor and everything, to see what's going on.

Her sodium is low; that's the number one concern I see with her.

When thinking about client concerns, nurses also use **setting priorities** to identify those things about their clients that do not worry them and thus are not a concern. This allows them to concentrate on the things that really are a concern and gives them less to think about at any one time. Here are some examples of this use of **setting priorities**:

The IV [being infiltrated] wouldn't worry me right then, because she still has another IV site.

I don't care about the rash on his trunk either.

I wouldn't be concerned about his anemia.

So, I don't see anything in her history that I would pinpoint as being very worrisome.

At this point, I wouldn't worry about her failure to gain weight.

Another way that nurses use **setting priorities** when thinking about client concerns is to distinguish among client data that which is more versus less worrisome, which, again, allows the nurse to concentrate on what is really important at the moment. This ability to distinguish between relevant and irrelevant information is well known in nursing (Baumann & Bourbonnais, 1982, 1984; Benner & Wrubel, 1982). Some examples of using **setting priorities** in this way follow:

The blood pressure is 140/80. Well, that's not really critical. I'm more worried about her blood sugar of 50.

Even if the fetal monitor shows a flat line, I'd be worried, but not real worried. The baby is doing fine, but mom takes priority at this moment because she can't breathe.

Improving the Thinking Strategy Setting Priorities

In their book *Diagnostic Reasoning and Treatment Decision Making in Nursing*, Carnevali and Thomas (1993) recommend that nurses strive to develop the habit of using a systematic method for **setting priorities**. One that these authors recommend is a 10-point urgency scale for **setting priorities** during data collection. Using this scale, data that a nurse believes should be collected immediately would be assigned the number 1, and they would assign the number 10 to the data judged to be the least urgent. Other data would be given a number somewhere in between, depending on how important they were judged to be. Practicing urgency scaling, as Carnevali and Thomas suggest, is one way for nurses to improve their ability to use the thinking strategy **setting priorities** in their practice.

In her text *Critical Thinking in Nursing: A Practical Approach*, Alfaro-LeFevre (1995) delineates a systematic approach that nurses can use to identify immediate priorities in practice. Using this approach, nurses would categorize problems into three levels of priority. The first level would consist of problems that were potentially life-threatening, such as airway and breathing problems. The second level would represent problems that should be addressed as soon as the first-level problems have been attended to. Second-level problems would include changes in mental status, abnormal laboratory findings, and risks for safety. The third level would represent health problems such as knowledge deficit, coping difficulties, fatigue, and activity intolerance.

Similarly, in their text *Critical Thinking in Nursing: An Interactive Approach*, Rubenfeld and Scheffer (1995) provide a summary of guidelines that they recommend nurses use for **setting priorities**, which ranges from life-threatening concerns (highest priority) to nursing priorities (lowest priority).

As is true of metacognition in general, the process of thinking about your thinking in regard to **setting priorities** will help you to improve your use of this important thinking strategy. In other words, the more often you think about and make yourself aware of how and why you set priorities in your practice, the more likely you are to improve in your use of this important cognitive skill.

References

Alfaro-LeFevre, R. (1995). *Critical thinking in nursing: A practical approach*. Philadelphia: Saunders.

Baumann, A., & Bourbonnais, F. (1982). Nursing decision making in critical care. *Journal of Advanced Nursing, 7*, 435–446.

Baumann, A., & Bourbonnais, F. (1984). *Rapid decision making in nursing: A case study method for nurses*. Ryerson, Toronto: McGraw-Hill.

Benner, P., & Wrubel, J. (1982). Skilled clinical knowledge: The value of perceptual awareness. *Nurse Educator, 7*, 11–17.

Carnevali, D., & Thomas, M. (1983). *Diagnostic reasoning and treatment decision making in nursing*. Philadelphia: Lippincott-Raven.

Jacavone, J., & Dostal, M. (1992). A descriptive study of nursing judgment in the assessment and management of cardiac pain. *Advances in Nursing Science, 15*, 54–63.

Rubenfeld, M. G., & Scheffer, B. K. (1995). *Critical thinking in nursing: An interactive approach*. Philadelphia: Lippincott-Raven.

Suchman, E. (1987). *Plans and situated actions*. Cambridge: Cambridge University Press.

Wilkinson, J. (1992). *Nursing process in action: A critical thinking approach*. Menlo Park, CA: Addison Wesley Nursing.

6 *Searching for Information*

For the purposes of this book, the thinking strategy **searching for information** is defined as mentally looking for missing or concealed information. Findings from the Thinking in Practice (TIP) Study revealed numerous types of data or information that nurses look for when using the thinking strategy **searching for information**: vital signs, logistical information, medication information, the plan, and test data.

Barrows (1990, p. 3) describes inquiry (**searching for information**) as "a skill central to clinical practice." He explains, "When clinicians first encounter a patient they will always need more information than is initially available" (p. 3). And since nurses focus on treating the human responses to actual or potential health problems equally as much as they focus on diagnoses and treatment, then it stands to reason that they will need even more information about their clients and that they will need that information, not just initially, but during the entire time that their clients are in their care.

Searching for Information about Vital Signs

One type of information that nurses search for when thinking and making clinical decisions is vital signs: temperature, heart rate, respiratory rate, and blood pressure. The following are examples from the TIP Study of nurses searching for this type of information:

The blood pressure . . . what was it before?

I don't have a temperature here.

But if she needs blood . . . the other thing would be her blood pressure. What's her blood pressure?

She's still breathing, right?

What was his pulse?

Does she have shortness of breath with it [chest pain]? I'd check her vital signs.

Knowledge about a client's current and past vital signs is essential information for nursing care. In the previous examples, the nurses seem to be **searching for information** for a variety of reasons. In the first example, the nurse is **searching for information** about a client's previous blood pressure, presumably to compare it to the current blood pressure value. Making such comparisons helps nurses to identify trends and assess status. Sometimes, nurses **search for information** about their client's vital signs because they need this information to further understand their client's therapy or to assist in understanding the meaning of their client's signs and symptoms. In the third example (*But if she needs blood . . . the other thing would be her blood pressure. What's her blood pressure?*), the nurse is **searching for information** about a client's blood pressure because it is important information if the client is going to be receiving blood and will thus need to have the blood pressure monitored frequently; additionally, knowing the client's blood pressure will help the nurse determine how urgently the client needs the blood. In the last example, the nurse is **searching for information** about the client's vital signs to provide further understanding about the significance of the client's chest pain.

Searching for Information about Assessment Findings

Nurses frequently **search for information** about the information that is obtained from examining a client. Examples of this use of **searching for information** follow:

What does she look like?

Is there bloody drainage?

Does he have short-term memory loss? Does he remember you from yesterday? Does he remember himself? Does he remember anything?

IV antibiotics . . . if this was just prophylactic . . . I'd like to know if she has any infection. What is her respiratory status?

I have to assess whether she hurt herself.

I'd like to know what her oxygen saturation is. Meanwhile, I'm in there with her, and I'm assessing her chest tightness.

Searching for Information

Mentally looking for missing or concealed information

Do we have any contractions? How bad are they? Do we have uterine irritability versus contractions? What sort of cervical dilatation has occurred? What position is the baby in?

Given information about a client case, the nurses in the previous examples are **searching for** additional **information**, all of which represent assessment findings that are relevant to the information that the nurse has already been given. In the fourth example (*IV antibiotics . . . if this was just prophylactic . . . I'd like to know if she has any infection. What is her respiratory status?*), the nurse considers the information that has already been given—the patient is on IV antibiotics. This leads the nurse to **search for information** about the assessment findings that would be relevant to this type of therapy—for example, does she have an infection, possibly respiratory? In the last example, the nurse is responding to information that has been given about an obstetric patient who may possibly be in labor. This information provides an incentive for the nurse to **search for** a cluster of additional **information** related to assessment findings.

Searching for Logistical Information

Nurses sometime use the thinking strategy **searching for information** to discover logistical data, that is, details related to a situation. Some examples follow:

Where's the nurse assigned to this patient? I don't know where his nurse is, but I'd see if I could offer my assistance. Maybe the patient's nurse stepped out of the room, because we're not always in the same room.

So, I've got six women in labor?

It looks like the acuity is high in the seven patients that I agreed to take, so I would want to know if there are any families around that I can count on to let me know if there is trouble.

Is there a lot of patient teaching that needs to be done today, a lot of drug teaching or teaching about respiratory care?

Logistical information assists nurses' thinking when they are confronted with a clinical dilemma by providing contextual facts about the dilemma. Dilemmas and their associated problems often appear to be relatively unstructured when first encountered. In other words, there is often more unknown than known information about the dilemma, making it appear to be an unwieldy, ambiguous situation. As nurses gain more information about a clinical situation, including the associated contextual information, the dilemma and its accompanying problems become easier to understand and thus resolve.

Searching for Information about Client History

Nurses in the TIP Study frequently used **searching for information** to discover more about their client's history. The following are examples of nurses using this thinking strategy for that purpose:

I want to find out if this guy has been on diuretics in the past and if possibly that was overlooked when he was discharged.

And also, find out if the physician has ever considered, if the client has a history of depression, has he ever had him on antidepressants? Has something happened besides just these little things that could be causing his depression?

Is he a diabetic?

I wonder when he was last on dialysis.

I'd like to know if she had preterm labor with her first baby, which is probably the best indicator of preterm labor with the second one.

I would want to know when she was burned, if they are new burns or healing injuries.

I want to know if her father is really a significant other in her family or if he is just someone who visits on occasion.

Medical, surgical, and socioeconomic information about a client's past (history) can frequently contribute rich contextual information to enhance understanding of the client's current problems. In the second example, the nurse is **searching for information** about the client's previous experience with depression; this information will provide a context for the current problem of depression, which will then help the nurse to determine the etiology of the depression and to identify the possible interventions and therapy that would assist in its resolution.

Searching for Information to Determine the Plan

Sometimes, nurses use **searching for information** to help them determine what will be the plan of care for their clients. The following are some examples of nurses **searching for information** for this purpose:

And I would also want to know his code status. If he has lymphoma and AIDS and maybe a pneumonia, and now he has a serious GI bleed, then does he want to be resuscitated?

And I would want to make sure that there are orders for at least five weekly PT [prothrombin time] draws at this time.

I'd want to see if they want to give him platelets.

And I'd call the doc to ask about blood cultures to see what he wants to do.

So, if I saw the physician, then I would ask him what the plan is, what does he think is going on?

I'd get him [the physician] in there [the client's room] and ask, what are we doing? If he's a no code, then are we going to help him along? How aggressive are we going to be with this guy? Are we going to help him stay comfortable and focus more on comfort care?

These examples demonstrate nurses using the thinking strategy **searching for information** to determine what the plan is for a particular client. Although a plan is intrinsic to the care that nurses provide to each of their clients, these examples suggest that nurses are not always sure that their understanding of the plan in a given situation is the same as the physicians' or the client's. In the first and last of the previous examples, the nurses do not seem to know what the plan is regarding their client's code status [whether to resuscitate] or how aggressive to be with therapy if the client's condition deteriorates. Not knowing this plan seems to be the impetus for the series of questions on the nurse's mind, all of which are examples of **searching for information** to determine the plan of care.

Searching for Information about Test Data

In addition, nurses search for information about test data, as the following examples demonstrate:

I want to know what her H&H [hematocrit and hemoglobin] is. I want to know what her white [blood cell] count is. I want to know what her PT [prothrombin time] and PTT [partial thromboplastin time] are.

I'd look for the differential [on her CBC] to see if she possibly has an infection.

I'd look for other things like his ammonia level. I would want to know if his ammonia level was high, to determine whether or not he's in a hepatic coma.

And have they done a chest x-ray? Did they do one in the ER? Have they done a blood gas?

I'd like to know what his Dilantin [phenytoin] level is.

Information from diagnostic testing can help nurses to generate and refine hypotheses regarding the etiology of problems. This seems to be the purpose of the nurses' use of the thinking strategy **searching for information** in all of the previous examples. The purpose of using **searching for information** in the last example (*I'd like to know what his Dilantin [phenytoin] level is.*) may be to obtain information to determine etiology, but the purpose may also be to modify or refine the Dilantin therapy.

Improving the Thinking Strategy Searching for Information

You can improve your ability to use **searching for information** by developing a habit of inquisitiveness in your practice. When you are in the clinical setting with your clients, your inquiries should be tuned to the client's problems as they unfold. When new information suggests new hypotheses and new problems or potential problems, your inquiry should produce additional information that will assist in confirming or disconfirming the new hypotheses and in refining your understanding of these new problems or potential problems. When urgent and clear-cut problems are manifested, your information search should be focused on these immediate and obvious problems. Barrows (1990, p. 4) reminds us that "effective and efficient problem related inquiry (searching) skills require a higher order of cognitive skills based on a good understanding of disease pathophysiology." He further cautions that these skills must be practiced and perfected throughout training under the guidance of the clinical teacher. Indeed, to become really good at using this and the other thinking strategies described in this book, you ought to practice and perfect them throughout your career whenever you encounter client problems.

Facione, Facione, and Sanchez (1994, p. 345) have proposed that inquisitiveness is an important attribute of "a nurse with ideal clinical judgment." Inquisitiveness has been identified by the American Philosophical Association (APA) (1990) as one of the seven attributes (dispositions) of an ideal critical thinker. The APA defines inquisitiveness as "curious and eager to acquire knowledge and learn explanations even when the applications of the knowledge are not immediately apparent" (Facione & Facione, 1992). The California Critical Thinking Disposition Inventory (CCTDI) is an instrument that measures inquisitiveness and the six other dispositions of the ideal critical thinker: open-mindedness, analyticity, cognitive maturity, truth seeking, systematicity, and self-confidence. Many schools of nursing and some health care agencies have begun to use this instrument as one means of measuring clinical judgment in nursing students and practicing nurses (Facione, Facione, & Sanchez, 1994). You might want to inquire if the CCTDI is available through your school or agency. Assessing your performance on this inventory will help you to identify both those dispositions that you might like to improve and those that are already well developed but that you might like to develop further.

Part of the skill embedded in **searching for information** is recognizing the pieces of information or data that are missing and persisting in trying to find those pieces. Alfaro-LeFevre (1995, p. 120) suggests that the ability to identify missing information can be improved by identifying assumptions, checking the accuracy and reliability of data, clustering related cues, recognizing inconsistencies, and identifying patterns.

References

Alfaro-LeFevre, R. (1995). *Critical thinking in nursing.* Philadelphia: Saunders.

American Philosophical Association (1990). *Critical thinking: A statement of expert consensus for purposes of educational assessment and instruction. The Delphi Report: Research findings and recommendations prepared for the committee on pre-college philosophy.* (ERIC Document Reproduction Service No. ED 315 423.)

Barrows, H. (1990). Inquiry: The pedagogical importance of a skill central to clinical practice. *Medical Education, 24,* 3–5.

Facione, N., Facione, P., & Sanchez, N. (1994). Critical thinking disposition as a measure of competent clinical judgment: The development of the California Critical Thinking Disposition Inventory. *Journal of Nursing Education, 33*(8), 345–350.

Facione, P., & Facione, N. (1992). *The California Critical Thinking Disposition Inventory.* Millbrae, CA: California Academic Press.

7 *Generating Hypotheses*

For the purposes of this book, the thinking strategy **generating hypotheses** is defined as asserting tentative explanations that account for a set of facts. Findings from the Thinking in Practice (TIP) Study revealed several distinct ways that nurses use this thinking strategy: to identify a disease or health problem, to make a determination of the client's status, to speculate about client needs, to decide on intervention and therapy, and to identify possible etiologies.

For some time, there has been considerable evidence in the literature from across the health professions that **generating hypotheses** is a dominant thinking strategy. A major finding of Elstein, Shulman, and Sprafka's (1978) classic research on physicians' clinical reasoning is that experienced physicians begin to generate diagnostic hypotheses within just a few minutes of a client encounter. Other research has also demonstrated that physicians frequently **generate hypotheses**, primarily about a diagnosis, usually in response to a limited amount of observation and a minimum number of diagnostic tests. These initial hypotheses provide a framework to guide subsequent assessment and data collection. In Elstein, Shulman, and Sprafka's (1978) study, the more experience that physicians had, the fewer the number of hypotheses that they generated and the more structured was their guiding framework. These findings have been supported by subsequent research with physicians (Kassirer & Kopelman, 1991; Kuipers & Kassirer, 1984; Pople, 1982) but have not been similarly confirmed in studies of nurses.

Generating Hypotheses to Identify a Disease Condition or Health Problem

One way that the nurses in the TIP Study used the thinking strategy **generating hypotheses** was to speculate about the possible diseases or health problems that their clients might have. In practice, nurses are confronted with an increasing amount of data about each client case from a variety of sources, including the chart, reports from tests and procedures, assessment findings, and data provided by the client, their families and friends, and other health care providers. This information stimulates nurses to **generate hypotheses** about the possible disease conditions and health problems that their clients might have. The following are examples of nurses' **generating hypotheses** in this way:

She could be in failure, too. If she's getting a lot of fluid and getting blood and she has crackles already and pitting edema, then she's in failure.

It sounds like he's a pretty long-term COPDer [chronic obstructive pulmonary disease], and because he's had two hospitalizations recently, he probably has a pneumonia. He had pneumonia a month ago, and he hasn't been taking his Augmentin [amoxicillin-clavulanate] or his prednisone.

Okay, so right then, when I see that someone has become increasingly short of breath, requiring three pillows at night in order to sleep, I know that is somebody who is probably in congestive heart failure.

Because she's had so many babies and a quick delivery, it could be uterine apnea.

If I were to guess what his opportunistic infection is, he probably has *Pneumocystis carinii* pneumonia.

In several of these examples, the nurses are also using the thinking strategy **recognizing a pattern**. This fits with evidence from the literature suggesting that **recognizing a pattern** is a powerful stimulus for **generating hypotheses**. Research has shown that physicians generate diagnostic hypotheses by recalling disease processes (**recognizing a pattern**) with similar features that they have encountered in the past (Kassirer & Kopelman, 1991); studies of nurses have demonstrated similar findings (Miller & Babcock, 1996).

Whereas **generating hypotheses** assists nurses in identifying probable diagnoses or problems, certainty about these diagnoses may be difficult to establish, especially early in a client encounter. Overconfidence in a particular diagnosis can lead to diagnostic errors and must be guarded against by nurses and other health care providers. One strategy suggested by Kassirer and Kopelman (1989b, p. 30) to assist in confirming a diagnosis is to ask yourself a series of questions, including "Are all the findings in the client explained by the working diagnosis(es)? Are all the clinical features pathophysiologically consistent? Are there still convincing competing hypotheses? Do predictions based on the hypothesis come to pass?" In addition, we must also not forget that sometimes our clients may have a more accurate understanding of their problems than the health care providers do. We

Generating Hypotheses

Asserting tentative explanations that account for a set of facts

must learn to carefully listen to our clients and to ask them for their understanding of their health problems.

Generating Hypotheses to Speculate about a Client's Status

The nurses in the TIP Study also used the thinking strategy **generating hypotheses** to speculate about their clients' status, that is, their bio-psycho-social state or condition. The following are examples of nurses' **generating hypotheses** about their clients' status:

Her platelets are low, so I think she's at risk to bleed.

I think he's going into shock because his pressure is so low.

I mean, he's probably clinically starving. Because, when you see a guy who has already got edema in his feet and his weight is down to 100 . . .

She might have family who are not nearby, but who might be able to come to stay with her.

So probably he's dehydrated.

He might be starting to get septic again.

I imagine that he is in fluid overload.

In these instances, the thinking strategy **generating hypotheses** is used to speculate about a client's status to provide direction for further assessment and intervention and to evaluate the client's condition. **Generating hypotheses** about a client's status helps nurses focus on cues (often subtle) that they might otherwise not have paid much attention to or might have missed entirely. For instance, in one of the previous examples, a nurse is **generating a hypothesis** about a client who is at risk to bleed (*Her platelets are low, so I think that she's at risk to bleed.*). This hypothesis provides direction for further assessment of the client to identify evidence of bleeding, including observing for blood in the urine and stool, determining if there is bleeding from the gums, checking for bruising of the skin, watching for bleeding from any wounds that the client might have, observing for signs of cerebral bleeding, monitoring pertinent laboratory data, and watching for subtle changes in the client's vital signs. **Generating hypotheses** to speculate about a client's risk of bleeding would also provide direction for choosing interventions that would lessen that risk or minimize its impact on the client's status should bleeding occur. Such interventions, depending on the context of the situation, might include maintaining a patent IV, maintaining fluid balance, keeping a supply of blood products on hold and administering them as needed, minimizing invasive procedures and trauma to the tissues, and so on.

Generating Hypotheses to Identify Clients' Needs

Sometimes, nurses generate hypotheses to identify their clients' needs, as demonstrated in the following examples:

. . . I think she needs blood.

She may need some insulin while she has the infection.

The patient probably needs some furosemide.

Maybe she just needs a little support.

Generating hypotheses about client needs provides direction for decisions, actions, and interventions. In the first three examples, the nurse might be prompted to investigate further to help clarify and confirm these needs, to consult with the other members of the health care team regarding these needs, or to obtain whatever additional data are necessary prior to initiating the therapy that appears to be needed. In the last of the examples, the nurse **generates a hypothesis** that *maybe she just needs a little support*. This clinical hunch would guide further inquiry to determine if, indeed, this is a need of this client, as well as to identify what sources of support are available to the client.

Generating Hypotheses about Interventions or Therapy

Nurses often **generate hypotheses** about interventions and appropriate therapy. Some examples follow:

If there are family members there, then I might want to discuss how aggressive they want to be.

At this time, we would probably want to have an ultrasound done to tell us what position the baby is in and to try to determine how we're going to deliver the baby.

I may even want to put a Foley catheter in her.

It probably wouldn't hurt to give her some oxygen.

We could start something like magnesium sulfate, which won't cause as many problems.

I'd probably take his blood pressure too.

This manner of **generating hypotheses** is common in other health care professions. Flemming's (1991) research demonstrated that occupational therapists more frequently **generate hypotheses** about treatment than they do about diagnoses. Moreover, as occupational therapists carry out interventions, they revise their hypotheses and plan of action according to the client's needs, wishes, body, abilities, and limitations.

Nurses' ability to **generate hypotheses** to make decisions about interventions and therapy is inextricably connected to two important variables: (1) their familiarity and experience with situations similar to the current client situation and (2) the context of the situation. There is ample research to demonstrate that skill in thinking and decision making is highly dependent on familiarity and experience with situations similar to the one that currently requires thinking and decision making. For example, Walton and Matthews (1989) demonstrated that individuals who reason well within an area of expertise possess rapid methods of achieving solutions to problems with which they are familiar, because of the experience they have gained after leaving formal education. A study by Fisher and Fonteyn (1995) examining the reasoning of highly experienced critical care nurses revealed that their skill in making decisions about interventions and therapy evolved over time after multiple encounters with similar client cases. This study also identified a distinct difference in the nurses' ability to make decisions about interventions and therapy when subjects with expertise in one area of critical care floated to a different critical care unit to care for client cases with which they had little familiarity or experience. In these situations, the nurses relied heavily on physician orders and that unit's standard protocols and were unable to independently **generate hypotheses** regarding interventions or treatment.

Generating Hypotheses to Determine Etiology

One additional reason that nurses **generate hypotheses** is to formulate clinical hunches about the etiology (cause) of their clients' problems. Examples of nurses **generating hypotheses** for this purpose follow:

Part of that can be because of fluid overload. But she's probably lost potassium from being on digoxin. My intuitive feeling would be, here's somebody that hasn't been taking their digoxin.

I would feel very differently if this was somebody that just came in for something else entirely, and yet their hemoglobin was low. But I see this patient's low hemoglobin as part of his pathology, leading to his need for surgery [to repair the source of the bleeding].

He may be unconscious from his encephalopathy.

I would look for the possibility that he's bleeding from esophageal varices.

She's obviously going into some type of respiratory distress, probably from the magnesium sulfate, which can cause pulmonary edema.

His symptoms could be from the amphotericin B [a parentally administered anti-fungal agent]; they may not be from an infection.

Skill in **generating hypotheses** to determine etiology is moderately dependent on one's ability to apply one's basic science and pathophysiologic knowledge, since such knowledge often forms the basis for hypotheses about etiology. Since formal knowledge has been shown to have a finite longevity (3–5 years), it is important for nurses to identify and develop a habit of using accurate and feasible resources to get the appropriate facts and answers needed to identify the cause of a client's signs and symptoms and to accurately interpret the results of a client's tests and procedures. Such resources might include current textbooks, journals, other health professionals, specialists, and a variety of computerized databases. Nurses need to learn how to use all of these resources appropriately and efficiently to become adept in using them to **generate hypotheses** in their area of practice.

Improving the Thinking Strategy Generating Hypotheses

The previous discussion has already provided many suggestions for improving your ability to **generate hypotheses** to guide your decisions and actions in practice. Additionally, your thinking can be improved when you **generate** successive **hypotheses**, test each hypothesis through further inquiry and investigation, and refine your initial hypotheses accordingly. Research has demonstrated the efficacy of this approach for producing sound critical thinking and for successful problem solving (Mathews, Stanley, Buss, & Chinn, 1985).

As you practice self-monitoring of your thinking (metacognition) by continuously reflecting on and reviewing your thoughts and decisions during client care, pay attention to the language that you are using to form your thoughts. Your use of the thinking strategy described as **generating hypotheses** may be associated with certain phrases that reflect some degree of tentativeness suggestive of uncertainty or hesitancy. The tentative language that the nurses in the TIP Study used when **generating hypotheses** included *probably, the possibility, may be, my intuitive feeling, might, I imagine, I think, might have, could be, it sounds like, possibly, it's likely, part of that can be, there's a possibility, I would suspect, that points to, if I were to guess,* and *I'm guessing.* Many further examples of the language that is associated with **generating hypotheses** can be found in Kassirer and Kopelman's (1989) intriguing article "The Luxuriant Language of Diagnosis."

The tentativeness that is often associated with **generating hypotheses** is particularly appropriate early in a client encounter when hypotheses serve as guides for further inquiry and data collection, for identifying the client's primary problems, and for making initial decisions about interventions and therapy.

Studies have shown that there is a strong tendency for individuals to look for additional information to confirm rather than disconfirm a hypothesis, even though both are of equal importance, and concentrating only on the former may lead to errors in diagnosis and treatment (Klayman & Young-Won, 1987). A strategy that would help guard against these errors has been defined by Elstein, Shulman, and Sprafka (1978) as the competing-hypotheses heuristic, which involves formulating a set of hypotheses that includes alternative explanations for a group of observations, findings, or datum. Numerous studies have demonstrated that entertaining multiple competing hypotheses is one of the main ways that sound thinkers avoid "becoming prematurely wedded to a favored, but possibly incorrect, hypothesis" (Elstein, Shulman, & Sprafka, 1978, pp. 179–180). For example, you might generate the competing hypotheses of orthostatic hypotension, transient ischemic attacks, and medication side effect as explanations for the etiology of your client's complaint of occasional dizziness. If you then identify positive orthostatic vital signs, it would still be important to continue to entertain the competing hypotheses until enough additional evidence is obtained to rule them out with confidence.

Asking the following questions suggested by Wilkinson (1996, p. 37) would help in hypothesis confirmation: "What assumptions am I making about the client? Are my data correct and accurate? What data are important, relevant? How reliable are my sources? What biases do I have that might cause me to miss important information? Am I listening carefully to get the client and family's perspective?" In addition, Barrows and Pickell (1991, p. 215) suggest, "Generate new hypotheses whenever your inquiry becomes unproductive or new data makes your present hypotheses less likely."

References

Barrows, H., & Pickell, G. (1991). *Developing clinical problem-solving skills.* New York: Norton.

Elstein, A., Shulman, L., & Sprafka, S. (1978). *Medical problem solving: An analysis of clinical reasoning.* Cambridge, MA: Harvard University Press.

Fisher, A., & Fonteyn, M. (1995). An exploration of an innovative methodological approach for examining nurses' heuristic use in clinical practice. *Journal of Scholarly Inquiry, 9*(3), 263–276.

Flemming, M. (1991). Clinical reasoning in medicine compared with clinical reasoning in occupational therapy. *The American Journal of Occupational Therapy, 45*(11), 988–996.

Kassirer, J., & Kopelman, R. (1989). The luxuriant language of diagnosis. *Hospital Practice, 24*(7), 36–49.

Kassirer, J., & Kopelman, R. (1991). *Learning clinical reasoning.* Baltimore: Williams & Wilkins.

Klayman, J., & Young-Won, H. (1987). Confirmation, disconfirmation, and information in hypotheses testing. *Psychological Review, 94*, 211–228.

Kuipers, B., & Kassirer, J. (1984). Causal reasoning in medicine: Analysis of a protocol. *Cognitive Science, 8*, 363–385.

Mathews, R., Stanley, W., Buss, R., & Chinn, R. (1985). Concept learning: What happens when hypothesis testing fails? *Journal of Experimental Education, 53*, 91–96.

Miller, M., & Babcock, D. (1996). *Critical thinking applied to nursing.* St. Louis: Mosby.

Pople, H. (1982). Heuristic methods for imposing structure on ill-structured problems. In P. Szolovits (Ed.), *Artificial intelligence in medicine*. Boulder, CO: Westview Press.

Walton, H., & Matthews, M. (1989). Essentials of problem-based learning. *Medical Education, 23*, 542–558.

Wilkinson, J. (1996). *Nursing process: A critical thinking approach*. Menlo Park, CA: Addison Wesley Nursing.

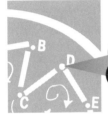

8 *Making Predictions*

For the purposes of this book, the thinking strategy described as **making predictions** is defined as declaring in advance. Findings from the Thinking in Practice (TIP) Study revealed numerous areas about which nurses **make predictions**: about interventions, about outcome, about a situation, about findings, about an event, about a response, and about needs.

Elstein, Shulman, and Sprafka (1978, p. 34) assert, "Much of our functioning on a day-to-day basis, whether as teachers, physicians, or parents, involves predictions of future events, based on data of variable quality or on interpretations of the efficacy of past actions or decisions based on records of past events." Jensen, Shepa, Gwyer, and Hack's (1992) study of physical therapists' reasoning found that the more experienced therapists had an elaborate framework for predicting client outcomes, which seemed to be associated with confidence in gathering and interpreting clinical data. In a study of coronary care nurses' decision making, Bourbonnais and Baumann (1985) describe how the nurses relied on their experience to anticipate (predict) emergencies that might occur. In a study of critical care nurses' clinical reasoning, Fonteyn (1991) found that subjects made predictions as a way of envisioning and then preparing for future clinical events. In their study of expert physicians' reasoning strategies, Patel, Evans, and Kaufman (1989, p. 306) postulate that predicting promotes problem solving: "Experts who were familiar with the presenting complaint employed prototype matching strategies [**recognizing a pattern**] with selective use of predictive reasoning to refine hypotheses." Carnevali and Thomas (1993) describe how nurses' prognostic judgments precede treatment decisions. They define prognosis as "a prediction of the possible or probable course of events and outcomes associated with a particular health status or situation under various circumstances, treatment options or lack of treatment" (p. 79). Being able to make prognoses thus requires skill in **making predictions**; in fact, Carnevali and Thomas (193, p. 89) describe a prognosis as "a prediction, an educated guess, a possibility." They suggest that skill in prognostic judgment involves the ability to combine client data, knowledge from previous experience, and formal knowledge to arrive at clinical judgments. They caution that "predicting the future is an uncertain process and carries some risk for error" (p. 101).

Making Predictions about Interventions

One way that the nurses in the TIP Study used the thinking strategy **making predictions** was to anticipate the interventions or therapy that they thought their clients were going to receive. The following are examples of nurses' **making predictions** about interventions:

What we'd do is give her D50 [50% dextrose], and then draw another blood sugar, maybe in a half hour, to see where we are, and then check her mentation and her other vital signs.

We'd be giving her both blood and platelets, so I'd start another IV to give her the blood in one site and the platelets in another.

And they'd end up taking her back to surgery because there's something bleeding in there.

And they'll give him treatments, and morphine, and steroids, and whatever they need to do to try to get him past this without having to tube [intubate] him.

If he's bleeding that bad, then they'd probably call for a vascular surgeon.

More than likely we'd probably just give him normal saline to expand the volume that he's losing, while we're getting the vascular surgeon to come repair the bleeding.

Being able to predict interventions and treatment in advance helps nurses to plan care for their clients. In one of the previous examples, the nurse is **predicting** the plan of care: *We'd be giving her both blood and platelets, so I'd start another IV to give her the blood in one site and the platelets in another.* Had this nurse not predicted that the client would receive these blood products, he or she would not have planned to start another IV, and precious time might have been wasted as the client was deteriorating.

Making Predictions about Outcome

The nurses in the TIP Study also made predictions about their clients' outcome. The following are examples:

And we're going to put her into more failure giving her the blood.

Making Predictions

Declaring in advance

He will starve to death in the bed while we watch.

. . . he'll start developing a lot of pain.

If he keeps progressing this along this way, with tachycardia at 150 and respirations at 44, then something's going to give out.

Since the days of Florence Nightingale, nursing has used outcome measures to evaluate nursing care (Marek, 1989). Naylor, Munro, and Brooten (1991, p. 210) define outcomes as "the end results of care, the changes in a patient's health status that can be attributed to the delivery of care." There is some research to support the notion that outcomes can be at least partially predicted (Nielsen, 1992). In the examples provided here, we see evidence of nurses' **making predictions** to anticipate client outcomes. In many of these examples, the nurse is **making predictions** about the client's physiologic status, which is one of the most commonly occurring categories related to outcome found in the literature (Marek, 1989). Several of the previous examples indicate how the nurses in the TIP Study **made predictions** about physiologic outcome: heart failure, starvation, bleeding, and pain. Although client outcomes cannot be fully predicted because of the complex nature of human physiology and psychology, it still is no doubt useful to nurses' thinking to anticipate physiologic outcomes, particularly if they are expected to be negative. By anticipating a possible negative outcome, the nurse prepares for it in advance and also tries to intercede with measures that might prevent such an outcome from occurring, or might, at least, lessen its impact on overall client morbidity, or might, if nothing else, prevent mortality.

Making Predictions about Findings

Nurses often make predictions to anticipate findings prior to further examination or investigation. Examples of this use of **making predictions** include the following:

So, with the dementing process, I would expect short-term memory loss, flat affect, maybe hallucinations, maybe psychotic kind of stuff. And with depression, I'm going to see the more vegetative symptoms.

If he has liver problems, then his PT [prothrombin time] is going to be elevated.

I would expect the baby's heart rate to be higher, around 180 to 190.

We've got the mom on magnesium sulfate, so I'd expect this baby not to have any variability [in heart rate].

Making predictions about findings helps focus nurses' thinking and alerts them to what data to look for, as seen in the second example: *If he has liver problems, then his PT is going to be elevated.* By predicting in this manner, the nurse alerts himself or herself both to watch for the PT results and to look to see if the PT is elevated. If so, then the working hypothesis that the client has liver problems is further validated; if not, then other competing hypotheses to better explain the client's signs and symptoms need to be pursued.

Predicting findings stimulates and guides further inquiry. In examples three and four, this way of **making predictions** makes the nurse watchful for specific assessment findings: a higher heart rate (around 180 to 190 beats per minute) for the baby in example three and no variability in the baby's heart rate in example four. If actual findings are different from those predicted, the nurse is more likely to investigate further to try to find an explanation for the variance.

Making Predictions about a Situation

Sometimes, nurses **make predictions** about a situation, as seen in the following examples:

This is going to be difficult, because he speaks Russian and she's deaf.

They're not going to be on a monitor at that point.

Let's see, cath [the cardiac catherization] lab would probably start calling for my two patients at this point.

So she needs to be there with her patient with somebody supporting her who has more experience and then she can get through the situation until the patient becomes more stable, and then we'd probably sit down and talk.

But at this time in the morning in labor and delivery, the physician's probably not going to be there, so I would start doing things and then call the physician.

That will be what happens, or other physicians will try to get in the way.

We know at this point that it's not going to be a good evening.

It could be as soon as tomorrow when this guy's mental status deteriorates, and I now have an unresponsive patient with no designated power of attorney, and that's not a good situation.

Making Predictions about Events

Nurses also make predictions about future events. Some examples of nurses **making predictions** in this manner follow:

It's good that she's been ruled out that she had a myocardial infarction, although I'm thinking with all this stuff going on she's definitely prone to them [myocardial infarctions] in the future.

This patient would probably come in and spit the baby out.

And there will be times that she cries.

But then there will be times when she'll need him, and that's okay.

Predicting situations and events helps nurses prepare for them, both mentally and logistically. For example, if an obstetric client is expected to come in and *spit the baby out*, that is, deliver very rapidly, predicting this event in advance would definitely help the nurse to prepare for it: "Are there personnel and space available for this event? What equipment will be needed? What complications might be anticipated?"

In the last example in the previous section, a nurse conjectures that a client may become unresponsive soon (possibly tomorrow). As it stands now, he would not have a designated power of attorney, which the nurse assesses as *not a good situation*. It seems reasonable to infer that the nurse intends to try to get this client to designate a power of attorney as soon as possible, before his mental condition deteriorates.

Making Predictions about Responses

Another reason that nurses **make predictions** is to anticipate responses. Examples include the following:

And the intern may say, "Oh, I haven't had time to look at his pain meds."

And she'll probably say yes, because she sounds overwhelmed.

Depending on what herbs she's taken, the magnesium sulfate probably won't interact that much, because magnesium sulfate is a normal part of our body makeup.

The physician will say, "Why are you asking for Demerol for someone who's not having pain?"

Several of these examples involve expecting a certain response from a physician when orders are requested. Perhaps anticipating a physician's response in this way would help nurses to be better prepared to provide their rationale for the requested orders. Fenton (1984) identified assertiveness with physicians as a factor that promotes success in advanced practice roles in nursing. The successful nurse will discuss client problems with physicians, ask them questions, and provide them with information that is important to the client's case. Perhaps **making predictions** to prepare for a physician's response would improve nurses' ability to be assertive with physicians when necessary for the good of the client.

The second example is from the thoughts of a home health nurse who is planning to ask the client's spouse if she would like a home health aide to come out to assist with her husband's care. The nurse predicts that *she'll probably say yes, because she sounds overwhelmed.* If she doesn't say yes, the nurse will no doubt want to try to determine why the predicted response did not occur. Is she not really as overwhelmed as she seems, or is there another reason that she wouldn't say yes, such as she doesn't want to seem weak and unable to care for her husband by herself? In that case, perhaps the nurse can encourage her to talk about some of these concerns and can then reassure her so that she might feel more comfortable about accepting help.

Making Predictions about a Need

A final area where nurses make predictions is regarding their clients' needs. Examples of nurses **making predictions** in this way include the following:

And I assume that he's going to need dialysis because that's a very high BUN [blood urea nitrogen].

The problem is he's got a clotted shunt, so there's going to have to be another access, like a catheter or something.

He's going to need fluids just for maintenance.

He's going to need extra fluids to get him hydrated.

She's going to need treatment for the infection, and she's going to need to be treated for hypoglycemia.

They're going to have to have better control of their blood sugar, so I'm going to have a consultation with her physician.

Probably she's going to need to receive some insulin to stay controlled until the infection is resolved.

In these examples, **making predictions** helps the nurses to prepare for methods (interventions and therapy) to meet their clients' needs. If, as in example three, a client is *going to need fluids*, then **making predictions** will help the nurse focus on how to prepare to meet these needs, which may lead to prediction of additional needs: an IV line may need to be started, a Foley catheter may need to be inserted to assist in monitoring output, intravenous solutions may need to be obtained, and so on.

Improving the Thinking Strategy Making Predictions

Since **making predictions** is used in so many different ways in nursing practice, developing and improving this strategy are important and necessary for sound thinking and efficient and accurate decision making. Carnevali and Thomas (1993, p.

91) suggest that nurses use the following approach when making prognostic (predictive) judgments:

- Identify the diagnosis (problem or condition) for which prediction is being made.
- Retrieve from memory information that will assist the prediction.
- Use this information as a guide for viewing the current situation and for establishing a database.
- Analyze the data collected.
- Make prognostic (predictive) judgments.
- If appropriate, discuss these judgments with the person involved.

Carnevali and Thomas (1993, p. 105) also propose that this strategy can be improved when nurses compare predicted outcomes to "desired outcomes" and when they identify ways that their predictions influence their evaluation of a client's response to nursing treatment.

Barrows and Pickell (1991) recommend that when practitioners are **making predictions**, they should try to recall past client experiences that are similar to the current one to identify what they can learn from the past that might make their current predictions more accurate. They also recommend that practitioners review the outcome of a case after it has been resolved and that they note the accuracy of their predictions and consider, after review, how they would have handled the problem or situation differently.

In her classic work *From Novice to Expert*, Benner (1984, p. 102) states, "One outstanding characteristic of expert nurses is that they spend a great deal of their nursing time thinking about the future course of a patient, anticipating what problems might arise and what they would do about them." This suggests that whenever you think ahead about the course that you believe your client will take, you not only can improve your skill in **making predictions**, but you also will be exhibiting a distinguishing characteristic of expert nursing practice.

Wilkinson (1996, p. 174) suggests that when nurses plan care for their clients, they should "use therapeutic judgment to determine [predict] which interventions have a high probability of achieving the desired outcomes." And when **making predictions** about client outcomes, Wilkinson (p. 191) suggests that nurses ask themselves, "Are the predicted outcomes realistic and achievable?" Because skill in predicting outcomes is directly related to the likelihood of achieving the outcomes predicted, nurses and other health care providers need to focus on outcomes that are realistic and achievable.

References

Barrows, H., & Pickell, G. (1991). *Developing clinical problem solving skills*. New York: Norton.
Benner, P. (1984). *From novice to expert: Excellence and power in clinical nursing practice* (pp. 262–274). Menlo Park, CA: Addison Wesley.

Bourbonnais, F., & Baumann, A. (1985). Crisis decision making in coronary care: A replication study. *Nursing Papers Perspective in Nursing, 17,* 4–19.

Carnevali, D., & Thomas, M. (1993). *Diagnostic reasoning and treatment decision making in nursing.* Philadelphia: Lippincott.

Elstein, A., Shulman, L., & Sprafka, S. (1978). *Medical problem solving: An analysis of clinical reasoning.* Cambridge, MA: Harvard University Press.

Fenton, M. (1984). Identification of the skilled performance of master's prepared nurses as a method of curriculum planning and evaluation. In P. Benner (Ed.), *From novice to expert: Excellence and power in clinical nursing practice.* Menlo Park, CA: Addison Wesley.

Fonteyn, M. (1991). *A descriptive analysis of expert critical care nurses' clinical reasoning.* Unpublished doctoral dissertation, University of Texas, Austin.

Jensen, G., Shepa, K., Gwyer, J., & Hack, L. (1992). Attribute dimensions that distinguish master and novice physical therapy clinicians in orthopedic settings. *Physical Therapy, 72*(10), 711–722.

Marek, K. (1989). Outcome measurement in nursing. *Journal of Nursing Quality Assurance, 4*(1), 1–9.

Naylor, M., Munro, B., & Brooten, D. (1991). Measuring the effectiveness of nursing practice. *Clinical Nurse Specialist, 5*(4), 210–215.

Patel, V., Evans, D., & Kaufman, D. (1989). A cognitive framework for doctor-patient interaction. In D. Evans & V. Patel (Eds.), *Cognitive science in medicine* (pp. 257–312). Cambridge, MA: MIT Press.

Wilkinson, J. (1996). *Nursing process: A critical thinking approach.* Menlo Park, CA: Addison Wesley Nursing.

9 Forming Relationships

For the purposes of this book, the thinking strategy **forming relationships** is defined as connecting information to further understanding. Findings from the Thinking in Practice (TIP) Study revealed numerous types of relationships that nurses form. Nurses **form relationships** to connect assessment findings with a variety of other information, including client history, other assessment findings, client problems, treatment, and client status. Nurses also **form relationships** to connect treatment information with other types of information, such as actions, problems, and other treatments. Nurses also **form relationships** to connect information about client history with information about client problems and client status. Another type of relationship that nurses form is between test data and context and between test data and client status. Two final reasons why nurses **form relationships** is to connect client problems with client status and to connect various types of organizational data.

In his classic work "The Structure of Ill-Structured Problems," Herbert Simon (1973, p. 187), the Nobel prize–winning cognitive scientist, proposes the notion that many of the problems that individuals attempt to solve are initially perceived as ill structured (i.e., poorly defined and unclear). Problems become well structured as part of the problem-solving process. Simon proposes, "There is merit to the claim that much problem solving effort is directed at structuring problems, and only a fraction of it at solving problems once they are structured." To illustrate his point, Simon uses the analogy of constructing a house. Initially, the construction of a house represents an ill-structured problem. As the architect sets goals with consideration of the intended overall layout of the house, the number of rooms, their size and location, and many other factors, eventually the structure of the house becomes clear in all its detail; it is then a well-structured problem for which there are standard guidelines for resolution. The thinking strategy **forming relationships** assists one's thinking by clarifying and defining ill-structured problems.

Fonteyn's (1991) research examining expert nurses' clinical reasoning demonstrated how subjects used their knowledge and experience to **form relationships** between elements of client data to identify and comprehend the nature of client problems, to plan care, and to make clinical decisions. In this study, Fonteyn identified three types of relationships that nurses formed between concepts when reasoning about an acutely ill, unstable client. These relationships were causal (forming relationships of cause and effect), connotative (forming relationships of meaning), and indicative (forming relationships that point out or suggest significance). **Forming** these types of **relationships** helped the nurse-subjects to change the ill-structured problems depicted in the client case to well-structured problems and, subsequently, to develop and refine a plan of care for the client.

Barrows and Pickell (1991, p. 3) also describe client problems as ill structured: "The lack of definite guidelines for working up the problem, the mutability of the problem, and the lack of assurance that the problem has been solved . . . are characteristic of ill-structured problems." They explain how new information that the clinician obtains about a client is associated with (related to) the information that is already known about the problem to progressively define (structure) it. They describe how physicians "assemble or synthesize the data they feel are important into an evolving mental image of the problem" (p. 5).

Like physicians', much of nurses' thinking focuses on understanding the problems that they encounter in their practice. The thinking strategy **forming relationships**, like many of the thinking strategies that nurses use in their practice, provides insight into and understanding of the nature of problems. Benner, Tanner, and Chesla (1996, p. 147) explain the relationship between problem clarity and nursing intervention: "Where patterns and trends are clear and there are definite actions associated with the clinical trend, the nurse can respond quickly and fluidly."

Frequently, the thinking strategy **forming relationships** becomes an inherent part of the thinking strategy **recognizing a pattern**. The patterns that nurses recognize in their practice represent schemata composed of related information. When **forming relationships**, nurses connect information that helps them to recognize the familiar patterns of similar problems that they have dealt with before in their practice.

Forming Relationships between Assessment Findings and Other Information

One of the primary ways that nurses gain a better understanding of clients' problems is by **forming relationships** between assessment findings and other information or data.

The following are examples of nurses' thoughts when **forming relationships** between information about assessment findings and client history:

Forming Relationships

Connecting information to further understanding

And what would worry me would be the 30 mL out the NG [nasogastric] tube in the last 3 hours, if her abdomen is firm and she's just had bowel surgery.

Okay, right then, complaining of feeling feverish and having an incision that is red and sore, that's a big red flag [indicating] that there's somebody who's diabetic and they're getting an infection.

The following are examples of nurses' thoughts when **forming relationships** between information about assessment findings and client treatment:

At 6 L of oxygen [per minute] via nasal cannula, and he already has scattered crackles throughout, I'm wondering whether he's going to need [an oxygen] mask if they [the physicians] really want to keep his saturation that high.

She's probably not feeling anxious; obviously the ritodrine hydrochloride has worked.

At [a temperature] of 103.8°F [39.89°C], I'd want to do something that's cooling, like wet clothes under the axilla.

The following are examples of nurses' thoughts when **forming relationships** between information about assessment findings and client problems:

If she's combative, that could be from her low blood sugar.

If I were to walk in to her [the client's] room and she was in respiratory distress, I'd look to see what her color was like, and if she could talk, what her mentation was, and what her vital signs were.

So, he's already got skin breakdown, which is serious trouble for somebody with AIDS.

If he's just had black stools, and he's vomited bloody emesis, then he could be bleeding acutely.

ST segment elevation and inversion of T wave, there's definitely ischemia going on.

The following are examples of nurses' thoughts when **forming relationships** between information about assessment findings and client status:

With the internal os being just a fingertip, you can't even put your finger through it, she's essentially got a closed cervix. Her cervix is 1 cm and soft, so she's probably about 50% effaced.

But his pulses are there and his blood pressure is okay, so he's getting profusion down there.

With a slightly bloody show, possibly her membranes are ruptured.

The following are examples of nurses' thoughts when **forming relationships** between various assessment findings:

Her heart rate is up a little; that's compensating for the little bit of drop in the blood pressure.

Her respirations are up, and her pressure could be higher, too.

His lips are dry and cracked, and his abdomen is tense, rigid, and boardlike.

He was anxious and dusky in appearance.

He's blue. He has a weak, thready irregular pulse, and rales.

Forming Relationships between Information about Treatment and Other Types of Information

Another type of relationship that nurses form is that between treatments and other types of information.

The following are examples of nurses' thoughts when **forming relationships** between treatments and nursing actions:

We're giving her blood and platelets, so I'd start another IV to give her blood in one site and platelets in another; because platelets you can push right in.

We've got orders to put her in Trendelenburg position. I'd listen to her heart and lungs to see if anything is going on.

The following are examples of nurses' thoughts when **forming relationships** between various types of treatments:

We'd probably be giving him fluids too; and he's probably going to be in Trendelenburg position.

Not only are we giving him furosemide, but he's also on oxygen.

You can put the monitor on the patient and be talking to them at the same time.

Oxygen and an IV—a lot of times these two things make the nurses and the doctors feel good.

Forming Relationships between Client History and Client Problems or Client Status

Nurses often connect information about client history with other data, including client problems and client status.

The following are examples of nurse' thoughts when **forming relationships** between client history and client problems:

It sounds like he's a pretty long-term COPDer [chronic obstructive pulmonary disease], and because he's had two hospitalizations recently, he probably has a pneumonia. He had pneumonia a month ago. And he hasn't been taking his Augmentin [amoxicillin-clavulanate] or his prednisone, so that's like a double whammy.

If he has lymphoma and AIDS and maybe pneumonia, and now he has a serious GI bleed, does this guy want to be resuscitated?

If I know that she has coronary artery disease and that she came in with chest pain, then I'd wonder if it's true cardiac pain versus perhaps GI pain.

Her lab report shows diabetes, which really increases her risk factors for coronary artery disease, I think more than two to one.

The following are examples of nurses' thoughts when **forming relationships** between client history and client status:

At 25 weeks' gestation and she seems to have had good prenatal care, we've got a good prognosis versus someone who comes in with no prenatal care and says, "Ehhh, I think I had a period a couple of months ago."

Yeah, she's got some risk factors such as poor nutrition, because that husband is unemployed and she's working as a seamstress, probably making ten cents an hour, so she's not going to get much food, living with elderly parents and trying to support them.

Forming Relationships between Test Data and Context or Status

The following is an example of nurses' thoughts when **forming relationships** between test data and context:

A blood sugar of 50 is rather worrisome, but being in the [intensive care] unit, I can check it and give something right away.

The following is an example of nurses' thoughts when **forming relationships** between test data and client status:

Her platelets are low; so I know she's at risk to bleed; and I think she needs blood.

Forming Relationships between Client Problems and Status

She has liver failure, and of course I'm going to wonder about a living will, depending on how bad it [the liver failure] is.

I'm not sure what the research has shown, but I know there's a tremendous amount of trouble with people going septic with central lines and TPN [total parenteral nutrition] when they have no immune system.

She hasn't gained enough weight, so that's not good because too little weight or too much weight corresponds to possible fetal development problems.

These examples also demonstrate how **forming relationships** helps nurses identify potential problems and anticipate treatment.

Forming Relationships among Organizational Data

It's very unlikely that, even though we're full [every client bed is occupied], there's not a couple of patients that we could group together, with one nurse taking one of another nurse's two patients, and another nurse taking the second patient; and then you have a nurse free.

Not only will he take up so much of my time, but also we don't have certain medications and certain medication drips that he might need; we aren't equipped to provide the one-on-one attention that he needs.

It's 2:00 A.M., so you have no doctors around.

And if I've got somebody [a float RN] from a general med-surg unit, she knows nothing about OB [obstetrics] and probably hates being there with me.

The reality is that this person has no place else for her 2-year-old to be, which leaves the mom to either go home and deliver her 30-week baby there or keep the 2-year-old with her in the hospital [where she can deliver her baby with help].

Benner, Tanner, and Chesla (1996, p. 142) describe expert nursing practice as being characterized by "increased intuitive links between seeing the salient issues in the situation and ways of responding to them." Mentally connecting organizational factors helps nurses to understand the contextual factors associated with a clinical situation.

Improving the Thinking Strategy Forming Relationships

There is evidence in the literature that increasing your metacognitive awareness of how you use the thinking strategy **forming relationships** will help you to improve your knowledge and expertise within an area of nursing practice. Thompson, Ryan, and Kitzman (1990, p. 2) have proposed that expertise is characterized by "the creation of a network of concept nodes interconnected by relational links, resulting in the ability to accurately perform the required mental or physical activity rapidly and with the fewest number of cues." Arseneau's (1995) and White and

Gunstone's (1992) work provide further support of the premise that expertise develops as new elements of knowledge are connected and linked to existing knowledge to further meaning and understanding. Arseneau (1995, p. 685) describes how individuals can "elaborate" their knowledge bases by focusing on the links among knowledge elements: "The greater the number of links to a piece of knowledge, the greater the number of ways to access that piece of knowledge." Van der Vleuten and Newble (1995, p. 1033) remind us that "it is not simply the knowledge, but the way the knowledge is stored, retrieved, and used that distinguishes the expert from the novice."

Some practical suggestions for developing your skill in **forming relationships** come from the literature on critical thinking in nursing. Alfaro-LeFevre (1995) suggests grouping or clustering data in a way that helps you to see the relationships among the data. Jones and Beck (1996) also suggest that nurses cluster cues. Another strategy is to struggle to distinguish similarities from differences in current and past situations. Rubenfeld and Scheffer (1995, p. 144) support the method of clustering and cluster analysis for improving the thinking strategy **forming relationships**: "To make sound conclusions, nurses must look beyond individual pieces of data and how they compare to norms, to the relationships among the data and among the clusters."

References

Alfaro-LeFevre, R. (1995). *A practical approach*. Philadelphia: Saunders.

Arseneau, R. (1995). Exit rounds: A reflection exercise. *Academic Medicine, 70*(8), 684–687.

Barrows, H., & Pickell, G. (1991). *Developing clinical problem-solving skills*. New York: Norton Medical Books.

Benner, P., Tanner, C., & Chesla, C. (1996). *Expertise in nursing practice: Caring, clinical judgment, and ethics*. New York: Springer.

Fonteyn, M. (1991). *A descriptive analysis of expert nurses' clinical reasoning*. Unpublished doctoral dissertation, University of Texas, Austin.

Jones, R., & Beck, S. (1996). *Decision making in nursing*. Albany, NY: Delmar.

Rubenfeld, M., & Scheffer, B. (1995). *Critical thinking in nursing: An interactive approach*. Philadelphia: Lippincott.

Simon, H. (1973). The structure of ill-structured problems. *Artificial Intelligence, 4*, 181–201.

Thompson, C., Ryan, S., & Kitzman, H. (1990). Expertise for expert system development. *Advances in Nursing, 13*, 1–10.

van der Vleuten, C., & Newble, D. (1995). How can we test clinical reasoning? *Lancet, 345*, 1032–1035.

White, R., & Gunstone, R. (1992). *Probing understanding*. London: Farmer Press.

10 *Stating a Proposition*

For the purposes of this book, the thinking strategy **stating a proposition** is defined as stating a rule governed by IF–THEN. Findings from the Thinking in Practice (TIP) Study revealed several different ways that nurses use this thinking strategy: to rule out or rule in a disease or health problem, to choose a plan of action, to speculate about possible etiology, to make judgments about intervention and therapy, to evaluate assessment findings and other data, and to clarify a policy or procedure.

Stating a Proposition to Rule In or Rule Out a Problem

One way that the nurses in the TIP Study used **stating a proposition** was to rule in or rule out possible problems that their clients might have.

The following are examples of nurses using **stating a proposition** to rule in problems:

If at the end of my shift he hasn't peed [urinated] yet, then we've got a problem.

If he's been having black stools, and he's vomited bloody emesis, then he could be bleeding acutely.

If this pain would not go away for 20 to 30 minutes, and it stayed at a high level like 7 to 9/10 and did not get better with nitroglycerin, then I'd have to wonder if she was actually experiencing a myocardial infarction.

If he has a liver problem, then his prothrombin time is going to be elevated.

The following are examples of nurses using **stating a proposition** to rule out problems:

If she were in failure with respiratory distress, then she'd be tachycardic.

63

But I would think that if he were bleeding from post-surgery, then blood would be dumping into the chest tube, so I'm not sure why he's got blood in his Foley [catheter].

If I know that she has coronary artery disease and that she has come in with chest pain, then I'd wonder if it's true cardiac pain versus perhaps GI pain.

If it were a drug-induced preterm labor, she would either have symptoms of being high or crashing.

Much of the thinking that nurses do in practice focuses on identifying actual or potential client problems. To do this, nurses collect data and interpret their meaning. IF–THEN rules, such as depicted in the previous examples, assist nurses' thinking by giving meaning to data concerning actual or potential client problems. By using an IF–THEN approach, client problems become easier to identify, their presence can be more readily verified, and the associated interventions and therapy can be initiated more quickly.

Stating a Proposition to Choose a Plan of Action

Another way that the nurses in the TIP Study used **stating a proposition** was to guide decisions related to a plan of action. The following are examples:

I mean, if this guy can't eat because the pain is too much, then I either need to get at why the pain is that bad and/or stop the pain.

If he's bleeding from both his stomach and his intestines, then we may want to change the IV to normal saline.

If he's having any kind of swallowing problems, then I'm going to request a speech therapy evaluation for him.

If there were family available, then I would encourage them to come in.

If the client's pulse is less than 60, and I don't know the doctor, then I'm going to ask the doctor about the anticipated normal range for this client's pulse.

But if he started to deteriorate, then I'd probably just go get the house staff and tell them, "You need to see him now."

Stating a Proposition

Stating a rule governed by IF–THEN

In these examples, IF–THEN propositions help the nurses to anticipate what action to take if certain events occur, certain signs and symptoms are manifested, or the client's status changes. This type of anticipatory planning has been shown to be associated with expert nursing practice. Benner (1984) describes expert nurses' ability to anticipate problems, plan for contingencies, rapidly match demands and resources in emergency situations, and perceive early warning signals prior to client deterioration.

Stating a Proposition to Determine Etiology

If she's combative, then that could be from her low blood sugar.

If she is difficult to arouse, then it could be her blood gases.

But I would think that if he were bleeding from post-surgery, then blood would be dumping into the chest tube.

In the above examples, the IF–THEN rules may assist in confirming or refuting etiology, in the same manner that such rules often assist in ruling in or ruling out actual or potential client problems. In the last of these examples, the nurse is struggling to identify the etiology of a client's bleeding and uses an IF–THEN rule to refute the hypothesis that the bleeding is occurring at the surgical site: IF that were the source of the bleeding, THEN blood would be dumping into the chest tube. But blood is not dumping into the chest tube; therefore, the nurse must continue to search for another cause of the bleeding.

Stating a Proposition to Make Judgments about Intervention and Therapy

If his last checkup was a year and a half ago, then you assume he's been on that medication for at least a year and a half.

If he's in congestive heart failure, then we might want to put him on one or two more meds besides his hydrochlorothiazide.

If I can get the oxygen saturation to 93% or above, then the cardiologists should be pretty happy.

And if he was requiring morphine very frequently, then that's a good reason to send him down to the intensive care [unit] for treatment.

If the physician feels like the digoxin is really needed, then most likely at least the first dose will be given IV.

If she weighs about 30 kg, then that would help me know that this was an appropriate dose of morphine.

Carnevali and Thomas (1993, pp. 134–135) remind us, "Decision making about nursing treatment is a complex task—probably even more complex than diagnosis. Yet the nurse is subject to the same constraints of memory limitations as were present in [other] cognitive tasks." The IF–THEN thinking strategy can assist nurses in overcoming these constraints by providing rules to guide treatment decisions.

Stating a Proposition to Evaluate Assessment Findings and Other Data

If she was lethargic and unresponsive, then that might be a worry.

If he has some very different spiritual and personal values, then he may not look depressed, and we may call in a psych[iatric] consult, because we don't think his affect is appropriate.

If it's regular, then I'm not too concerned about his pulse. If it's lower than 50, then I'd start to worry.

And if his ammonia turns out to be high and his blood sugar is all right, assuming it is, then I would worry about him still not being arousable.

If she's underweight, then I would guestimate the baby, the fetus, to be a little bit smaller than normal.

A major component of nurses' reasoning in practice involves collecting and interpreting assessment findings. Carnevali and Thomas (1993, pp. 53, 55) explain, "Nurses will begin early in data collection to cluster cues and to sense or recognize problem areas. . . . The selected cue cluster in working memory becomes a signal for retrieval of possible diagnostic explanations from long term memory."

Stating a Proposition to Clarify a Policy or Procedure

If the patient still needs to be in the unit [intensive care], then they [the insurance company] approve another 3 or 4 days.

Now if she's [an RN] just starting in the unit, but she's had a year of medical surgical nursing, but she hasn't had any critical care experience, then she'd go through a 6- to 8-week orientation.

If administration really needs me to be there [at a meeting], then I need to have a day off or a management day.

If we're not at the county hospital, then we don't have an interpreter—there's only me, the nurse.

Using IF–THEN rules to clarify a policy or procedure seems to assist nurses' thinking by defining the context of a given situation and thus framing or structuring the associated problems.

Improving the Thinking Strategy Stating a Proposition

The process of making a generalization from a finite body of data often takes the form of IF–THEN rules. These IF–THEN rules help individuals to assess the relationship between pieces of information and to draw conclusions about the meaning of these relationships (Kassirer & Kopelman, 1988). Kassirer and Kopelman (1991, p. 41) have proposed that one way knowledge is stored in our memory is as production rules. They explain that a production rule is "a compiled form of categorical knowledge in the form of an IF–THEN statement, with the IF part of the statement representing some semantically meaningful condition . . . and the THEN part of the statement representing some action to be implemented whenever the IF condition is satisfied." For example, IF the client is short of breath and has crackles on auscultation, THEN consider that the client may have heart failure. Kassirer and Kopelman (1991, p. 65) assert that "much of the clinical reasoning we do from day to day probably involves this kind of already compiled, rule-based reasoning." Research on human cognition has demonstrated that individuals use simple logical rules to reason and problem solve (Medlin, 1986; Nosofsky, Clark, & Shin, 1989; Ward & Scott, 1987). This research suggests that the rules that humans form (and store in their memory as knowledge) during problem solving are imperfect and often are contradictory or do not apply in a given situation. However, these exceptions derived from experience when a rule fails to work are also believed to be stored in memory and are applied to other problem-solving situations that are encountered after the exceptions have been learned.

Although research has shown that the particular rules and exceptions that individuals use during problem solving are highly idiosyncratic (Nosofsky, Palmeri, & McKinley, 1994), there has nonetheless been some effort to replicate these rules to use them in the development of computerized decision support or expert systems. Production rules in the form of IF–THEN statements are developed by computer scientists from the knowledge obtained by studying one or more human experts who have extensive knowledge and experience (and thus have developed many rules and exceptions) in the area that is represented by the expert system (Frenzel, 1987). MYCIN was one of the first expert systems to use such production rules. It was developed at Stanford University to assist physicians to diagnose and treat infectious blood diseases.

Miller and Babcock (1996) describe the thinking strategy **stating a proposition** as possibility thinking. They contend that such thinking is an important component of nurses' thinking in practice. Propositional thinking helps nurses to explicate what is implicit (implied but not directly expressed) in their thinking. Propositions in the form of IF–THEN statements include a premise or premises and a conclusion. Bandman and Bandman (1995, p. 46) describe this type of thinking as inductive arguments "in which the premises give some evidence, but not conclusive evidence, for the truth of the conclusion."

Stating a proposition is a thinking strategy that you may have gotten used to using in your thinking without even realizing it. The propositions that you think about may be sound or unsound. By thinking about your thinking (using metacognition) on a regular basis, you should be able to gradually become aware of the IF–THEN rules that you use to guide your reasoning and decision making, as well as the exceptions that you have developed regarding these rules. Whenever you find yourself using an IF–THEN rule or identifying an exception to a rule, stop to consider whether the rule or exception is valid for the situation in which you are using it. To improve your ability to make inferences that are valid, Alfaro-LeFevre (1995) suggests that you try to avoid making inferences based on only one cue (and its associated rule) but rather verify the correctness of your inferences by gathering more information. She also recommends developing the habit of perceiving inferences as suspicions or hypotheses rather than as facts; this will help you to avoid jumping to conclusions prematurely.

References

Alfaro-LeFevre, A. (1995). *Critical thinking in nursing: A practical approach.* Philadelphia: Saunders.

Bandman, E., & Bandman, B. (1995). *Critical thinking in nursing* (2nd ed.). Norwalk, CT: Appleton & Lange.

Benner, P. (1984). *From novice to expert: Excellence and power in clinical nursing practice.* Menlo Park, CA: Addison Wesley.

Carnevali, D., & Thomas, M. (1993). *Diagnostic reasoning and treatment decision making in nursing.* Philadelphia: Lippincott.

Frenzel, L. (1987). *Understanding expert systems.* Indianapolis: Howard W. Sams & Company.

Kassirer, J., & Kopelman, R. (1988). Intuitive and inspirational or inductive and incremental? *Hospital Practice, 23*(9), 21–27.

Kassirer, J., & Kopelman, R. (1991). *Learning clinical reasoning.* Baltimore: Williams & Wilkins.

Medlin, D. (1986). Commentary on "memory storage and retrieval processes in category learning." *Journal of Experiential Psychology: General, 115,* 373–381.

Miller, M., & Babcock, D. (1996). *Critical thinking applied to nursing.* St. Louis: Mosby.

Nosofsky, R., Clark, S., & Shin, H. (1989). Rules and exemplars in categorization, identification, and recognition. *Journal of Experimental Psychology: Learning, Memory and Cognition, 15,* 282–304.

Nosofsky, R., Palmeri, T., & McKinley, S. (1994). *Psychological Review, 101*(1), 53–79.

Shortliffe, E. (1976). *Computer-based medical consultations: MYCIN.* New York: Elsevier.

Ward, T., & Scott, J. (1987). Analytic and holistic modes of learning family-resemblance concepts. *Memory and Cognition, 15,* 42–54.

11 *Asserting a Practice Rule*

For the purposes of this book, the thinking strategy **asserting a practice rule** is defined as asserting a truism that has been shown to consistently hold true in practice. Findings from the Thinking in Practice (TIP) Study revealed that nurses use this thinking strategy when calling to mind formal rules, such as policies or procedures established by their agency, and when considering the informal rules, or maxims, that they have learned through their practice experience.

Asserting a Practice Rule about Policy

One way that the nurses in the TIP Study used **asserting a practice rule** was to call to mind the policies that employees or members of an institution or organization are expected to follow. The following are examples of nurses' using **asserting a practice rule** in this way:

We [nurses] initiate conversation with the patient about durable power of attorney. In fact, it's on the nursing database: "Who is your durable power of attorney and who do you want us to contact in case of emergencies?"

Also, staff are not allowed to sign or witness on durable power of attorneys.

There's a whole system set up; we have a disaster list.

We have a form that we fill out when we have a disaster drill; they want to know who are the sickest patients and who are ambulatory.

The police will discuss things [in the case of suspected child abuse] with the nurse on the units, certainly social service and the physicians.

But when you're dealing with children, they are still children of the state until they're 18 years of age. Since they are minors, other rights get superseded, including the right of privacy and the right to handle your own life.

Asserting a Practice Rule about Procedures

Another way that the nurses in the TIP Study used **asserting a practice rule** was to reflect on procedures, the steps to be followed in establishing some course of action. The following are examples:

Usually, we do blood cultures every 48 hours.

Anybody who is on chemo [chemotherapy as treatment for cancer] is immediately put on chemotherapy precautions.

We can give random type O blood in an emergency.

The standard procedure for administering nitroglycerin is that they can have up to three tablets 5 minutes apart, and if it's necessary to take a third one, it's time to call 911 and get in to the hospital.

Cardiac pain has pretty much been established in this patient already, so usually there will be a prn order for nitroglycerin.

Whoever did the surgery would have been called way back when we first thought she was bleeding.

Policies and procedures make the rules of practice explicit; a major strategy for decreasing conflict in organizations is to formalize rules in this way (Benner, 1984). From these examples, we can see that formalized rules guide nurses' thinking in practice.

Rubenfeld and Scheffer (1995) propose that nurses who use sound critical thinking interpret practice rules in the context of a given situation. Because much of the context in an organization is determined by its policies and procedures, when nurses use the thinking strategy **asserting a practice rule** to call to mind a policy or procedure, they are delineating the context of the clinical dilemma that they are trying to resolve.

One way that **asserting a practice rule** facilitates thinking may be that it stimulates use of other thinking strategies that will assist in resolving the dilemma. In the last example, for instance, the nurse states a procedural rule: *Whoever did the surgery would have been called way back when we first thought she was bleeding.* In other words, the procedure to follow on that unit when a fresh postoperative client might be bleeding is to call the surgeon as soon as it is suspected that the client might be

Asserting a Practice Rule

Asserting a truism that has been shown to consistently hold true in practice

bleeding. Thus, this nurse tries to put the situation depicted in the dilemma of a postoperative client who is showing signs of bleeding into context by asserting the rule (procedure) that this situation brings to mind. **Asserting** this **rule** may then lead to the use of other thinking strategies, such as **searching for the information** to determine if, indeed, the surgeon has been called. Another thinking strategy that might be used in this situation is **making choices** about interventions or therapy that will slow down or stop the bleeding or replace the lost volume while awaiting further intervention by the surgeon.

Kassirer and Kopelman (1991) describe how physicians develop rules of procedure that guide their decision making. They caution, however, that situations will often arise in which the patient or clinical setting is in some way atypical. Although procedural rules are often useful in practice, in atypical situations these rules may not assist in guiding decisions. For example, the procedure of having a prn order for clients with cardiac pain *(Cardiac pain has pretty much been established in this patient already, so usually there will be a prn order for nitroglycerin)* would not be useful to guide decisions in the atypical situation in which a client is allergic to nitroglycerin or taking nitroglycerin is contraindicated for some other reason.

Asserting a Practice Rule That Is a Maxim

Nurses also use the thinking strategy **asserting a practice rule** when considering the informal rules that they have learned from their experience in nursing practice. Some examples follow:

I mean, his CO_2 is probably a hundred, and you hate to intubate these patients [with chronic obstructive pulmonary disease]. You do everything that you can not to, because you never get them off the ventilator.

I mean, people can die from blood transfusions.

We could just put the next unit of blood on a pump. There's like 250 to 300 mL in a bag of blood, and we can pump it in 15 to 20 minutes. And sometimes we might have two bags running, if we're just trying to replace the volume with the blood. Now, in an older person, you just might put them into failure [if you run the blood in that fast]; you're kind of walking a thin line.

Skin signs don't lie.

Skin care is nursing care.

It's a nursing judgment to just slap a protective dressing like Duoderm on this guy's buttock.

I'm a firm believer in not playing doctor, so I let the doctors be the doctors.

One thing I do when I go to a house [for a home health visit] is a home check. I check out the bathroom, I check out the bedroom.

I usually ask my male patients that [if they get up at night to urinate].

I've learned that digoxin isn't held that often for a pulse less than 60 anymore. We usually give it if the pulse is at least in the 50s.

Benner (1984, p. 10), calls these informal rules of practice maxims. A maxim is a succinct formulation of a fundamental principle, a general truth, or a rule of conduct (*The American Heritage Electronic Dictionary*, 1992). Benner (p. 11) conceptualizes maxims as part of the "wealth of untapped knowledge [that] is embedded in the practices and the know how of expert nurse clinicians." The maxims that guide experienced nurses' thinking in their practice should not be confused with the "rule-governed behavior" that Benner explains as being typical of the novice nurse. Rather, thinking that is guided by maxims reflects a breadth of nursing experience and a depth of contextual understanding of a given situation. To understand this distinction, consider the last example: *I've learned that digoxin isn't held that often for a pulse less than 60 anymore. We usually give it if the pulse is at least in the 50s.* In nursing school, we are taught that digoxin should be held for a pulse that is less than 60 beats per minute, and this rule would thus guide novice nurses early in their practice. The thoughts of this more experienced nurse, however, indicate that her behavior is no longer governed by this rule. Rather, she has learned that *digoxin isn't held that often for a pulse less than 60 anymore,* and thus her thinking is guided by a maxim that states that digoxin is usually given if the pulse is at least 50. Note that the nurse qualifies (modifies, limits, or restricts by giving exceptions) this maxim by the term *usually,* suggesting that she would consider the context of each situation prior to applying this rule.

This tendency to qualify a maxim reflects the deep contextual understanding that is associated with expert nursing judgment. Another of the previous examples depicts the same tendency to qualify a maximum: *Now, in an older person, you just might put them into failure [if you run the blood in that fast]; you're kind of walking a thin line.* Thus, the maxim that you will put an older person into failure if you run blood in too fast is qualified by the phrase *just might,* again implying that this nurse would consider the context of each situation prior to applying this rule in practice.

Other of the previous examples do not contain such qualifiers. The maxim *skin signs don't lie,* for example, has no qualifiers attached to it, suggesting that this nurse believes that in every case, the signs that are manifested by the skin (e.g., color, temperature, presence or absence of diaphoresis, and so forth) are never falsely represented. They can be believed, as they are manifested in every case. Following this maxim would not, however, prevent nurses from misinterpreting or overlooking certain skin signs.

Some of the examples reveal nurses' use of maxims to guide their thinking about the distinctions between nursing and medical practice: *Skin care is nursing care. It's a nursing judgment to just slap a protective dressing like Duoderm on this guy's buttock. I'm a firm believer in not playing doctor, so I let the doctors be the doctors.* In their text *Expertise in Nursing Practice: Caring, Clinical Judgment, and Ethics,* Benner, Tanner, and Chesla (1996, p. 281) refer to the "blurring of boundaries between medicine and nursing," and they recommend (p. 306) that "both medical and nursing education could benefit from greater clarity about the relationship between the two disciplines in patient care."

Improving the Thinking Strategy Asserting a Practice Rule

As you gain experience in nursing practice, you will develop a repertoire of maxims to use to guide you. You may also learn these informal rules from your nursing colleagues. Benner (1984, p. 10) says, "Expert nurse clinicians can learn much from the maxims they are able to pass on to one another. . . . The outside observer and less expert nurse can also gain clues about areas of clinical knowledge—particularly perceptual knowledge—that are cloaked in maxims." Pyles and Stern (1983) also propose that less experienced nurses can learn much about practice from more experienced nurses, who serve as mentors. When you work with nurses whose judgment you admire and respect, look for evidence of the maxims that they use when thinking about their practice. Ask them to explain what they mean when you hear them use a maxim, and ask them how they came to know the maxim. Ask how confident they are in the maxim. Does it hold true in every case, or are there exceptions to it? Then, look for situations to apply these maxims to your own practice; see if the rule holds true for client cases that you encounter; and watch also for exceptions for the maxims that you have learned. Additionally, as part of the development and refinement of your thinking in practice, be aware of the maxims that you develop from your experiences; examine their validity and reliability in the same manner that you examine the maxims that you learn from others.

References

Benner, P. (1984). *From novice to expert: Excellence and power in clinical nursing practice.* Menlo Park, CA: Addison Wesley.

Benner, P., Tanner, C., & Chesla, C. (1996). *Expertise in nursing practice: Caring, clinical judgment, and ethics.* New York: Springer.

Kassirer, J., & Kopelman, R. (1991). *Learning clinical reasoning.* Baltimore: Williams & Wilkins.

Pyles, E., & Stern, P. (1983). Discovery of nursing gestalt in critical care nursing: The importance of the gray gorilla syndrome. *Image: The Journal of Nursing Scholarship, 15,* 51–57.

Rubenfeld, M., & Scheffer, B. (1995). *Critical thinking in nursing: An interactive approach.* Philadelphia: Lippincott.

12 *Making Choices*

For the purposes of this book, the thinking strategy **making choices** is defined as selecting from a number of possible alternatives, to decide on and pick out. Findings from the Thinking in Practice (TIP) Study indicate that much of nurses' thinking while reasoning about a clinical dilemma focuses on **making choices**. Nurses in the TIP Study made choices about the following: nursing interventions, actions, treatments, and test data. These choices depict a range of nursing autonomy: independent—choices that do not require the supervision or direction of another; interdependent—choices made in collaboration with others; and dependent—choices that are reliant on another health professional.

The nursing process is a systematic method of planning and carrying out nursing care that consists of five phases: assessing, diagnosing, planning, implementing, and evaluating. Implementing is the phase where nurses put the plan of care into action (Kozier, Erb, Blais, & Wilkinson, 1995). A thinking strategy that is common to this phase of the nursing process is **making choices**. In Fonteyn's (1991) study of expert critical care nurses' reasoning about a critically ill, unstable client, subjects frequently verbalized their choice of nursing action or treatment. Those subjects who had more experience with cases similar to the one depicted in the study (i.e., domain expertise) **made choices** more often than those subjects with less case-specific expertise. Similarly, Benner, Tanner, and Chesla (1996, p. 167) found that the nurses in their study who exhibited expert judgment were nurses characterized by "having interventions and responses linked with a good clinical grasp."

Making Choices about Nursing Interventions

Carnevali and Thomas (1993, p. 109) stress that "nurses' diagnostic and prognostic judgments are not ends in themselves, only steps, but crucial steps toward determining what actions to take." They thus imply that a primary reason for nurses' diagnostic reasoning is to **make choices** about nursing actions or interventions.

Often, nurses in the TIP Study used the thinking strategy **making choices** to identify nursing interventions that they would use to care for the clients described in the clinical dilemmas. *Nursing intervention* is defined as "any act by a nurse that implements the nursing care plan or any specific objective of that plan" (Anderson,

Anderson, & Glanze, 1994, p. 1088). Examples of nurses' **making choices** about nursing interventions follow.

In the first example, a nurse from a cardiac unit is reasoning about a client who has just been admitted to the unit from the emergency department with crushing chest pain, "almost like I can't breathe," that radiates to his left arm. In response to this information, the cardiac nurse thinks aloud in the following manner:

I'll want to check his oxygen saturation every shift, get daily weights, and keep him on a low sodium diet. Those are all nursing measures. He needs pillows to sleep in an upright position, and I'll elevate the head of his bed for comfort.

In the second example, a psychiatric nurse is reasoning about a client who is agitated and angry. He says, "Don't anybody touch me!" The nurse thinks aloud:

I would say, "Michael, I'm not going to touch you." I'd say, "Okay, why don't you sit there, and let's talk." And I would just wait and see. Just sit for awhile. I'd let him stay over there, and I'd sit by the door on the floor so that I would not be so imposing.

In a third example, an obstetric nurse is thinking aloud about a 31-year-old married Asian woman, at 25 weeks' gestation, who was briefly seen in the emergency department for cramping and spotting and was subsequently admitted to labor and delivery for observation and further evaluation. She doesn't speak English. She practices herbal medicine and has continued to do so throughout her pregnancy.

We should have a fetal monitor on her before we get any medication going. I need to see if she understands some English phrases; if not, I would point or gesture, or I might use pictures. There are such things as cervical dilation charts that I could use to show her: "You're open this much, and it's too early for the baby." Also, before starting the medicine, I would try to explain to her what's going to happen. Once she is no longer NPO [nothing by mouth], I will be encouraging her to take her traditional herbs and foods. If taking the herbal medicine is something that she finds supportive, then I would tell her that's good for the baby.

In the final example, a pediatric nurse is thinking aloud about a 6-month-old girl who is admitted from the emergency department for seizure disorder. Her ambulance ride was unremarkable, but she seized as soon as she arrived in the emergency department.

Making Choices

Selecting from a number of possible alternatives

I would want to order an apnea and bradycardia monitor for this patient. I certainly would want to follow the oxygen saturation. I would set up suction at the bedside and set up a bag and mask to be ready to ventilate this child should she need it. I would want these things prepared so that I could monitor and care for this patient. As I'm doing things, I would explain to the mom what I was doing, but I would want to get my house in order . . . before I spoke to the mom. I would say something to the mom like "It's going to take me a few minutes to orient myself to your daughter and to check her over; as soon as I'm finished, I'll sit down to talk to you."

Making choices about nursing interventions seems to consistently be an independent nursing activity. Although nurses would certainly want to keep other members of the health care team apprised of their plan of care and associated nursing interventions, they do not require the supervision or direction of other health professionals to carry them out.

Making Choices about Actions

Nurses in the TIP Study also often used the thinking strategy **making choices** to determine what action to take in response to a clinical dilemma depicting a client case within their area of domain expertise. *Action* is defined in *The American Heritage Dictionary* (1994) as "the state or process of acting or doing." Suchman (1987, p. viii) states that "purposeful actions are inevitably situated actions, actions taken in the context of particular, concrete circumstances." The following examples of nurses' **making choices** about actions seem to support the contextual nature of such actions.

In this first example, a nurse from the HIV/AIDS unit thinks aloud about a client who was just admitted with AIDS-related (non-Hodgkin's) lymphoma and dehydration. He has been suffering from diarrhea and weight loss for the past week and has been experiencing persistent esophageal pain, nausea, dizziness, and lightheadedness. He has had difficulty swallowing and can only keep down liquids. He has general weakness and esophageal and throat pain. His abdomen is tense, rigid, and boardlike on palpation. Bowel sounds are present in all quadrants.

I would report a lot of the physical findings to the physician. I would call him and tell him, "you know, this guy's tummy is tight as a board." I would get the intern's attention and say, "Look, this is what's going on." I'd let him do the diagnostic workup. If he wouldn't respond, I'd say, "Look, you make the time, or I'll call your supervisor." I could say, "Should I beep the attending?"

In a second example, a nurse from home health thinks aloud about a client who is a 75-year-old woman who is 3 days postoperative for surgical repair of a fractured hip. She has been discharged.

She lives alone in a house above street level that can only be accessed by a flight of stairs (15 steps). You arrive at her house, and when you ring the doorbell, you hear a lady yell that "the door is open!" As you enter the house, you notice that there is no carpet; instead, there is only wood flooring. When you enter Lucy's bedroom, you notice that she is in an old-fashioned bed that is at least 42 inches high. There are dirty clothes all around the bed. Next to the bed you observe a stack of unpaid bills. As you begin to do your assessment of Lucy, she tells you that the phone has been disconnected and that the power company is threatening to cut off its service to her.

Number one, I'm going to definitely order physical therapy. In this case, I would also immediately page the social worker. I would tell the social worker that the patient's case is marginal and unsafe; the power might be cut off. If I had to, I would call the power company from the patient's house and explain that the patient is bed-bound, has just gotten out of the hospital, and that we have a social worker that will be working on this case.

In this next example, a critical care nurse is thinking aloud in response to a description of a dilemma of a patient in critical care who suddenly experiences acute shortness of breath. Auscultation of his lungs reveals diffuse crackles.

I'd just tell his physician, "We did a chest x-ray; you need to write an order." I'd tell him, "He needs some furosemide, so how much do you want me to give? Go look at his chest x-ray, and tell me how much furosemide you would like."

In a final example, an oncology nurse thinks aloud in response to a description of a dilemma in which a client has AIDS and probable opportunistic pneumonia.

On entering his room, you note that his oxygen mask is off and lying on the bed. His oxygen saturation is 77%, his heart rate is 150 beats per minute, and his respiratory rate is 44 breaths per minute. At this time, the client is difficult to arouse.

I'd get the physicians in there, and I'd ask, "What are we doing?" I'm thinking maybe it's time to get him to the intensive care unit. I think I'd probably have another nurse in the room.

In some of these examples, the actions about which the nurses are **making choices** seem at least interdependent, if not dependent. In the second of the previous examples, the home health nurse **makes the choice** to order physical therapy for her client. This action will ultimately require a physician's order for reimbursement purposes; it will also require collaboration with the physical therapist. In the subsequent example, the critical care nurse is **making choices** about getting an x-ray and giving furosemide, both of which actions, she seems to realize, will require a physician's order. So the nurse mentally calculates how she will obtain the order without delaying the actions. Benner, Tanner, and Chesla's (1996, pp. 167–168) study of expert practice showed how "experiential learning allows the practitioner to come to terms with boundaries, limits, and possibilities. . . . Having a good clinical grasp and having interventions and responses linked with that clinical grasp, sets up the possibility for expert nurses to take strong positions with other nurses and physicians to get what they believe the patients need." We will see more examples of nurses' ability to work with and through others when they **make choices** about treatments.

Making Choices about Treatment

Nurses in the TIP Study used the thinking strategy **making choices** to determine what treatments should be used to assist the clients described in the clinical dilemmas. *Treatment* is defined as "pharmacological or procedural therapy" (Anderson, Anderson, & Glanze, 1994, p. 1582).

In the first example, a nurse from the AIDS/psychiatric unit responds to a clinical dilemma describing a client who is paranoid and agitated.

Since this guy has been screaming, "Don't touch me," has been drinking a lot, and doesn't look well, and since I have an Ativan [lorazepam] order for agitation, I would use my nursing judgment and give it, knowing that actually Ativan will help him if he's going into the deep detox. I'd give him his medications, make sure he's safe, let him crash.

In a second example, the critical care nurse thinks about how she'd recruit the intern to help her handle a case of hypoglycemia (blood sugar of 50 mg/dL.).

I think her problem is low blood sugar, so I'd get the intern to give her a bolus of dextrose 50% [D50] and then repeat it in maybe an hour or two. I'd just grab him and push him into the room and say, "We're going to give some D50."

In the next example, that same nurse is thinking aloud about a clinical dilemma involving a client with a hematocrit of 21.4% hemoglobin of 6 gm/dL, and platelets of 58,000/mm^3. The physician has ordered two units of packed red blood cells and one six-pack of platelets. The patient's oxygen saturation drops to 89% on 6 L of oxygen. Her respirations increase to 32 breaths per minute, and her abdominal dressing is noted to have a new spot of drainage. The patient becomes difficult to arouse. Her other vitals are blood pressure, 98/58 mm Hg; heart rate, 140 beats per minute. The nasogastric tube output volume is increasing and is now draining bright red blood.

I'd increase her oxygen concentration. She obviously needs blood, so I'd start the blood. After I got the blood started, then I would start another IV, in case we needed to give her fluids or administer some other kind of drug. In the meantime, we'd be giving her blood and maybe starting her on some vasopressors, dopamine, to see if that brings her blood pressure up.

In another example, an obstetric nurse is reasoning about a clinical dilemma depicting a client who is in premature labor and is on 150 µg/min of ritodrine. She calls the nurse into her room and says anxiously, "I'm having really bad chest pain, and it feels like someone is standing on my chest. I need to sit up."

I'm probably turning off the ritodrine so I can get the drug out of her system. We've got orders to put her in Trendelenburg position, but we might have to get her head raised. I'd listen to her heart and lungs to see if there's anything going on. It probably wouldn't hurt to give her some oxygen.

In the final example, an oncology nurse thinks aloud about a dilemma describing a client with a white blood cell count of 1200/mm³, hematocrit of 34.6%, and platelet count of 29,000/mm³. His temperature is 102°F [38.9°C]. He is shaking after receiving a dose of amphotericin B to combat fungal infection.

I'd want to see if the physician wants to give him platelets. And while I'm on the phone, I'd say, "Can I get blood cultures, sputum cultures, urine cultures, and could I also get an order for 25 mg of meperidine?"

In the next to the last of these examples, we see further evidence of an experienced nurse **making a choice** not to carry out the treatments that were ordered: the ritodrine and Trendelenburg position. Instead, the nurse tentatively **makes** other **choices**: *I'm probably turning off the ritodrine. . . . We've got orders to put her in Trendelenburg position, but we might have to get her head raised.* Here again, Benner, Tanner, and Chesla (1996, p. 168) provide insight about this way of thinking: "The expert demonstrates taking a moral stance, in the case of the exceptional and unexpected, at odds with convention and other expectations. . . . It is personally and ethically untenable to experience helplessness in the face of medical emergencies when lives are at stake."

Making Choices about Test Data

A final way that nurses in the TIP Study used the thinking strategy **making choices** was to consider what test data should be ordered for a particular client. *Test data* is defined as "a procedure intended to detect, identify, or quantify information to aid in the management of disease" (Anderson, Anderson, & Glanze, 1994, p. 1880).

In this first example, a nurse from the obstetric unit responds to a dilemma describing a client who was brought to the emergency department by her husband at 2:00 A.M. after complaining of cramping and spotting for 2 days.

In the emergency department, she received a 4-gm loading dose of magnesium sulfate IV piggy back over 30 minutes. You enter Mrs. T.'s room to evaluate her and find the following: Vital signs are oral temperature, 38°C; heart rate, 116 beats per minute; respirations, 28 breaths per minute; and blood pressure, 86/40 mm Hg. Fetal heart rate is 166 beats per minute, with no periodic changes. She is awake and very restless, moving from side to side, trying to get out of the bed. Her skin is pale, cool, and clammy; nail beds are cyanotic. There is bilateral neck vein distention, and her pulses are bounding. There are bilateral rales in her lower lobes, and she is complaining of dyspnea. She has hypoactive bowel sounds; her abdomen is soft. There is no leakage of blood, fluid, or mucus from the vagina.

At this time, we would probably want to have an ultrasound done to tell us what position the baby is in and to try to determine how we're going to deliver the baby. The mom's heart rate is at 116 [beats per minute], which is a lot more concerning at this point. I'd probably be calling for some baseline blood gases and calling for some help. I certainly don't want the contractions to increase, but I would have to turn off the magnesium sulfate and get a magnesium level from the lab.

In a second example of **making choices** about test data, the obstetric nurse is responding to a dilemma describing a client who hemorrhages after delivery.

At this point, where I'm massaging her fundus and looking at the bleeding, I want to get her typed and crossmatched.

Here again, the nurse is **making choices** that in reality cannot be made autonomously, since they will require a physician's order. Yet, we do not see evidence that the nurse thinks about obtaining an order when **making a choice** to obtain these laboratory tests. Benner, Tanner, and Chesla's (1996, p. 285) study of expert practice revealed a phenomenon that they called the blurring of disciplinary boundaries between nursing and medicine: "Nursing has assumed much more responsibility for medical decision making without the corollary explicit recognition of this contribution." Thus, it is not surprising to see that nurses often think about **making choices** about interdependent or dependent actions when, in the reality of today's practice, these choices could not be made without collaboration with physicians. Perhaps this is an indication that actual clinical practice has not kept pace with ideal clinical practice, at least regarding how experienced nurses think about their practice.

Improving the Thinking Strategy Making Choices

Fagin (1992) recommends that nurses be given greater authority to act on matters within their area of clinical competence, such as modifying medications when appropriate, ordering tests, and so on. Until such changes come about, you can strive in your own practice to foster positive relationships with physicians and other health care providers. Indeed, several studies have identified a positive relationship between optimal client outcomes and positive nurse-physician relationships (Knaus, Draper, Wagner, & Zimmerman, 1986; Mitchell, Armstrong, Simpson, & Lentz, 1989).

When **making a choice** in your practice, always consider the purpose of your choice and the intended goal or outcome. Alfaro-LeFevre (1995) recommends that nurses practice identifying those nursing actions that will increase the likelihood of achieving positive client outcomes and will decrease the likelihood of doing harm to clients and, by doing so, develop a safe and efficient plan of care. To do this, you should clarify the specific client problems for which you are **making choices**, determine the desired client outcomes, tailor choices to increase the likelihood of achieving those outcomes, and fine-tune your choices to maximize client benefit and minimize harm.

References

Alfaro-LeFevre, A. (1995). Critical thinking in nursing: A practical approach. Philadelphia: Saunders.

Anderson, K., Anderson, L., & Glanze, W. (Eds.). (1994). *Mosby's medical, nursing, and allied health dictionary* (4th ed.). St. Louis: Mosby.

Benner, P., Tanner, C., & Chesla, C. (1996). *Expertise in nursing practice: Caring, clinical judgment, and ethics*. New York: Springer.

Carnevali, D., & Thomas, M. (1993). *Diagnostic reasoning and treatment decision making in nursing*. Philadelphia: Lippincott.

Fagin, C. (1992). Collaboration between nurses and physicians: No longer a choice. *Academic Medicine, 67*, 295–303.

Fonteyn, M. (1991). *A descriptive analysis of expert critical care nurses' clinical reasoning*. Unpublished doctoral dissertation, University of Texas, Austin.

Knaus, W., Draper, E., Wagner, D., & Zimmerman, J. (1986). An evaluation of outcome from intensive care in major medical centers. *Annals of Internal Medicine, 104*, 410–418.

Kozier, B., Erb, G., Blais, K., & Wilkinson, J. (1995). *Fundamentals of nursing: Concepts, process, and practice*. Redwood City, CA: Addison Wesley.

Mitchell, P., Armstrong, S., Simpson, T., & Lentz, M. (1989). American Association of Critical Care Nurses Demonstration Project: Profile of excellence in critical care nursing. *Heart and Lung, 18*, 219–237.

Suchman, L. (1991). *Plans and situated actions. The problem of human-machine communication*. Cambridge: Cambridge University Press.

13 *Judging the Value*

For the purposes of this book, the thinking strategy called **judging the value** is defined as forming an opinion or evaluation about worth in terms of usefulness, significance, or importance. Findings from the Thinking in Practice (TIP) Study revealed several types of data of which nurses **judge the value**: assessment findings, treatments, and test data.

Evaluation is one of the phases of the nursing process and is recognized by regulatory agencies and the Nurse Practice Act as an essential component of nursing practice. Evaluation occurs whenever nurses make judgments about their clients' status or progress, their treatment plan, or about the meaning of the clinical data that are associated with a particular client case. Thus, **judging the value** is an important thinking strategy for nurses to develop, refine, and improve.

Judging the Value of Assessment Findings

A primary reason that nurses use the thinking strategy **judging the value** is to interpret the meaning of their clients' assessment findings. The following are examples from the TIP Study of nurses' using **judging the value** for this purpose:

Her heart rate's up a little; that's compensating for the little bit of drop in the blood pressure. Her respirations have increased to 28. They were 24; now they're up a little bit. [Blood pressure of] 98/58 is still not that bad. It's bad; it's low for her. And if she is difficult to arouse, it could be her blood gases [her arterial carbon dioxide level may be abnormally high].

A fetal heart rate of 150 [beats per minute] is within normal range.

She's having very mild contractions, and the rest of her assessment is within normal range. But, if she's having contractions every 10 minutes, then she may be having up to six contractions an hour, which is too much. We want her to have three or less, but very mild.

A fever of 103.8°F [40°C] in an asthmatic child who is 9 months old is not that high. It's high for an adult, but it's not all that unexpected in a child.

60 mL of bright red drainage immediately post-op is worrisome. I would think that's a lot. And the fact that her right arm is swollen after a lumpectomy would worry me also. I'd probably call the physician to assess it.

In this last example, we can see how using the thinking strategy called **judging the value** directs the nurse regarding what to do next: *I'd probably call the physician to assess it.* Here again, consideration of context is important in that the nurse **judges the value** of 60 mL of bright red drainage within the context of other assessment findings (*and the fact that her right arm is swollen from a lumpectomy would worry me also*) and of time since surgery (*immediately post-op is worrisome.*)

Judging the Value of Treatments

Another reason that nurses use the thinking strategy **judging the value** is to evaluate their clients' treatments in terms of significance, usefulness and appropriateness, and cost. The following are examples from the TIP Study of nurses' using **judging the value** to evaluate the medications that their clients are receiving:

TPN [total parental nutrition] is also incredibly expensive, and that may cloud the picture at a county hospital. It's really expensive stuff.

He has Lasix [furosemide], 80 mg ordered IV twice a day. That's good because it will help get rid of some of that extra fluid.

Ritodrine tends to cause a lot more problems, increased heart rate and palpitations and things like that, than magnesium sulfate. Yeah, the side effects of ritodrine can be worse than what we're actually using it to treat. So we have her on 150 µg/min of ritodrine, and 300 to 350 µg/min is the maximum amount that you're going to give somebody. We've got her halfway up to that amount.

Several of these examples demonstrate the nurses' consideration of risk versus benefit when **judging the value** of the medication treatment that their client is receiving. In the first example, the nurse is **judging the value** of TPN therapy in light of the fact that this type of therapy is *incredibly expensive*; clients at a county hospital (who are often poor or indigent) may not be able to afford this therapy for very long, if at all. In the last of these examples, the nurse is **judging the value** of ritodrine by weighing the benefits of this particular medication against the risk of the

Judging the Value

Forming an opinion or evaluation about worth in terms of usefulness, significance, or importance

client experiencing side effects from the medication, particularly when it is given at an increasingly high dose. Kassirer and Kopelman (1991) advise that treatment decisions should always include a consideration of both the benefit-cost and benefit-risk ratios.

In the other of the previous examples, the nurse **judges the value** of furosemide as *good* and then goes on to explain: *because it will help get rid of some of that extra fluid.* The nurse thus identifies an expected outcome of the furosemide therapy. If this outcome is not achieved within the anticipated length of time, the nurse may then **judge the value** of the therapy differently (i.e., as ineffective or inadequate). Nielsen (1992, p. 69) reminds us that "outcomes can be partially predicted . . . [but] they can never be fully predicted because of human physiology and psychology." According to Nielsen, when an expected outcome is not met, the therapy should be reviewed and reconsidered to enhance the likelihood of achieving the desired outcome.

Judging the Value of Test Data

Another reason that nurses use the thinking strategy **judging the value** is to evaluate the meaning of their clients' test data. The following are examples from the TIP Study of nurses' using **judging the value** to evaluate this type of data:

The sodium is slightly low; the potassium is borderline low. His glucose and total cholesterol are decent. But his potassium is at the borderline level, so he might need [to receive] a little extra potassium, whether just for the interim or ongoing, once a day.

Her platelets are only 58,000/mm³, so they're dropping. Her platelets are low, so I know she's at risk to bleed, and I think she needs the blood [transfusion].

In the following example, the nurse is thinking aloud in response to information about a client whose red blood cell count is 2.9 million/mm³, whose hemoglobin is 9.6 gm/dL, and who is scheduled for an exploratory laparotomy in the morning: *His red blood cell count is not okay. It's too low for somebody who's going to surgery. His hemoglobin is not okay. My concern is if he goes to surgery with his hemoglobin being low.*

In this next example, the nurse is thinking aloud in response to information about the laboratory values of a 72-year-old man who is on renal dialysis three times per week: [his] international normalized ratio (INR) is 1.6; blood urea nitrogen (BUN), 57 mg/dL; creatinine, 5.9 mg/dL; and potassium, 5.0 mEq/L: *The INR is too low. His BUN is high. His creatinine is sky-high for somebody who is on dialysis, and his potassium is high.*

Tests serve several functions in clinical practice: they provide information for diagnostic purposes, they assist in monitoring a client's physiologic status, and they assist in the evaluation of the effectiveness of therapy. For this reason, nurses as well as other health practitioners are frequently involved in carrying out and interpreting the results of their clients' tests. Corbett (1996, p. 7) describes the nurse's role in regard to laboratory data: "In addition to using laboratory data to formulate nursing diagnoses, nurses must determine if the results of a test need to be reported immediately to a physician or if the report is not urgent. The nurse may also need to alert other health care workers or the client and family about symptoms to watch for or precautions to take."

In the previous examples of nurses' using the thinking strategy **judging the value** to evaluate test data, it seems clear that the values obtained from tests are being judged against reference values. Most reports of laboratory tests include the normal (numerical) reference values on the report, in addition to the values that were obtained for the particular client who was tested. It is interesting to note, however, that when nurses think about and **judge the value** of test results concerning a particular client's case, they use non-numerical and rather qualitative terms, such as those in the previous examples: *slightly low, borderline low, low, pretty low, too high,* and *sky-high.* Findings from Fonteyn's (1991) dissertation research revealed that there is a relationship between the qualitative nature of the nurses' evaluative language and their understanding of the context of a client case. An illustration of this contextual evaluation can be seen in the third of the previous examples, where the nurse evaluates the client's red blood cell count and hemoglobin level within the context of his impending surgery.

Improving the Thinking Strategy Judging the Value

Evaluation has been identified as an important component of sound critical thinking. Beginning in 1988 and ending in 1989, a Delphi methodology was used to conduct a systematic inquiry into the state of critical thinking and critical thinking assessment. A panel of 46 scholars with expertise in teaching or evaluating critical thinking developed a consensus statement regarding the conceptualization of critical thinking and the characteristics of the ideal critical thinker (Facione, 1992). Evaluation, which included the ability to assess the credibility and the contextual relevance of information, was identified by the panel as a core critical thinking strategy.

Additionally, the expert panel described the dispositions, or habits of mind, that are conducive to sound critical thinking. Among the dispositions identified were fair-mindedness in evaluation and prudence in making judgments. Two multiple-choice instruments have been developed as a result of the findings from this Delphi study, the California Critical Thinking Skills Test (Facione, 1990) and the California Critical Thinking Dispositions Inventory (Facione & Facione, 1992). Both instruments assess individuals' ability to judge and evaluate information, and they are being used by increasing numbers of nursing schools to evaluate their students' ability to think critically as well as to evaluate their disposition to do so (Facione, 1992).

Wilkinson (1996, pp. 280–281) suggests that using an evaluation checklist during each step in the nursing process will help nurses improve their use of this important thinking strategy. The checklist would consist of several key questions that are designed to evaluate each unique step. Some questions to ask during the assessment step, for example, would include the following: "Were the assessment data incomplete or inaccurate?" "Are there data that still need to be validated?" "Has the client's condition changed?" Some questions to ask during the diagnosis step are the following: "Is the diagnosis irrelevant or unrelated to the data base?" "Is the diagnosis inadequately supported by data?" "Has the nursing diagnosis been resolved?"

In a similar manner, Richard Paul (1993, p. 530) recommends that individuals develop a habit of asking themselves a series of questions to determine if an evaluation has a logic: "Are we clear about what precisely we are evaluating?" "Given our purpose, what are the relevant criteria or standards for evaluation?" "Do we have sufficient information?" "Have we applied our criteria accurately and fairly to the facts as we know them?" Paul (p. 54) reminds us that sound critical thinking adheres to established intellectual standards, among them "the ability to evaluate information for its relevance."

Alfaro-LeFevre (1995) advocates that nurses practice distinguishing between normal and abnormal data and assessment findings as a means to improve their ability to evaluate data. She reminds us that evaluating is an ongoing process for nurses throughout their care provision.

References

Alfaro-LeFevre, R. (1995). *Critical thinking in nursing.* Philadelphia: Saunders.

Corbett, J. (1996). *Laboratory tests and diagnostic procedures with nursing diagnoses.* Stamford, CT: Appleton & Lange.

Facione, P. (1990). *The California Critical Thinking Skills Test—College Level* (Technical Reports Nos. 1–4). (ERIC Document Reproduction Service Nos. ED 327 549, ED 327 550, ED 325 584, ED 327 566.)

Facione, P. (1992, November). *Empirical methods of theory and tool development for the assessment of college level critical thinking and problem solving.* Paper presented at the Conference on Collegiate Skills Assessment, U.S. Department of Education, Washington, DC.

Facione, P., & Facione, N. (1992). *The California Critical Thinking Dispositions Inventory (CCTDI) and the CCTDI test manual.* Milbrae, CA: California Academic Press.

Fonteyn, M. (1991). *A descriptive analysis of expert critical care nurses' clinical reasoning.* Unpublished doctoral dissertation, University of Texas, Austin.

Kassirer, J., & Kopelman, R. (1991). *Learning clinical reasoning.* Baltimore: Williams & Wilkins.

Nielsen, P. (1992). Quality of care: Discovering a modified practice theory. *Journal of Nursing Care Quality, 6*(2), 63–76.

Paul, R. (1993). *Critical thinking: How to prepare students for a rapidly changing world.* Santa Rosa, CA: Foundation for Critical Thinking.

Wilkinson, J. (1996). *Nursing process: A critical thinking approach* (2nd ed.). Menlo Park, CA: Addison Wesley Nursing.

14 *Drawing Conclusions*

For the purposes of this book, the thinking strategy called **drawing conclusions** is defined as reaching a decision or forming an opinion. Findings from the Thinking in Practice (TIP) Study revealed that nurses primarily **draw conclusions** about their clients' status or condition, but they also draw conclusions about situations.

A primary purpose for nurses' thinking in practice is to make decisions or form opinions; thus, it is not surprising that the thinking strategy called **drawing conclusions** was frequently used by the nurses in the TIP Study.

Drawing Conclusions about a Client's Condition or Status

One reason that nurses use the thinking strategy **drawing conclusions** in their practice is to form an opinion about their clients' condition or status. The following are examples from the TIP Study of nurses' using **drawing conclusions** for this purpose:

A nurse who is reasoning about laboratory findings concludes: *She's anemic, with an RBC [red blood count] at 3 million/mm³, hemoglobin at 10 gm% [gm/dL], and hematocrit at 32%.*

A nurse who is reasoning about an obstetric client who is in premature labor and has been receiving magnesium sulfate to stop her contractions concludes: *She's obviously going into some type of respiratory distress, probably secondary to the mag-sulfate, which causes pulmonary edema.*

A nurse who is reasoning about a client's perfusion status concludes: *But his pulses are there and his blood pressure is okay and his heart rate is okay, so he's getting profusion down there [to his lower extremities].*

A nurse who is reasoning about the etiology of a client's chest pain concludes: *But she has every other risk factor, so chances are this is chest pain caused by myocardial ischemia. The chest pain was precipitated by moving furniture and a lot of [strenuous] activity. So, I'd probably believe that it was some kind of true cardiac event, just because of all the risk factors she has.*

An oncology nurse who is reasoning about a client with pneumonia whose respiratory rate is up to 40 breaths per minute and is labored, blood pressure is 92/60 mm Hg, heart rate is 140 beats per minute, and temperature is 38°C concludes: *Now I'm getting concerned that he's going into sepsis. He's getting septic. He has an increased heart rate and decreased blood pressure. That is a major sign right there.*

In all of the previous examples, the nurses explain their reasons for their conclusions, and in doing so, they mentally justify the validity of these conclusions. This justification is an indication of the nurses' self-confidence in their thinking. Facione and Facione (1996, p. 131) describe critical thinking self-confidence as an important disposition, or habit of mind, of the ideal critical thinker: "The ideal critical thinker is trustful of reason."

Nurses in the TIP Study, however, did not always explain or justify their conclusions. Often, the nurses seemed to use the thinking strategy **drawing conclusions** to offer a tentative explanation for information or data that they were given in a dilemma. The following are examples of nurses' using **drawing conclusions** in this manner:

A psychiatric nurse who is reasoning about a mentally disturbed client who is HIV-positive concludes: *This is a human being, and he's probably not having a good day.*

A cardiac nurse who is reasoning about a client who has been admitted with the diagnosis of R/O MI (rule out myocardial infarction) concludes: *So far, he's not having any chest pain or anything like that.*

A critical care nurse who is reasoning about a client who continues to complain of severe chest pain and shortness of breath, who is becoming increasingly agitated and restless, and whose skin is cool, ashen, and diaphoretic concludes: *It sounds like he's going into cardiogenic shock . . . the patient is in bad shape.*

A nurse who is reasoning about a client who was found unarousable, is suspected of having encephalopathy with associated jaundice, and has elevated liver enzymes concludes: *I don't know what's going on. He's jaundiced. He's got elevated liver enzymes. I'm thinking it's hepatic encephalopathy.*

In all of these examples, we note a tentativeness in the nurses' conclusions. Language such as *probably, so far, it sounds like,* and *I'm thinking* indicates some degree of uncertainty regarding the conclusions that the nurses reach. This uncertainty is

Drawing Conclusions

Reaching a decision or forming an opinion

not necessarily a bad thing, nor is it indicative of poor reasoning or unsound critical thinking. Indeed, being tentative regarding one's conclusions, especially early in a client encounter when there is limited data available with which to draw firm conclusions regarding client status, may be indicative of possessing several of the dispositions for ideal critical thinking: maturity, systematicity, and truth-seeking.

Facione and Facione (1996, p. 131) define the disposition toward critical thinking called cognitive maturity as "prudence in making, suspending, or revising judgment; an awareness of multiple solutions may be acceptable and that reaching closure may be necessary even in the absence of complete knowledge." They propose that cognitive maturity is critical to the development of expertise as a clinician (Facione, Sanchez, Facione, & Gainen, 1995).

The disposition toward critical thinking called systematicity is defined as "valuing organization, focus, and diligence in the approach to complex problems" (Facione & Facione, 1996, p. 131). Studies of critical thinking have revealed that organized approaches to problem solving and decision making are hallmarks of a thoughtful person regardless of the problem domain being addressed (Facione, Sanchez, Facione, & Gainen, 1995).

The disposition toward critical thinking called truth-seeking is defined as "a courageous desire for the best knowledge in a context, even if such knowledge fails to support or undermines one's preconceptions, beliefs, or self-interests" (Facione & Facione, 1996, p. 131). Research has demonstrated that the truth seeker is one who remains receptive to giving serious consideration to additional facts, reasons, or perspectives even if this should necessitate changing one's mind on some issue (Facione, Sanchez, Facione, & Gainen, 1995).

When nurses are tentative in their conclusions, it may be indicative of their possessing the previously described dispositions toward critical thinking. Rubenfeld and Scheffer's (1995, pp. 83–84) description of **drawing conclusions** as a process helps explain the tentative nature of many nurses' conclusions: "Conclusions are part of all phases of the nursing process. Most conclusions are like rest stops on a journey; they provide guidance for travel along the nursing process path. . . . The conclusions represent the nurses' thinking about the information at hand."

Drawing Conclusions about a Situation

Another reason that nurses use the thinking strategy **drawing conclusions** is to make decisions or form opinions about a situation. The following are examples from the TIP Study of nurses' using the thinking strategy **drawing conclusions** for this purpose:

A nurse reasoning about an AIDS client concludes: *I have a very complex situation on my hands, and it's hard to know what to do.*

A nurse reasoning about a central line placement that is scheduled to be done on the critical care unit later in the day on a client who is HIV-positive concludes: *And if the central line placement is scheduled for 1:30 P.M., then it'll probably never happen right at that time. Things never seem to go according to schedule in the unit. It's either that they're putting in a line in an emergency-type situation, or if it's not an emergency, then they do it when they have a spare moment. And I think it's kind of risky because the patient is HIV-positive, so we'd have to be extra careful.*

A nurse who is orienting a registered nurse who is new to the critical care unit reasons about how well she is coping with a crisis situation and concludes: *The nurse is probably totally overwhelmed by now. And we're kind of in a pseudo-code situation here, so maybe I'll have her record things so that she's still there getting the experience and seeing what's going on.*

An obstetric nurse reasons about a client who is in premature labor and is tearful. She is placed on a fetal monitor that shows an irritability pattern, and her vaginal examination reveals 2-cm dilation, 50% effacement, and a slightly bloody show. The nurse concludes: *Obviously, something is going on here.*

Drawing conclusions about a situation in practice helps nurses to understand the contextual information that may influence their thinking and decision making. Baker (1996) suggests that an improved awareness of clinical context facilitates nurses' critical thinking. Miller and Babcock (1996, p. 20) agree: "Thinking critically includes being sensitive to the context in which thinking occurs . . . the entire situation, background, or environment relevant to a particular situation."

Understanding the context of a situation assists us in making sense out of data and incorporating it into a line of reasoning (Kassirer & Kopelman, 1988). In his classic treatise *The Reflective Practitioner*, Schön (1983, p. 40) tells us, "Problem setting is a process in which, interactively, we *name* the things to which we will attend and *frame* the context in which we will attend to them." Schön reminds us of the value of being aware of the manner in which we frame the problems that we encounter in our practice: "When a practitioner becomes aware of his frames, he also becomes aware of the possibility of alternative ways of framing the reality of his practice."

Framing errors can occur when data are provided in a misleading fashion. Sonnenberg, Kassirer, and Kopelman (1986) provide an example of this by describing a clinical case of a benign urinary tract lesion that was misdiagnosed as a malignancy in part because of the language that the radiologist used in describing what he saw as a "mass" rather than as a "space-occupying lesion." It was felt that the clinicians might have been less inclined to believe the client had cancer if the radiologist's description had been different. Thus, it is important for practitioners to be aware of the context in which they are **drawing conclusions**, both conclusions about their clients as well as conclusions about practice situations.

Improving the Thinking Strategy Drawing Conclusions

You can improve your ability to think critically and reflectively by monitoring your thought processes and critically assessing your conclusions. Ennis (1996) provides a list of some words that we often use when we are **drawing conclusions**: *therefore,* *hence, thus,* and *so.* "These indicators are not always present," says Ennis (p. 19), "but when they are present, you should take advantage of them." Becoming aware of those times when you are **drawing conclusions** helps improve your thinking through metacognition, thinking about your thinking.

According to Paul (1993), conclusions that result from sound critical thinking are deep, reasonable, and consistent. **Drawing conclusions**, says Paul (p. 199), "is part of a broader process of reasoning things through. The particular inferences made have a specific logic that can be assessed, and the total process of reasoning things through has a general logic that also can be assessed." The skilled critical thinker maintains an awareness of the circumstances that led to his or her conclusions, their implications and consequences, and the assumptions on which they are based.

Alfaro-LeFevre (1995, p. 113) cautions that the ability to **draw conclusions** that are valid requires "problem specific knowledge and knowledge of cultural influences." Her suggestions for improving this ability include, "Avoid making inferences based on only one cue" and "Once you've made an inference, verify whether it's correct by gathering more information."

References

Alfaro-LeFevre, R. (1995). *Critical thinking in nursing: A practical approach*. Philadelphia: Saunders.

Baker, C. (1996). Reflective learning: A teaching strategy for critical thinking. *Journal of Nursing Education, 35*(1), 19–22.

Ennis, R. (1996). *Critical thinking*. Upper Saddle River, NJ: Prentice-Hall.

Facione, N., & Facione, P. (1996). Externalizing the critical thinking in knowledge development and clinical judgment. *Nursing Outlook, 44*(3), 129–136.

Facione, P., Sanchez, C., Facione, N., & Gainen, J. (1995). The disposition toward critical thinking. *JGE: The Journal of General Education, 44*(1), 1–25.

Kassirer, J., & Kopelman, R. (1988). The case presentation: I. Principles. *Hospital Practice, 23*(7), 21–29.

Miller, M., & Babcock, D. (1996). *Critical thinking applied to nursing*. St. Louis: Mosby.

Paul, R. (1993). *Critical thinking: How to prepare students for a rapidly changing world*. Rohnert Park, CA: Center for Critical Thinking and Moral Critique.

Rubenfeld, G., & Scheffer, B. (1995). *Critical thinking in nursing: An interactive approach*. Philadelphia: Lippincott.

Schön, D. (1983). *The reflective practitioner: How professionals think in action*. New York: Harper Collins.

Sonnenberg, F., Kassirer, J., & Kopelman, R. (1986). An autopsy of the clinical reasoning process. *Hospital Practice, 23*(12), 21–29.

15 *Providing Explanations*

For the purposes of this book, the thinking strategy **providing explanations** is defined as offering reasons for actions, beliefs, or remarks. Nurses in the Thinking in Practice (TIP) Study used this thinking strategy to suggest reasons for therapy, tests, nursing interventions, and actions and to explain their concerns and predictions.

Providing the reasons in support of an action or conclusion is seen as an important component of sound critical thinking, including critical thinking in clinical practice (Ennis, 1996; Facione, Sanchez, Facione, & Gainen, 1995; Fonteyn, 1991; Paul, 1993).

Ennis (1996) describes the various types of explanation associated with critical thinking: describing a process, stating a meaning, justifying something, and explaining by a hypothesis or a conclusion that accounts for something that is or was. Facione and Facione's (1996, p. 131) description of the cognitive skills of the ideal critical thinker (derived from the American Philosophical Association's Delphi Study) includes the cognitive skill **explanation**, defined as "to state the results of one's reasoning; to justify that reasoning in terms of the evidential, conceptual, methodological, criteriological and contextual considerations upon which one's results were based; and to present one's reasoning in the form of cogent argument." Fonteyn (1991, p. 78) identifies **explain**, which she defines as "providing a rationale for a choice of treatment or action," as one of the cognitive processes inherent in expert nurses' clinical reasoning. Paul (1993, pp. 160–161) proposes that "good reasoners assert a claim only when they have sufficient evidence to back it up, can articulate and therefore evaluate the evidence behind their claims, and draw conclusions only to the extent that they are supported by the data."

Thus, there is considerable evidence in the literature to support the premise that **providing explanations** is an important component of sound thinking.

Providing Explanations for Therapy

According to Barrows and Pickell (1991, p. 162), "The therapeutic decision is the whole purpose of your encounter with the patient." Thus, much of thinking in practice will focus on therapeutic decisions. **Providing explanations** for these decisions is important to sound thinking about them. Additionally, Barrows and Pickell (1991, p. 208) propose that the ability of clinicians "to continuously reflect on their thinking about therapy and to review their thoughts and decisions during a client encounter is critical to self-improvement."

The following are examples of nurses in the TIP Study **providing explanations** for therapy:

She obviously needs the blood, so I'd start the blood.

We would be giving her the blood and maybe starting her on vasopressors, dopamine, to see if that brings her blood pressure up.

He's going to need fluids, just for maintenance. He's also going to need extra fluids to get him hydrated.

We'll get him started on the morphine drip to keep him comfortable because right now he's not comfortable.

One purpose of **providing explanations** for therapy may be to identify the goals of the therapy. In the first of these examples, the nurse's **explanations** assist in identifying two of the purposes of this therapy: as a necessary replacement for blood loss and to bring her blood pressure up. In the second example, the nurse's **explanations** of the purpose of the fluid therapy are both to hydrate the client and then to maintain hydration. Additonally, in the last example, **providing an explanation** for the morphine drip clarifies the purpose: *to keep him comfortable*.

Providing Explanations for Tests

Kassirer and Kopelman (1991, p. 17) describe diagnostic testing as "an information gathering task" intended to "reduce diagnostic uncertainty" and to "selectively distinguish among competing hypotheses." We see evidence of these inten-

Providing Explanations

Offering reasons for actions, beliefs, or remarks

tions in the following examples of nurses using the thinking strategy **providing explanations** for tests:

And I'd want to get another EKG [electrocardiogram] to see if she's had any changes since this episode. Because we already know that she came out positive on her stress test.

With that glucose of 500 [mg/dL], I would think the physician would order frequent blood sugar checks, to make sure his level comes down.

I'd look at the differential [on the complete blood count report] to see if she possibly has an infection.

So I would want to see if his ammonia level was high, to determine whether or not he's in a hepatic coma.

But we need to have her typed and crossmatched, and as we start an IV, we need to get a stat hematocrit and hemoglobin, to see where we're coming from.

In the third of these examples, we see evidence of the nurse's **providing an explanation** for a test (*the differential*) intended to assist in verifying a hypothesis (*if she possibly has an infection*). In the fourth example, the nurse's explanation indicates that the purpose of a test (*ammonia level*) is to help rule in or rule out the hypothesis that *he's in a hepatic coma.* Kassirer and Kopelman (1991) remind us that although tests can be useful for refining diagnostic hypotheses in the light of new data, clinicians should struggle to weigh the benefits of tests for diagnosis and therapy against their inherent risks (physiologic, psychological, and economic). For example, "when a disease is highly unlikely, further tests to disprove the diagnosis often are not needed" (p. 24).

Providing Explanations for Nursing Interventions

Providing explanations for their interventions is one way that nurses can ensure that they will follow high professional standards. There are numerous agencies involved in establishing standards and regulations to guide nursing care, including federal, state, and local governmental agencies, accrediting bodies, and professional nursing organizations. Although the standards delineated by such agencies and organizations certainly are useful in guiding our practice, our own self-awareness of our thinking associated with choosing and implementing nursing interventions is perhaps our surest and most consistent guide. Alfaro-LeFevre (1995, p. 62) cautions, "Never perform an action if you don't know why it's indicated, why it works (the rationale), and whether there are risks of harm." The following examples of nurses' **providing explanations** (rationales) for their nursing interventions illustrate self-awareness in their thinking:

He needs pillows to sleep in an upright position, and I'll elevate the head of his bed for comfort, to help with lung expansion.

After I got the blood started, then I would start another IV, in case we needed to give her fluids or administer some other kind of drug.

I'd want to keep watching her monitor to make sure that there aren't any more changes.

So I'd probably make sure that somebody got in there to see this patient because it sounds like somebody should take a look at him. And I'd also check to see if his nurse is comfortable in that situation.

So what I'd want to do now is turn off the nitroglycerin because his blood pressure is so low.

She may or may not understand the vaginal exam, but hopefully I can be talking about it as I do the exam and kind of show and tell to see if that will help her feel a little bit more comfortable.

Alfaro-LeFevre (1995, p. 130) proposes that "identifying specific interventions designed to increase the likelihood of achieving the [intended] outcomes and decrease the likelihood of harm is essential to developing a safe and efficient plan." In several of the previous examples, nurses use the thinking strategy **providing explanations** to identify the desired outcome associated with the specific interventions that they propose. In the first example, the nurse explains the purpose of using pillows and elevating the head of the client's bed: *for comfort, to help with lung expansion*. In the last example, the nurse explains that the purpose of talking as she does during the vaginal examination is to help the client *feel a little bit more comfortable*. The three middle examples depict nurses' **explanations** of interventions that are intended to maintain the client's stability or to prevent further deterioration in the client's status. In all three of these examples, the language of the nurses' thoughts (*in case*, *to make sure*, and *I'd probably make sure*) reveals the strategy of being prepared in advance for the possibility of a change in the client's status.

Providing Explanations for Actions

Rubenfeld and Scheffer (1995, p. 196) submit that part of a care plan "consists of the rationales for the nursing actions," and they caution that "all nursing actions must be based on sound nursing principles." In the following examples of nurses' thoughts about actions, we see evidence of their providing a rationale for their actions:

I can only be in one place at one time, so sometimes I just have to say, "Listen, I've got this other patient who's crumping down the hall. I need to be down there, so you need to handle things here."

I'd get the supervisor up [here] and get some help because I can't do everything. I can do a lot, but not all of this. And the liability there is phenomenal.

First of all, I'm going to call for help here, too, because I can't start an IV and massage her uterus at the same time.

I'd call the doctor to see if he knows about the 28,000 [/mm³] platelets.

And I'd call the doc to ask about the blood cultures and to see what he wants to do.

The first three examples depict nurses' **providing explanations** of actions that involve calling for help with a particular situation. Benner, Tanner, and Chesla (1996, pp. 167–168) identify this type of activity as characteristic of expert practice: "Recognizing the unexpected requires persuading and marshaling appropriate responses from others. . . . Experiential learning allows the practitioner to come to terms with boundaries, limits, and possibilities. . . . Part of nursing expertise lies in strengthening and working with others so that no one is overburdened and all possible resources are brought to bear in difficult situations." In the last two of the previous examples, the nurses' **explanations** for calling the doctor are to exchange important information about the client case and then to reach a decision about what to do about the information. In clinical practice, clients rely heavily on nurses' acting as their advocates to keep their physicians informed and to solicit their advice and actions whenever necessary.

Providing Explanations for Concerns

Chapter 5 described how concerns about clients are a frequent focus of nurses when using the thinking strategy **setting priorities**. In the following examples, we see evidence of **providing explanations** for their focus of concern:

I'm focusing on that hip, and I don't really care about anything else right now because for all I know she might have broken her hip.

So, the patient with Vtach [ventricular tachycardia] would be the first [to be evacuated] because he could have a cardiac arrest.

I'm a little concerned that her cervix is 2 cm dilated, since this is her first pregnancy.

If it's anterior, I'm going to be more worried about her because the cervix has come around to the front, getting her ready to go.

In the first example, the nurse indicates that her only concern at the moment is *that hip*, **explaining** her concern that the client *might have broken her hip*. As mentioned in Chapter 5, a characteristic of highly experienced nurses' reasoning is their ability to zero in on the most significant symptoms (Jacavone & Dostal, 1992). In the second example, a nurse is responding to a clinical dilemma depicting a fire on her unit, necessitating the evacuation of all of the clients and staff. She **provides an explanation** for her decision to evacuate the patient with ventricular tachycardia (a life-threatening dysrhythmia) first: *because he could have a cardiac arrest*. Here again, we see evidence of experienced nurses' ability to identify strategies to prevent deterioration in their clients.

Providing Explanations for Predictions

The following are examples from the TIP Study of nurses **providing explanations** for their predictions, thus substantiating the premise that nurses who think well in practice consistently provide rationales for their thinking:

And they'd end up taking her back to surgery because there's something bleeding in there.

This is going to be difficult because he speaks Russian and she's deaf.

If this baby's breech, and the mom is dilating, and her contractions don't stop, she may go for a C-section [cesarean section] because we're going to try to save that head from going through the cervix and getting compressed.

So probably with a 14-year-old who is not real well developed or anything like that, the baby is not going to fall out, so you have a little time to think about some of the things you're going to do and to get ready for them.

The previous examples demonstrate how **providing explanations** helps nurses to justify and thus lend credibility to their predictions.

Improving the Thinking Strategy Providing Explanations

Higgs and Jones (1995) discuss the close relationship between strong self-monitoring skills and proficiency in clinical reasoning. Hasselbrock, Jonas, and Bauer (1993) propose that self-monitoring is important to planning, controlling, and evaluating one's knowledge and strategies during clinical reasoning. The thinking strategy **providing explanations** can facilitate your self-monitoring skills by raising your awareness of the rationale for your beliefs, decisions, and actions, and ultimately increasing your self-confidence in your ability to think well in practice. Facione, Sanchez, Facione, and Gainen (1995, p. 8) describe critical thinking self-confidence as an important disposition toward critical thinking: "[Critical thinking] self-confidence allows one to trust the soundness of one's own reasoned judgments and to lead others in the rational resolution of problems." Another disposition toward critical thinking that is fostered by using the thinking strategy **providing explanations** is analyticity: "prizing the application of reasoning and the use of evidence to resolve problems, anticipating potential conceptual or practical difficulties, and consistently being alert to the need to intervene" (Facione, Sanchez, Facione, & Gainen, 1995, p. 7). There is a growing consensus that developing sound critical thinking skills must include cultivating the dispositions toward critical thinking (Facione, Sanchez, Facione, & Gainen, 1995).

References

Alfaro-LeFevre, R. (1995). *Critical thinking in nursing.* Philadelphia: Saunders.

Barrows, H., & Pickell, G. (1991). *Developing clinical problem-solving skills: A guide to more effective diagnosis and treatment.* New York: Norton Medical Books.

Benner, P., Tanner, C., & Chesla, C. (1996). *Expertise in nursing practice: caring, clinical judgment, and ethics.* New York: Springer.

Ennis, R. (1996). *Critical thinking.* Upper Saddle River, NJ: Prentice Hall.

Facione, N., & Facione, P. (1996). Externalizing critical thinking in knowledge development and clinical judgment. *Nursing Outlook, 44*(3), 129–136.

Facione, P., Sanchez, C., Facione, N., & Gainen, J. (1995). The disposition toward critical thinking. *JGE: The Journal of General Education, 44*(1), 1–25.

Fonteyn, M. (1991). *A descriptive analysis of expert critical care nurses' clinical reasoning.* Unpublished doctoral dissertation, University of Texas, Austin.

Hasselbrock, F., Jonas, A., & Bauer, L. (1993). *Metacognitive aspects of medical problem solving.* Paper presented at the meeting of the American Educational Research Association, Atlanta, GA.

Higgs, J., & Jones, M. (1995). Clinical reasoning. In J. Higgs and M. Jones (Eds.), *Clinical reasoning in the health professions.* Oxford, England: Butterworth-Heinemann.

Jacavone, J., & Dostal, M. (1992). A descriptive study of nursing judgment in the assessment and management of cardiac pain. *Advances in Nursing Science, 15*, 54–63.

Kassirer, J., & Kopelman, R. (1991). *Learning clinical reasoning.* Baltimore: Williams & Wilkins.

Paul, R. (1993). *Critical thinking: How to prepare students for a rapidly changing world.* Santa Rosa, CA: The Foundation for Critical Thinking.

Rubenfeld, G., & Scheffer, B. (1995). *Critical thinking in nursing: An interactive approach.* Philadelphia: Lippincott.

16 *Other Thinking Strategies*

Although the thinking strategies described in the previous chapters predominated in the thoughts of the nurses in the Thinking in Practice (TIP) Study, several other thinking strategies were used by the nurses to a lesser extent. These strategies include **pondering, making assumptions, posing a question, qualifying,** and **making generalizations**.

Pondering

For the purposes of this book, the thinking strategy called **pondering** is defined as mentally pausing to reflect on the meaning of a piece of information. The following are examples of instances when nurses from the TIP Study used the thinking strategy **pondering**:

Well, let's see . . .

We'd end up . . . let's see . . . I'm trying to think.

Let me see . . . a pungent smell from the kitchen . . . I'd go see what it was.

Let me see . . . he's not on any blood pressure medications.

Let's see . . . we've already been told that she stopped taking her nitroglycerin because it gives her a headache.

In all of these examples, the nurses seem to be using the thinking strategy **pondering** to pause briefly to collect their thoughts before continuing. In his classic

Pondering

Mentally pausing to reflect on the meaning of a piece of information

work *The Reflective Practitioner: How Professionals Think in Action* (1983, p. 62), Schön provides insight regarding the possible utility of this thinking strategy: "A practitioner's reflection-in-action may not be very rapid. It is bounded by the action-present, the zone of time in which action can still make a difference to the situation. . . . The pace and duration of reflection-in-action vary with the pace and duration of the situations of practice."

Barrows and Pickell (1991, p. 25) describe **pondering** as a component of metacognition, entailing "putting conscious effort into thinking. . . . Besides **pondering** or reflecting over a perplexing situation, the clinician should be asking himself how well he is doing in thinking through the problem: does he need help, advice, more information?" Barrows and Pickell (p. 26) further recommend, "Whenever something does not seem right—the symptoms or signs are not typical, something the patient says cannot be readily understood, the laboratory findings do not make sense, or whatever—you must stop, review, and deliberate."

Posing a Question

For the purposes of this book, the thinking strategy called **posing a question** is defined as asking for answers without really expecting to receive them. The following are examples of instances when nurses from the TIP Study used the thinking strategy **posing a question**:

What are they doing approving a transfer?

Well, why is the nurse calling me to report on a patient who is already on the way?

So, how sick is this guy?

Is he going to hit me, or is he going to hit somebody else? Is anybody going to get hurt in the next 2 minutes?

And now I start wondering, well, has he been stumbling around? Has he been intoxicated? Has he been in fights? Has he been on the streets? Is he so out there that he can't take care of himself?

Who knows what his whole history is? Does he have a sleep disturbance? Is he ruminating about suicide?

I would wonder how I could have possibly hung a hundred times the dose. I

Posing a Question

Asking for answers without really expecting to receive them

would wonder if I should have had that much responsibility, given a seven-patient assignment, five of whom were pretty high acuity. I would wonder why I didn't ask someone else to watch my patient while I took the time to investigate exactly the morphine dose and checked all my tubing.

Standing in this room, I'd be wondering what happened.

And if I were thinking that I had to start his IV, I'd be wondering what his IV access would be like, since he was an IV drug user.

The order for Ativan [lorazepam] would make me wonder what type of IV drugs he is using, or if he is shooting speed.

I'd be wondering why the antibiotics haven't been started yet.

Facione, Sanchez, Facione, and Gainen (1995) identify inquisitiveness as an important disposition toward critical thinking. They define inquisitiveness as "one's intellectual curiosity and one's desire for learning even when the application of the knowledge is not readily apparent" (p. 6). They propose that "a deficit in inquisitiveness would signal a fundamental limitation of one's potential to develop expert knowledge and professional practice ability" (p. 6).

Making Assumptions

For the purposes of this book, the thinking strategy called **making assumptions** is defined as taking for granted or supposing. The following are examples of instances when nurses from the TIP Study used the thinking strategy **making assumptions**:

In this day and age, when the patient presents with KS [Kaposi's sarcoma], I would assume that he's had HIV on board for probably—not definitely, but probably—10 years.

Assuming she's still on the monitor, I'd check her monitor.

We're assuming that she had chest pain when she hit the floor, but what if she hit the floor first and that brought on the chest pain? We don't know that for sure.

Hopefully, the cardiologist should be in the house because he's scheduled to be doing a cardiac cath[eterization] on this person who is having Vtach [ventricular tachycardia]. So, I'm taking it for granted that he's on his way up to see the patient.

Making Assumptions

Taking for granted; supposing

I assume that he probably has a therapeutic dose of Coumadin [warfarin].

She's evidently been on digitalis for her congestive heart failure.

I assume that they would have given him glucose in the emergency department to see if he's hypoglycemic. I assume they would have given him Narcan [naloxone]. I assume they would have probably given him glucose also.

But since she's already 2 weeks post-op, I'm assuming she's probably doing fine.

Well, at 33 years old and you're diagnosed with leukemia and had no idea that it was coming down the line, it has to be terrifying.

Qualifying

For the purposes of this book, the thinking strategy called **qualifying** is defined as modifying, limiting, or restricting, as by giving exceptions. The following are examples of instances when nurses from the TIP Study used the thinking strategy **qualifying**:

But still, it's a weak diagnosis for admission into an acute care psych unit.

Although, we all know that the primary symptom of acute alcohol withdrawal, the number one symptom, is anxiety.

That doesn't necessarily mean he's very sick.

By and large, though, [many] people with KS do have HIV. It does happen, but it used to be everybody [who was HIV positive] had KS, and that's no longer the case.

And I can sit near him, but not too close.

So, I don't know if that would make a lot of sense right now to have him on that, unless he's got a pneumonia going in the middle of all this, too.

A lot of times, there is depression [ST] from angina or cardiac pain, although you might see a little different portrayal if it was an actual MI [myocardial infarction].

His creatinine is sky-high for somebody who is on dialysis.

That's too low [hemoglobin and hematocrit] for somebody who is going to surgery.

Qualifying

Modifying, limiting, or restricting, as by giving exceptions

And if his ammonia turns out to be high and his blood sugar is all right, assuming it is, I would worry about him still being unarousable.

For someone who's had a documented MI, he's a little tachycardic.

It would depend on how bad the building was or how bad the earthquake.

It would depend on how much we got her calmed down first, as far as her heart rate and things like that.

Depending on the bruises too, if they're still real purple.

Making Generalizations

For the purposes of this book, the thinking strategy called **making generalizations** is defined as inferring from many particulars. The following are examples of instances when nurses from the TIP Study used the thinking strategy **making generalizations**:

Staff frequently have adverse feelings about people with drug and alcohol problems. [People with alcohol problems] tend to roll into the ER drunk in the evenings and at night. Very rarely can they afford [alcohol or drugs] at the end of the month. They tend to come into the hospital in an acute detox on day 3, 4, or 5 of the month.

I'm not sure what the research has shown, but I know there's a tremendous amount of trouble with people going septic with central lines and TPN [total parenteral nutrition] when you have no immune system.

Most people who are bleeding, especially someone that's been bleeding during four to five different episodes over the last night (so we're going to figure 12 hours of bleeding), are probably dry.

A lot of people complain of shoulder pain when in fact they have a ruptured spleen.

Patients usually don't take nitroglycerin routinely unless they're having chest pain.

Making Generalizations

Inferring from many particulars

A lot of cardiologists feel that digoxin doesn't have a strong effect on the heart rate as we've all learned. Once you start to know the cardiologist, they always say even if the pulse is 58 or 56, give it.

And it happens very fast; the patient loses blood very quickly, and you end up taking a woman like this for a hysterectomy, or you have a woman going into shock and DIC [disseminated intravascular coagulation].

Sometimes when you're talking with families, you have to ask them their wishes regarding code status in very nonclinical terms.

References

Barrows, H., & Pickell, G. (1991). *Developing clinical problem-solving skills: A guide to more effective diagnosis and treatment.* New York: Norton Medical Books.

Facione, P., Sanchez, C., Facione, N., & Gainen, J. (1995). The disposition toward critical thinking. *JGE: The Journal of General Education, 44*(1), 1–25.

Schön, D. (1983). *The reflective practitioner: How professionals think in action.* New York: Harper Collins.

THREE

Thinking about Clinical Dilemmas

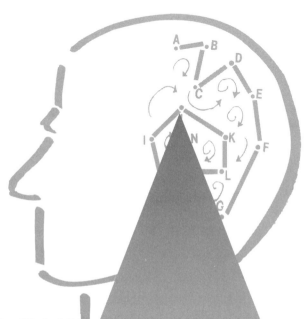

17 *Clinical Dilemmas in Obstetric Nursing*

The nurse who thinks aloud in response to the dilemmas in this chapter is a perinatal clinical nurse specialist who has had over 20 years of practice experience concentrated in high-risk labor and delivery.

Clinical Dilemma One

SCENE ONE

You are working the night shift in the labor and delivery department of a large city hospital. It is 2:00 A.M. Mrs. Joy Tam is a 31-year-old, married, Asian woman, gravida 1, para 0, at 25 weeks' gestation. She was briefly seen in the emergency department for cramping and spotting and was subsequently admitted to labor and delivery for observation and further evaluation.

Mrs. Tam and her husband, who is currently unemployed, live with her elderly parents in a small apartment in the Chinatown district of San Francisco. Neither she nor her husband speaks English, although they do understand some English phrases.

Joy is employed as a seamstress in the local garment district. She has continued to work 16-hour shifts throughout her pregnancy. Since her third month of pregnancy, she's been followed for prenatal care at Health Center Four. Her progress has been satisfactory, with the exception of her nutritional status—a failure to gain the amount of weight anticipated for 25 weeks' gestation. She has no known allergies and takes no medications except a daily prenatal vitamin. She uses herbal medicine and has continued to do so throughout her pregnancy. She was taken to the emergency department by her husband at 2:00 A.M. after complaining of cramping and spotting for 2 days.

Admitting orders are as follows: Admit to obstetric (OB) service for observation.

Diagnosis: urinary tract infection (UTI) and preterm labor secondary to UTI. Straight catheter for urinalysis and culture and sensitivity, then begin tocolytic therapy. Start an IV of 500 ml of D5W at 20 ml/hr. Administer a 4-gm loading dose of magnesium sulfate IV piggyback over 30 minutes, then give maintenance dose of 1 gm/hr. Restrict oral fluids to 1000 ml/24 hr. Strict bed rest.

The Nurse's Response

We're probably looking at preterm labor here. This is her first baby, and she's at 25 weeks' gestation. And yes, we have a viable baby here, probably 500, maybe 600 gm in weight. It's 2:00 A.M., so I have no doctors around. There's only me, the nurse, and if we're not at the county hospital, then I have no interpreter. All those factors in her economic situation have probably led to the preterm labor. She's on her feet doing hard work for 16-hour days.

And I'd want to know what herbal medicine she is taking, since many of them can have an impact on pregnancy and delivery. There are some herbs that are known to cause contractions, some that prevent contractions. She could also be taking something to improve anemia status and things like that, so all of this could be part of her nutritional status and could contribute to her failure to gain the appropriate amount of weight, which can be a problem in preterm labor.

She's obviously not getting a whole lot of help from the Health Center . . . the fact that this is a preterm labor, which is probably an admission for prevention.

The first question I would have is why would somebody give a pregnant woman D5W? Usually we don't give dextrose until we've done a diabetic screen, which she should have had between 24 and 28 weeks. I'm going to question the doctor's orders a little bit. The 4-gm loading dose of magnesium sulfate is fine, as is the 1 gm to 2 gm/hr of mag-sulfate; but, I have no information here to determine whether this is the appropriate medication to give this patient. What I'd be concerned about is her uterine activity. We should have an external fetal monitor on her before we even get any of these medications going. I would be saying, "Ehhh, let's see about this."

Do we have any contractions? How bad are they? Do we have uterine irritability versus regular contractions? What sort of cervical dilation is there? If she has a closed cervix, I would be questioning the orders to say, "Is this what you want?"

If I can get an interpreter . . . but, if I'm not in a large county hospital, I don't have one. If not, I would point or gesture and things like that. And I would need to see if she does understand some phrases. Most of the OB units also have some written information in her language. She may not have much education, either. In fact, she may not be able to read, or she may be very, very smart, and so I would see if she could read. Or I might use pictures and things like that. But there are such things as cervical dilation charts that I could use to show her: "You're open this much; it's too early for the baby." Most patients usually understand that.

Also, before starting the medicine, I would try to explain to her what's going to happen. I'd tell her that she'll feel really high and really sick and yucky. So I'd try to explain that before I start pushing her medication. At this point, I wouldn't worry about her failure to gain weight. If she's in the hospital with a problem of UTI and preterm labor, I'm more worried about saving the baby. She hasn't gained enough weight, so that's not good because too little weight or too much weight each corresponds to possible fetal development problems. If she's underweight, I could probably guestimate the baby, the fetus, to be a little bit smaller than normal.

At this time, we would probably want to have an ultrasound done to tell us what position the baby is in and to try to determine how we're going to deliver the baby. We can get some type of ultrasound done at 2:00 in the morning, although it's not as accurate. But it certainly can tell us what position the baby's in. Because if this baby's breech, and the mom's dilating, and the contractions don't stop, she may have to go for a C-section [cesarean section] because we're going to try to save that head from going through the cervix and because we will try to save this baby. At 25 weeks' gestation, and she seems to have had good prenatal care, we've got a good prognosis versus someone who comes in with no prenatal care and says, "Ehhh, I think I had a period a couple of months ago."

Depending on what herbs she's taken, the magnesium sulfate probably won't interact that much because magnesium sulfate is a normal part of our body makeup. It would be nice if . . . sometimes some people bring in their osteopath when they've been on herbal medicine, and they'll say, "She's taking two drops of this herb here," and they'll show you on the charts. If it's something that's helpful, I would not discourage her from taking it. They get these herbs from Chinese people, from those herb stores. They cook it and bring it to the hospital, and they're really superstitious about it; they strongly believe that it will help them. At this time, she's going to be NPO [nothing by mouth], so I'm going to be watching that people aren't bringing in their Chinese food during the night.

Once she is no longer NPO, I will be encouraging her to eat her traditional foods and things like that. I think there's a real protocol in their culture about what to take and not to take for pregnancy. This may not be helpful with other diseases, like diabetes, but in pregnancy, most traditional food is really helpful. It's just that we need to know that we're not giving them some medicine that may interfere with the traditional medicine that they're taking. Right now, with the magnesium sulfate being ordered, it would be best for her to only take what we give her. But once we get her stabilized and everything, I would actually encourage her to take her traditional herbs and food and to feel that this is a good thing for the baby, because most women in preterm labor think it's their fault: "I did something wrong for this baby to come." Yeah, she's got some risk factors such as poor nutrition, because the husband is unemployed, and she's working as a seamstress, probably making 10 cents an hour, so she's not going to get much food; living with elderly parents and trying to support them . . . so, she may blame herself, and that's going to be something we need to get an interpreter for, to say, "No, you were doing everything right." And if taking the herbal medicine is something that the client finds supportive, then I would tell her that's good for the baby. You know, this may even be what's keeping the baby in her uterus longer.

Commentary

The nurses' initial response to the information in this first scene is to attempt to frame the problem by delineating the context of the dilemma. To do this, she uses the thinking strategy **generating a hypothesis** (*We're probably looking at preterm labor here*), then **drawing a conclusion** (*And yes, we have a viable baby here*), and then **generating a hypothesis** (*probably 500, maybe 600 gm in weight*). Then she **draws** another **conclusion**: *It's 2:00 A.M., so I have no doctors around. There's only me, the nurse, and if we're not at the county hospital, then I have no interpreter* (**stating a proposition**).

Framing a problem provides a context that helps make sense out of data and helps the problem-solver incorporate it into a line of reasoning (Kassirer & Kopelman, 1988). A frame is a set of associated facts or ideas about a central concept. Frames vary in the type and amount of information they contain and in how that information is organized (Evans, Block, Steinburg, & Penrose, 1986, p. 1027). Framing a problem assists us in using a hypothesis-directed line of reasoning as a principal strategy and to pursue a single line of reasoning.

In his classic treatise *The Reflective Practitioner*, Schön (1983, p. 40) describes this process as problem setting: "a process in which, interactively, we *name* the things to which we will attend and *frame* the context in which we will attend to them."

Framing errors can occur when data are provided in a misleading fashion. Sonnenberg, Kassirer, and Kopelman (1986) provide an example of this by describing a clinical case of a benign urinary tract lesion that was misdiagnosed as a malignancy in part because the radiologist described what he saw as a "mass" rather than as a "space-occupying lesion." It was felt that the clinicians might have been less inclined to believe the client had cancer if the radiologist's description had been different.

Schön (1983, p. 40) reminds us of the value of being aware of the manner in which we frame the problems that we encounter in our practice: "When a practitioner becomes aware of his frames, he also becomes aware of the possibility of alternative ways of framing the reality of his practice."

Thinking Activities

1. Review the nurse's response to the information provided in scene one. Provide additional examples of thinking that helps her to frame the problems depicted in this first scene.

2. Identify the thinking strategies that the nurse uses in the examples that you have found.

3. Think about your own practice. What thinking strategies assist you in framing the problems that you encounter in your practice?

SCENE TWO

It is now 2:30 A.M. Your admission assessment revealed the following: Initial vital signs are oral temperature, 37.8°C; heart rate, 80 beats per minute; respiratory rate, 20 breaths per minute, shallow and even; and blood pressure (BP), 96/48 mm Hg. Fetal heart rate is 150 beats per minute by Doppler. The patient is tearful, awake, and oriented. She denies headache or visual disturbance. She has no edema. Her skin is warm, pink, and dry. Her lungs are clear, and she denies shortness of breath or dyspnea. Her abdomen is soft, nondistended, with active bowel sounds. The urine obtained from the straight catheter is cloudy and pink tinged. She is placed on a tocodynamometer, which shows an irritability pattern. A vaginal examination reveals 2 cm dilated, 50% effaced, and slight bloody show.

The Nurse's Response

Her temperature is somewhat elevated. I'm wondering if these vital signs were taken before or after she received the magnesium sulfate. I'm going to assume they were taken before. At 25 weeks, we expect the patient's blood pressure to be a little lower, and given her size and considering her ethnic background, I'd expect to see a blood pressure like this. What I would be concerned about is that one of the side effects of magnesium sulfate is that it may cause the blood pressure to go lower. But it's fine if she's breathing and percolating, and all those things, I wouldn't be too worried.

A fetal heart rate of 150 is within normal range, although I would expect it to be higher. I would expect to see a fetal heart rate around 180 to 190. And I would expect her pulse to be higher, also. The patient is tearful, awake, and oriented. She denies headaches or visual disturbances. Usually, we see that patients are tearful as a side effect of the magnesium sulfate. Her lungs are clear. I worry about the magnesium sulfate causing problems there. Since her urine is cloudy, I would also question if she has a kidney infection going on, which is very common. I would check to see if she has pain in either of her kidneys, which may indicate more is going on.

She is tearful and awake . . . all right, hopefully she's able to understand some of what we're doing to her. As I apply the toco monitor [tocodynamometer], I would be explaining that we're monitoring the baby. She may or may not understand the vaginal exam, but hopefully I can be talking about it as we do it and doing kind of a show-and-tell to see if that will help her to feel a little bit more comfortable. Since her cervix is 2 cm dilated, I'm a little concerned, since this is her first pregnancy. Obviously, something is going on here, but she's not effacing that much; it's only halfway effaced. The other thing I'd probably chart is the position of her cervix—if it's still in a low posterior position or if it's come up to an anterior position.

If it's anterior, I'm going to be more worried about her because the cervix has come around to the front, getting her ready to go. And I'm not sure from this description of the findings from the vaginal exam if the baby's head is down or not. I don't want to examine her again, but if I've got an intern or somebody inexperienced doing the exam . . . I mean, this is not a good patient for us to train an intern on. You really need to do hundreds of vaginal exams before you develop the art of knowing what you're feeling. The interns in OB have some chances to do some vaginal exams and to determine different dilatations. It's easier to learn the art if somebody before you has done it so you can follow, go in with your fingers and say, "Okay, this is what I'm feeling. This is where I'm finding the cervix." In my 20+ years in obstetrical practice, I've probably done a few million vaginal exams. But still, every once in a while there's a cervix that. . . . It took me probably a year before I felt a closed cervix in labor and delivery. I said, "What's this thing?" To feel a cervix that's closed and not dilated or not effaced much either, it's like, "What's this lump here?" And I still have problems feeling face presentations. I think I've felt two actual face presentations where I could feel the head coming. So it's like, "This feels funny here. Would somebody come and see what this is?" So, I still occasionally go, "Feel this." I had a patient a few weeks ago where the physician went in to feel the position of the baby after I had done a vaginal exam, and the patient had ruptured her membranes. She was at term and in very early labor; usually we don't check in those circumstances. The physician came in and said, "Oh, this is a breech." Actually, the patient was just barely dilated 2 cm, and the cord was over the baby's head—I could feel it pulsating. So, yeah, I deal with these things all the time. I can't tell from reading this, with her having a slight bloody show, if possibly her membranes are ruptured.

Usually while I'm doing the vaginal exam, I try to do it very gently, especially on a preterm mom, and I can feel whether the membranes are there intact or not. So, if they weren't intact, of course that would influence our decision about what we're going to do for this woman. We may or may not try to stop the labor at that time. The other thing I would be questioning is giving her a shot of betamethasone at this point to help prevent hyaline membrane disease. Some of the research has shown that it's not that effective, but it's kind of nice. With an irritable pattern and a cervix that's only 2 cm, probably we can hold her off for another 48 hours before she delivers. We could also put her in a slight Trendelenburg position, put her head down a little bit, to get the weight off the cervix.

Commentary

In making sense out of the additional information provided in this second scene, the nurse frequently uses the thinking strategy **setting priorities** to identify the major concerns about this client:

What I would be concerned about is that one of the side effects of magnesium sulfate is that it may cause the blood pressure to go lower.

I worry about the magnesium sulfate causing problems here.

Since her cervix is 2 cm dilated, I'm a little concerned, since this is her first pregnancy.

If it's anterior, I'm going to be more worried about her because the cervix has come around to the front, getting her ready to go.

After identifying the major concerns regarding this client, the nurse **generates** several **hypotheses** about what can be done for the client (*We may or may not try to* *stop the labor at that time. . . . Probably we can hold her off for another 48 hours before she delivers. . . . We could also put her in a slight Trendelenburg position).*

Generating hypotheses about what to do in an urgent situation such as the one the nurse is confronted with in this dilemma helps the nurse brainstorm about how to best intercede to assist the client. As time permits, initial hypotheses can then be reconsidered and refined, particularly in light of additional data that will be obtained as time passes.

◀ **SCENE THREE**

It is now 4:00 A.M. You enter Mrs. Tam's room to evaluate her and find the following: Vital signs are: oral temperature, 38°C; heart rate, 116 beats per minute; respiratory rate, 28 breaths per minute; BP, 86/40 mm Hg. Fetal heart rate is 166 beats per minute, with no periodic changes. She is awake and very restless, moving from side to side, trying to get out of the bed. Her skin is pale, cool, and clammy; nail beds are cyanotic. There is bilateral neck vein distention, and her pulses are bounding. There are bilateral rales in her lower lobes, and she is complaining of dyspnea. She has hypoactive bowel sounds; her abdomen is soft. There is no leakage of blood, fluid, or mucus from the vagina.

The Nurse's Response

Her temperature has gone up a little bit. Obviously, we didn't start her on antibiotics. Her heart rate's up. The fetal heart rate is at 166, with no periodic changes. That probably isn't something I'd like to get real concerned about with a 25-weeker with UTI, but I might expect it to be 180. The mom's heart rate's at 116, which is a lot more concerning at that point. There are no periodic changes, no accelerations, no decelerations. That's probably not something I would expect to see at 25 weeks. And that's the point where you also can't say anything about variability in the long term. So even if the fetal monitor shows a flat line, I'd be worried, but not real worried. The other part is that we've got her on the magnesium sulfate, so I'd expect this baby not to have any variability.

Given all the other urgent things that are going on with her, I'm not sure I would have taken the time to listen to her bowel sounds. There's no leakage of blood, fluid, or mucus from her vagina, but the baby's falling out. She's obviously going into some type of respiratory distress, probably secondary to the mag-sulfate, which causes pulmonary edema. Fortunately, she's in the labor room. I'd give her lots of oxygen. I'd have her sitting up in bed, which of course then is going to put pressure on her cervix, which may cause more dilatation, which may worsen the problem of the baby coming out. But, if you have a mom that doesn't breathe, whether the baby is in or out at that point doesn't matter. So, you've got to get the mom going. I'd probably be calling for some baseline blood gases and calling for some help, getting some people in there to help me, and turning off the mag-sulfate. I certainly don't want to increase the contractions at this point, but turning off the mag-sulfate . . . also getting a magnesium level with it.

I may even want to put a Foley catheter in her. She's got a urinary tract infection going on, but you want to keep some record of her intake and output too, so I may want to put a Foley catheter into her at this point. The baby is doing fine, so we're not really worried about that, but mom takes priority at this moment because she can't breathe. I would not do another cervical exam to see if she's dilating further. I'd be more worried about her breathing. I mean, if the baby's going to fall out . . .

Commentary

Here again, the nurse's response to the additional information that she is given in scene three is to **generate hypotheses**, as we see in the following examples:

Generating hypotheses *about the significance of assessment findings:*

The fetal heart rate is at 166, with no periodic changes. That probably isn't something I'd like to get real concerned about with a 25-weeker with UTI. . . . There are no periodic changes, no accelerations, no decelerations. That's probably not something I would expect to see at 25 weeks.

Generating hypotheses *about etiology:*

She's obviously going into some type of respiratory distress, probably secondary to the mag-sulfate.

Generating hypotheses *about interventions:*

I'd probably be calling for some baseline blood gases and calling for some help . . . and turning off the mag-sulfate.

Thinking Activities

1. Throughout the nurse's thoughts about the three scenes that compose this dilemma, we find a predominant use of the thinking strategy **generating hypotheses**. Why do you think that she used this particular thinking strategy so often?

2. What does the tentativeness inherent in this thinking strategy suggest about the nurse's understanding of the information described in the dilemma?

3. Do you believe that frequent use of the thinking strategy **generating hypotheses** reflects greater or lesser soundness of thinking? Justify your answer.

Clinical Dilemma Two

SCENE ONE

It is 6:00 A.M. You are the charge nurse on the labor and delivery unit on the night shift. It's been a hellish night. Your unit has had six admissions and three deliveries. The census on your unit is full, and you'll need to discharge three patients before you can admit the three pending deliveries. Your night shift has been short one registered nurse (RN), and one of your staff is an RN who has been floated to your unit from a general medical-surgical unit. Miss Shirley Jones is a 42-year-old, single, white woman, gravida 7, para 5, who just experienced a very precipitatious labor and birth (1 hour and 45 minutes total) of a healthy female infant.

No episiotomy was performed, and no lacerations were found. She did not receive analgesia during delivery and has no IV in place. You are completing the first postpartum evaluation in the recovery room, where the patient has been placed until a room is available.

As you approach the patient, she is shaking all over and says, "I'm so cold." Her vital signs are oral temperature, 37.0°C; heart rate, 120 beats per minute; respiratory rate, 32 breaths per minute, shallow and even; and BP, 87/46 mm/Hg. Her skin is pale, cold, and clammy. Her pulses are thready. Her fundus is boggy and 2 cm above the umbilicus at midline. Lochia findings are as follows: large amount of rubra lochia, two OB peripads soaked; chucks saturated; no clots. The perineum is nonedematous, with large protuberant hemorrhoids. There is constant oozing of blood from the vagina.

The Nurse's Response

So, I've got six in labor? No, we've already had three deliveries that are sitting there. Okay, so I only have three more deliveries then. And it's me and this RN who has been floated from the medical-surgical unit to the delivery area. So, it sounds like I've done three deliveries! I can't believe it! I'd be on the phone to the supervisor saying, "Get your butt up here, and give me some help." Because you'd probably only have two nurses working on a night shift. So, I'd have a little problem with that. I'd get the supervisor up and get some help because I can't do everything. I can do a lot, but not all of this. And if I've got somebody from a general med-surg unit, she knows nothing about OB and probably hates being there with me. And the liability there is phenomenal. If I haven't done the paperwork and called the supervisor and gotten some competent help or tried to at least 10 times already . . . yeah, this person is a med-surg nurse and knows nothing about birthing babies. So, I'm not sure what she's doing except probably recovering patients after they have delivered. She certainly can take vital signs. I'd certainly teach her to find the fundus and massage the uterus and to assess how much bleeding was normal after delivery. That would be about the only things she'd be trained to do. This Shirley Jones patient probably came in and spit the baby out.

Since she's a gravida 7, I'd be a little worried at this point because she can conceive that many babies that quickly. It doesn't say how big her baby was so, you know, she may also have a pretty large uterus, which could lead to problems. As you approach the patient, she is shaking all over and says, "I'm so cold." That could be due to a couple of things. One is that it's not unusual for somebody who had either a long or a precipitous birth to have the shakes and feel cold. And probably I'd check her before going to get her a blanket. She may have more bleeding to come.

There's constant bleeding from the perineum. She could have a small tear or bleeder inside that has been missed. First of all, I'm going to call for help here too, because I can't start an IV and massage her uterus at the same time. It's hard to do. I've tried it, and I can't do it. And I would probably want to get the uterus massaged down. At this point I'd be massaging and looking at the blood and everything else saying, "Oh, please! Someone get up here to help me!"

The medical-surgical nurse can definitely start an IV. Also, if she came in this fast and everything happened so quickly, there may not have been time to have any blood drawn. I want to get her typed and crossmatched. We usually know, at least with most pregnant women who've had some prenatal care, what their blood type is. But, we need to have her typed and crossmatched, and we need to get a stat hematocrit and hemoglobin, when we put in the IV, to see where we're coming from.

Massaging is going to bring her uterus down the best, but at the same time I'm also going to be getting a hold of a physician to examine her. The other thing I would worry about is that during the delivery, maybe little pieces of the placenta got left in there. Or, because she's had so many babies and a quick delivery, it could just be uterine apnea. You know, just let the uterus fall out here. Yes, I'd like to have women come in and deliver naturally, but I do also like to at least have an IV in place because this happens all the time. And it happens very fast; the patient loses blood very quickly, and we'll end up taking this woman for a hysterectomy, or you have a woman going into shock and possibly going into DIC [disseminated intravascular coagulation].

Hopefully, if the physician is there, I'm going to get the orders. But at this hour of the morning in labor and delivery, the physician's probably not going to be there, so I would start doing things and then call the physician. Because he will say, "Okay, sounds good to me. Sounds like a plan."

I would start emergency procedures because basically the law says let a nurse do these things in an emergency. I feel pretty comfortable with that, you know. Starting an IV, starting with a typical dose of Pitocin [oxytocin]. I mean, I wouldn't try to put 80 U of Pitocin into the IV when the usual dose is 20 to 40 at the most. Then I would have to be liable. In some hospitals, you can call the emergency room physician. So, they'll come up and say, "Oh, it looks like you're doing a good job. You deliver the baby, and I'll watch!" And then they'll say, "Now what would you like to give her?" But certainly, although I wouldn't order blood or anything like that, I would start an IV.

Commentary

The main problem depicted in this dilemma is that a 42-year-old single woman, gravida 7, para 5, who just experienced a very rapid labor and delivery, is bleeding excessively and is manifesting signs of hypovolemic shock. This is an urgent, possibly life-threatening situation that requires quick thinking and rapid, efficient decision making. In response, the nurse's thoughts are predominated by the thinking strategies **making choices** and **making predictions**.

The choices that she makes include getting some help, getting the uterus massaged down, getting the physician involved, getting the client typed and cross-matched, starting an IV, and giving intravenous oxytocin. The discussion in Chapter 12 of the **choices** that nurses **make** in their practice regarding actions, interventions, and therapy revealed that the degree of autonomy ranged from independent to interdependent to dependent. We see evidence of this entire range in this OB nurse's choices. Getting some help and getting the uterus massaged down seem to be independent choices. Getting the physician involved and starting an IV are interdependent choices, in that they require collaboration with others. In the first instance, the physician must be willing and able to get involved, and in the second instance, the unit may provide a protocol to cover nurses' starting an IV without an order, but ultimately the nurse will need to collaborate with the physician regarding what intravenous solution to run into the vein. Getting the client typed and crossmatched and giving intravenous oxytocin are both dependent choices, in that they require a physician's order. In reality, however, many highly experienced nurses feel comfortable in initiating these actions prior to obtaining the actual order, especially in an emergency situation.

Another thinking strategy that seems to predominate in the nurse's thoughts about this dilemma is **making predictions**. These predictions include: *She may have more bleeding to come. . . . And it happens very fast; the patient loses blood very quickly, and we'll end up taking this woman for a hysterectomy, or you have a woman going into shock and possibly going into DIC.* The nurse also makes a series of predictions that indicate her belief that the physician will support all of the actions that she has taken and will defer to her expertise in deciding what else she would like to give the client.

Thinking Activities

1. Comment on what you see as the relationship between the urgency of the situation described in this dilemma and the type of **choices** that the nurse **made**.

2. Think about your own practice. Describe a situation where you might be inclined to **make** dependent **choices** independently.

3. List the possible consequences of **making** dependent **choices** independently in the situation that you described.

4. List the possible consequences of not **making** dependent **choices** independently in the situation that you described.

Clinical Dilemma Three

SCENE ONE

It is 12:00 noon. You are a staff nurse who has worked on this particular OB unit for the past 5 years. This is your sixth day in a row, and you're tired and not feeling well. You regret having agreed to work a double shift today because you won't be getting off duty until after midnight. Miss Mary Johnson is a 14-year-old, single, black female, gravida 2, para 1 at 30 weeks' gestation. She has just been admitted after seeing an obstetrician at the 3rd Street Clinic to rule out preterm labor. Miss Johnson has felt intermittent abdominal cramping for the last 3 days, which is worse with activity.

She lives with her mother, a known drug addict, and her abusive stepfather. She had been attending high school classes regularly, leaving her 2-year-old son at the day care associated with her school. Her mother works nights, and her stepfather is not a reliable caretaker, so she has brought the 2-year-old to the hospital. She was accompanied to the unit by a staff person from the referring clinic, but he is unable to stay. The patient is assigned to you, and you enter her room to perform your initial assessment.

The Nurse's Response

Oh joy! I know at this point it's not going to be a good evening. Yes, I've been there a lot in my younger days, working night-day doubles, which when you're 20 you can do, but not when you're over 30. It's true! Because I think as you get older, you also know your limitations in everything. You may think, "Oh I can do this." And that's when you get into jeopardy. I see that with nurses all the time—that they make the wrong decisions, they take on too much.

But this is my patient now: Mary Johnson, 14-year-old, single black female, gravida 2, para 1 at 30 weeks' gestation. Usually the teenagers are 17 when they have their second one. She's been admitted after seeing an obstetrician at the 3rd Street Clinic to rule out preterm labor. I give her a lot of credit for attending high school regularly. This is not one of our typical children that we get, especially with this type of family.

It says she's brought her 2-year-old son to the hospital with her. The reality is that this person has no place else for her 2-year-old to be, and her only other choice is go home and have a 30-week baby there, which will cause more problems than keeping a 2-year-old here. And that's why I'd call a social worker, because it is only 12:00 P.M. [noon] instead of 12:00 A.M. [midnight], although I get to work till midnight. I'll call social services and say, "Look, we better make some arrangements." I'd like to know if she had preterm labor with her first baby, which is probably the best indicator for preterm labor with the second one.

Because if she has a history of it, she probably knows what to expect versus not having preterm labor on the first one. And, if there's a father involved, whether it be the father of the first baby or the second one, then how involved are they?

Commentary

In response to the information provided in the first scene of this dilemma, the nurse **recognizes the lack of fit with a pattern** that she is accustomed to seeing in her area of practice: *This is not one of our typical children that we get, especially with this type of family. . . . Usually they're 17 when they have their second one [this client is only 14 and she has a 2-year-old son].* While reasoning about the information in this first scene, the nurse also uses the thinking strategy **searching for information**: *I'd like to know if she had preterm labor with her first baby. . . . And, if there's a father involved, whether it be the father of the first baby or the second one, then how involved are they?* She also uses the thinking strategy **forming relationships**: *The reality is that this person has no place else for her 2-year-old to be, and her only other choice is go home and have a 30-week baby there, which will cause more problems than keeping a 2-year-old here.* Both of these thinking strategies may help her to **recognize** other **patterns** that are a better fit and thus to transform an ill-structured problem into a well-structured one, with routine approaches for intervention and treatment.

SCENE TWO

It is now 12:30 P.M. As you begin your assessment, you review the admission orders, which are as follows: Admit to general obstetric service for tocolysis. Diagnosis—preterm labor. Strict bed rest; place in Trendelenburg position; begin IV of 1000 mL of Ringer's lactate TKO; begin an infusion of ritodrine via pump at 50 μg/min. Keep NPO.

The Nurse's Response

Ritodrine tends to cause a lot more problems than magnesium sulfate—increased heart rate and palpations, and things like that. So, along with getting vital signs and determining if there's a live baby in there, because we don't know that yet, we're probably also going to get an EKG [electrocardiogram] and have lab work drawn, including a serum potassium and a serum glucose level. So, if they haven't ordered those things, I'll see that they do.

I'd also want—and usually most of your hospitals will have this—a ritodrine protocol that includes all those orders so that I can just say, "This is what we need," and have the physician sign it.

And of course, I would have continuous monitoring of the patient for both uterine contractions and the fetal heart rate. From the initial assessment, it sounds like she's a pretty put-together kid, going to school and everything, and trying to keep up with the clinic, trying to raise a 2-year-old with this mom and stepfather who's—where did you find those people? So, yeah, this patient's pretty put together.

If this were a drug-induced preterm labor, she would either have symptoms of being on a high or crashing. I think a lot of nurses might look at her and think, "Oh God, it's a kid. She doesn't know anything. Let's just plop her in the bed and do our thing here."

We've got somebody that was escorted from the clinic, from a nurse-managed center, where she had received very good care and follow-up that enabled her to keep her life together, even though she's only 14. I would complete the physical first, to make sure the baby and she were okay. I'm more comfortable with doing some of the physical things, and as I'm doing it, I'll talk to the patient and do some other assessments at the same time. Or I can put the monitor on the patient and be talking at the same time. You're doing the physical activity and showing her that you care at the same time.

With preterm labor in drug-addicted patients, they are in a lot of pain. So, if they're writhing in pain there, and the placenta is ripping off in the uterus—we're going to get that person delivered. But, this person comes walking in stating, "Ehhh, I've been doing this for about 3 days." I look at her and go, "Let's have a little talk about preterm labor precautions." Because, I think all the new studies out indicate that with preterm labor, the key to prevention is in education. She's 14; she may not know an awful lot about her body.

Commentary

In thinking about the additional information presented in this second scene, the nurse begins to **recognize** familiar **patterns**: *From the initial assessment, it sounds like she's a pretty put-together kid, going to school and everything, and trying to keep up with the clinic, trying to raise a 2-year-old with this mom and stepfather who's—where did you find those people? So, yeah, this patient's pretty put together. . . . We've got somebody that was escorted from the clinic, was leaving from a nurse-managed center, where she had received very good care and follow-up that enabled her to keep her life together, even though she's only 14. . . . With preterm labor in drug-addicted patients, they are in a lot of pain. So, they're writhing in pain there, and the placenta is ripping off in the uterus—we're going to get that person delivered.* Notice how **recognizing** these familiar **patterns** provides a focus for problem resolution. The nurse will try to stop the premature contractions, and if that doesn't work, is going to get this person delivered.

SCENE THREE

It is now 12:45 P.M. You begin your initial assessment of Miss Johnson and find the following: Vital signs are: oral temperature, 36.9°C; heart rate, 88 beats per minute; respiratory rate, 22 breaths per minute; and BP, 110/76 mm Hg. Fetal heart rate is in the 140s, with 3 to 5 beats per minute long-term variability and occasional accelerations. Vaginal examination indicates the following: external os, 1.5 cm dilated; internal os, fingertip; cervix, 1 cm, soft, anterior position; fetal head engaged; and bag of waters intact. Uterine contractions are every 10 minutes, lasting for 30 seconds, with +1 intensity. The remainder of a systems' assessment was within normal limits.

The Nurse's Response

She's had a baby before. She's had a vaginal delivery (I assume she had a vaginal delivery), or even if she had a C-section and she failed to progress or something like that, the first time her cervix dilated . . . it's not unusual for a woman who's had at least one baby to have the external os dilated a little bit. With the internal os being just a fingertip, you can't even put your finger through it, then she's essentially got a closed cervix. Her cervix is 1 cm and soft, so she's effacing, probably about 50% effaced. This is a little bit of a problem. The cervix is in the anterior position, so it has come around; she's been doing it, having these contractions, for 3 days. The head is engaged. We don't really know what stage the baby's head is at. It could be engaged. It's not really in the pelvis or anything like that. There's a head down there, but her bag of waters is intact.

She's having very mild contractions; the rest of her assessment is normal. I really would question starting ritodrine. If she's having contractions every 10 minutes, she may be having up to six contractions an hour, which is too much. We want her to have three or less, but very mild . . . I would probably put her on bed rest, get some hydration going, and see within an hour if her situation is going to change. If it doesn't change, yeah, then we need to start her on ritodrine or something like that, but the side effects of the medication can be worse than what we're actually using it to treat.

Commentary

The nurse's reaction to the assessment finding is to **draw conclusions** about them: *She's essentially got a closed cervix. Her cervix is 1 cm and soft, so she's effacing, probably about 50% effaced. This is a little bit of a problem. . . . She's having very mild contractions; the rest of her assessment is normal.*

Now the nurse seems to have a definite focus for problem resolution, with the goal being to decrease, or eliminate, the client's contractions: *We want her to have three or less, but very mild.* Consequently, we hear her **making choices**: *I would probably put her on bed rest, get some hydration going, and see if within an hour her situation is going to change. If it doesn't change, yeah, then we need to start her on ritodrine or something like that, but the side effects of the medication can be worse than what we're actually using it to treat.* The use of ritodrine in this case seems to concern the nurse; in fact, she had earlier thought, *I really would question starting ritodrine.*

SCENE FOUR

It is now 2:00 P.M. Miss Johnson is on 150 μg/min of ritodrine, and she calls you into her room. She says anxiously, "I'm having really bad chest pain, and it feels like someone is standing on my chest. I need to sit up."

The Nurse's Response

They didn't listen to me. So, we have her on 150 μg/min; usually we go up to . . . 300 or 350 is the maximum amount of ritodrine you're going to give somebody. We've got her halfway up to that amount. Chest pain is not an uncommon side effect with ritodrine, to have some chest pain, but it also could mean a big problem in a 14-year-old. So she's probably not having a heart attack, but rather experiencing one of the side effects of ritodrine, chest pain. Also, patients on ritodrine can go into pulmonary edema and things like that. I want to listen to her heart and lungs. While I'm doing that, I'm probably turning off the ritodrine at the same time, so I get that drug out of her system.

She's had an EKG, and she also had her potassium, glucose, hemoglobin, and hematocrit drawn, so I would check to determine that they are all within normal range for a 14-year-old. She may have cardiac disease—she has a history of a type of cardiac disease.

I'd get her calmed down. She speaks English, so that's a little bit easier. She can be in a strange place, and nobody can really help her. I mean, if I was single—is she Chinese?—I can't imagine trying to have a baby all alone, especially if something has gone wrong.

We've got orders to put her in Trendelenburg position, but I'd get her head raised. I'd listen to her heart and lungs to see if there's anything going on. It probably wouldn't hurt to give her some oxygen. Oxygen and an IV—a lot of times these two things make the nurses and the doctors feel good. We use them in a number of situations.

And I would probably, not frantically, call for help and have the physician come in to check her out. Also, I would be looking at the fetal monitor at that time to see what's the baby doing with this, and does the patient have any contractions? With ritodrine, she probably doesn't have any contractions, and baby should be responding fairly well to it.

Commentary

In response to this urgent situation, the nurse's thoughts focus on **making choices**: *I want to listen to her heart and to her lungs. While I'm doing that, I'm probably turning off the ritodrine at the same time. . . . I'd get her calmed down. . . . I'd get her head raised. I'd listen to her heart and lungs to see if there's anything going on. It probably wouldn't hurt to give her some oxygen. Oxygen and an IV—a lot of times these two things make the nurses and the doctors feel good. . . . And I would probably, not frantically, call for help and have the physician come in to check her out. Also, I would be looking at the fetal monitor at that time to see what's the baby doing with this, and does the patient have any contractions?*

SCENE FIVE

It is 5 minutes later. You complete a hasty assessment that reveals the following: Vital signs are heart rate, 136 beats per minute, irregular; respiratory rate, 30 breaths per minute; and BP, 90/50 mm Hg. The patient's skin is pale, cool, and clammy. The fetal heart rate is 194 beats per minute, with no long-term variability and no periodic changes. There is no leakage of fluid, blood, or mucus from the vagina. Uterine contractions are one to two per hour, lasting 30 to 45 seconds, with + 1 intensity.

The Nurse's Response

Usually, 140 [beats per minute, maternal heart rate] is what we consider abnormal. At about 120, we stop the ritodrine. At 136, we're getting pretty far up there. It's not uncommon for the blood pressure to be down with the ritodrine. Her respiratory rate is 30 [breaths per minute]; she's anxious; she's got something going on. Her skin is pale, cool, and clammy. The fetal heart rate is 194 [beats per minute], with no long-term variability and no periodic changes.

I don't know why the fetus would respond. . . . The patient has no other risk factors. She came in with preterm labor; it had nothing to do with a urinary tract infection. She hasn't had fever or anything like that. The fetal heart rate shouldn't be up that far. Probably what I would do would be to either readjust the monitor to see if it's accurate (sometimes the machines can inaccurately record the heart rate). And then I would also pull out a Doppler to listen to the fetal heart tones, to see what's going on.

And if that was what was going on—fetal heart rate of 194—we'd have to stabilize the mom first and then think of getting that baby out of there right away. There's no leakage of fluid, blood, mucosa (or baby) from the vagina. And uterine contractions one to two per hour, 30 to 45 seconds, + 1 intensity. She's probably not feeling anxious; obviously, the ritodrine has worked.

The only other assessment I would have checked is respiratory; I would've assessed her lung sounds to see if she's developing pulmonary edema. That could be a side effect from the medicine. It's not unusual for the heart rate to climb. It's not unusual for patients to feel palpations or that "somebody's standing on my chest"; any of those are not that unusual with ritodrine . . . it doesn't necessarily mean something's going on, but she could be going very quickly into pulmonary edema.

So this 14-year-old has got good kidney function. She's got good lung function. If she had these problems and I turned off the ritodrine, and it didn't work, the contractions kept coming at six or more a minute, we'd probably do a couple things. We could think about another drug that is real similar to ritodrine. And it would depend on how much we got her calmed down first, as far as her heart rate and things like that. The other drug would probably cause probably the same problem. We could start her on something like magnesium sulfate, which won't cause as many problems. But, if we're looking at something like pulmonary edema, we're just going to make it worse.

Just because she's having contractions doesn't mean she's necessarily going to deliver. So we could also be checking if there's cervical changes. We may have to consider that she's going to deliver because we can't risk the mom's health for the sake of the baby. We may not be able to stop it, and we may have to let that baby deliver. And we've done that with real sick moms when everything got away from us. And yeah—gravida 2, para 1, 30 weeks' gestation, we're probably talking about a 3½-pound baby. With a 14-year-old whose not real well developed or anything like that, the baby's probably not going to just fall out, so I have a little time to think about some of the things I'm going to do to get ready for it.

Commentary

In the nurse's thoughts about this final scene, we see repeated use of the thinking strategy **generating hypotheses**: *She's probably not feeling anxious; obviously, the ritodrine has worked. . . . That [respiratory rate 30 breaths per minute; heart rate up to 136 beats per minute] could be just a side effect from the medicine. It's not unusual for the heart rate to climb. . . . She could be going very quickly into pulmonary edema. . . . The other drug would probably cause the same problem. We could start her on something like magnesium sulfate, which won't cause as many problems. But, if we're looking at something like pulmonary edema, we're just going to make it worse.* **Generating hypotheses** about what is causing the sudden change in the client's condition (the nurse indicates that the client is probably experiencing a reaction to the ritodrine) and about alternative therapy (*We could start her on something like magnesium sulfate*) help the nurse to quickly assess the situation and to narrow down her choices regarding what to do about it.

She then **generates** several additional **hypotheses**: *We may have to let that baby deliver. . . . We're probably talking about a 3½-pound baby. The baby's probably not going to just fall out, so I have a little time to think about some of the things I'm going to do to get ready for it.*

The hypotheses that the nurse generates help her come to the conclusion that she has a little time to think about how to prepare for the now seemingly inevitable delivery. In his recent text *Critical Thinking*, Ennis (1996, pp. 4–5) reminds us that sound critical thinking is reasoned and reflective: "The first thing to do in approaching any situation is to figure out the main problem. Ask yourself: 'what is going on here, what really matters here, what's this all about?'. . . You should also try to get a fairly good idea of the reason or reasons." The nurse exemplifies sound critical thinking by first figuring out what the main problem is and then recognizing that she has *a little time to think about some of the things I'm going to do to get ready for it.* Pyles and Stern (1983, p. 55), in their classic study examining the cognitive process used by experienced nurses in making assessments and judgments, described this phenomenon as the nursing gestalt: "the accurate perception and identification of cues as well as the ability to assign valid meanings to feelings; knowledge and experience are inherent in these processes."

References

Ennis, R. (1996). *Critical thinking.* Upper Saddle River, NJ: Prentice Hall.

Evans, D., Block, M., Steinburg, E., & Penrose, A. (1986). Frames and heuristics in doctor-patient discourse. *Social Science Medicine, 22*(10), 1027–1034.

Kassirer, J., & Kopelman, R. (1988). The case presentation: I. Principles. *Hospital Practice, 21*(7), 21–29.

Pyles, S., & Stern, P. (1983). Discovery of nursing gestalt in critical care nursing: The importance of the gray gorilla syndrome. *Image: The Journal of Nursing Scholarship, 15,* 51–57.

Schön, D. (1983). *The reflective practitioner: How professionals think in action.* New York: HarperCollins.

Sonnenberg, F., Kassirer, J., & Kopelman, R. (1986). An autopsy of the clinical reasoning process. *Hospital Practice, 23*(12), 21–29.

18 *Clinical Dilemmas in Oncology Nursing*

The nurse responding to the clinical dilemmas in this chapter has over 13 years of experience in oncology nursing practice.

Clinical Dilemma One

SCENE ONE

You are an oncology nurse who has returned to work on the morning shift after having several days off. It is 7:30 A.M. You have been assigned to care for four clients today. One of your clients, Jane D., is a 55-year-old married woman who was admitted last night with the diagnosis of breast cancer. Jane is scheduled for a lumpectomy at 10:00 A.M.

As you enter the room, Jane is sitting on the end of the bed sobbing. When you ask why she is crying, she tells you that she is very confused. She is not sure if she made the right choice. She asks you to explain the difference between mastectomy and lumpectomy. She begins to cry, saying that she is so afraid of dying, and if she lives, she wonders if she'll be able to tolerate the pain.

The Nurse's Response

My first question would be to ask her if her physician has given her all the information that she needs. Hopefully, she was given the option of a mastectomy versus lumpectomy. Without seeing her x-rays or reading through her chart or anything, I'd be wondering how advanced is her disease. If there were any suspicion that she was having local metastasis or something, they'd probably do a mastectomy. So hopefully, they explained that to her. And maybe she just hasn't worked through it.

So, I'd either sit down on the bed with her or pull up a chair, getting as close as I could to her, and then I'd talk to her about dying, that it's a legitimate fear. If someone who is having surgery hears the word *cancer*, then it's terrifying. And the pain . . . I can usually guarantee people that there's a lot that can be done to relieve the pain. If they are in pain, then we can always change their medications; we can increase them or alter them if they're still uncomfortable, so that they can be as comfortable as possible. I think what's more important is my taking the time to talk with her, sitting down, and maybe holding her hand or rubbing her arm, and answering any questions that she has. If I don't know the answers, then I can go out and get the answers from the physician.

Commentary

When thinking about the information in this first scene, the nurse frequently uses the thinking strategy **stating a proposition**, a type of rule-based thinking that is frequently manifested when an individual has expertise in a specific area. This nurse has a repertoire of IF–THEN rules that she relies on when reasoning about dilemmas related to her area of practice expertise (oncology). In this situation, she uses these rules to assist in deciding how to respond to this patient's fears and concerns.

In the nurse's thoughts about what is described in this first scene, we also see evidence of her use of the thinking strategy **searching for information**, indicating that she needs additional information to adequately respond to the situation.

In addition, we see evidence of caring and compassion in the nurse's thoughts about this client. She thinks about what she would do to comfort the client: *either sit down on the bed with her or pull up a chair, getting as close as I could to her, and then I'd talk to her about dying, that it's a legitimate fear. If someone who is having surgery hears the word* cancer, *then it's terrifying. I think what's more important is my taking the time to talk with her, sitting down, and maybe holding her hand or rubbing her arm, and answering any questions that she has.* Thus, thoughts expressing caring seem to predominate in the nurse's response to the dilemma. There is an abundance of literature to support the premise that caring is an important and prominent characteristic of nursing practice, and there is also literature to support the notion that caring thinking is an important component of critical thinking. Lipman (1995, p. 12) proposes that caring thinking is a major aspect of higher-order thinking, claiming, "Without caring, higher-order thinking is devoid of a values component. . . . I suspect we feel emotions when we have choices and decisions to make, and these choices and decisions are the leading edges of judgment."

Thinking Activities

1. Review the nurse's thoughts about scene one. Locate the instances when she uses the thinking strategy **stating a proposition**.

2. What relationship do you see between this type of rule-based thinking and the nurse's expertise in oncology nursing practice?

3. Provide several examples of IF–THEN rules that you use in thinking about your nursing practice.

4. What relationship do you see between these rules and your expertise in an area of nursing practice?

5. Describe how caring influences your thinking in nursing practice.

6. What relationship do you see between caring thinking and critical thinking?

SCENE TWO

By the end of the conversation, Jane's spirits have lifted, and she seems better equipped to deal with the surgery and follow-up therapy. It is soon 12:00 noon. Jane returns from surgery wearing a 4 × 4 dressing over her incision and a self-suction drain in place. On assessment, the dressing is bright red, and the drain has collected 60 ml of bright red fluid. Jane's right arm is swollen. She is moaning and asking for a pain pill.

The Nurse's Response

60 mL of bright red drainage immediately post-op is worrisome. I would think that was a lot. And the fact that her right arm is swollen from a lumpectomy, that would worry me also. I'd probably call the physician right away and ask him to please come up to assess it. A lot of times they'll just say, "Well, you know, that's the way it's supposed to be." If it looked really bad to me and if I was really concerned, then I'd have her surgeon come up to look at it.

If she's having a lot of pain, then she should be getting her medication. And hopefully, the pain medication will be effective. I'm just hoping that the client has an order for a drug such as IV or IM Demerol [meperidine] or morphine. If not, I'd probably call up about that also to see if I could get one.

Commentary

In her thoughts in response to scene two, the nurse demonstrates use of another thinking strategy, **hoping** (to expect or desire): *And hopefully, the pain medication will be effective. . . . I'm just hoping that the client has an order for a drug such as IV or IM Demerol [meperidine] or morphine.* **Hoping** was a thinking strategy that was occasionally used by subjects in the TIP study. In these examples, **hoping** seems to assist the nurse in identifying an important client outcome: the relief of pain. In today's nursing practice, there is increased focus on the identification and evaluation of client outcomes (Naylor, Munro, & Brooten, 1991; Waltz & Sylvia, 1991). Thus, it is not surprising to find evidence of a focus on outcomes in the nurse's thoughts. Identifying the type of thinking strategies associated with nurses' thoughts about client outcomes may assist our thinking in this area.

Thinking Activities

1. Think about your own nursing practice. Do you ever use **hoping** in your thinking? If so, give an example of how you use this thinking strategy.

2. Using the examples that you have provided, describe the utility of this thinking strategy.

3. Discuss how using **hoping** might assist you in identifying client outcomes.

SCENE THREE

It's now 2:30 P.M. You feel completely drained, and you can't wait to get home, put your feet up, and put in a videotape. Jane's husband approaches you in the hall and asks if you have time to talk. Your answer is "Yes, of course I have time." He tells you that he is very worried about his two teenage daughters' getting cancer and that he is afraid he will cause the cancer to come back if he touches his wife's breasts during lovemaking. Finally, he wants to know when she can leave the hospital.

The Nurse's Response

As far as his teenage daughters go, I probably would have gotten some information on self-breast exam and I'd really encourage his daughters to start doing that on a regular basis. And if he felt uncomfortable talking to them, then maybe the next day he could bring them in and I would sit down, or he'd give Jane the information and she could pass it along to her daughters.

In regards to his concern that the cancer could come back when he touches his wife's breasts during lovemaking . . . I don't know . . . I mean, the subject of sex comes up with clients, but for me, I find it very uncomfortable. And I think it's because I'm usually the younger person speaking to older people. I mean, that's just not the way I was brought up.

But I would just try to give him as much encouragement as possible that nothing he could do could cause her any harm and that right now, with her altered body image, his affection and caring are probably the most important thing that he can provide for her and to just be there for her. And there will be times that she cries. If she's going to be getting chemo, there will be times that she just feels sick and disgusting and doesn't want to be touched. But then there will be times for him too, she'll need him, and that's okay.

Commentary

In this scene, the nurse confronts a dilemma that involves having to discuss the subject of sex with her client's spouse, which makes her feel *very uncomfortable*. There are many situations that nurses encounter in practice that make them feel uncomfortable, including: discussions about sex such as the one described in this dilemma, having to touch people's bodies, seeing clients without their clothes on, and so on. When confronted with these situations, nurses' thinking may take on an emotional component, known as affective thinking (Lipman, 1995). Use of the thinking strategy **providing explanations**, as this nurse utilized, may assist self-understanding and value clarification during affective thinking.

We note that despite the nurses' expressed discomfort, she will nonetheless try to help the client's spouse deal with his concerns. She uses the thinking strategy **making choices** to select interventions that will assist him in this endeavor.

Thinking Activities

1. Reflect on your practice. How do you use the thinking strategy **providing explanations**?

2. Describe a situation in practice when you used affective thinking.

3. Distinguish between affective thinking and other types of thinking that you use in practice.

Clinical Dilemma Two

SCENE ONE

You are a charge nurse for the morning shift on an oncology unit. Your caseload is light except for one client who could be quite challenging. Joe has been diagnosed with acute myelocytic leukemia. He is a 33-year-old single man who has lived in northern California all his life. His father died approximately 5 years ago. Joe is an entrepreneur who owns a restaurant, nightclubs, and commercial property and consequently has many friends. He does not smoke or use drugs. He has yearly physical examinations and maintains excellent physical conditioning through regular exercise and a sensible diet. Joe had been feeling well before his diagnosis. He sought medical attention when he noticed severe ecchymoses on the backs of his thighs. When you greet Joe in the morning to take his vital signs, he says to you, "I felt in perfect health before I came to the hospital. Next thing I know, my doctor tells me I have 20 minutes to go home, pack my things, and come in!"

The Nurse's Response

Well, at 33 years old and you're diagnosed with leukemia and have no idea that it was coming down the line, it has to be terrifying. I think that this would be another time that I'd stop what I was doing, pull up a chair, and sit down next to him, to see if I could get him to express himself some more. I'd come right out and ask him if he was afraid. I'd say, "If I were in your situation, that would terrify me. How do you feel?" or "That would really scare me." or "You must feel very overwhelmed right now." And sometimes that's enough to get people to open up. Sometimes it's enough of an opening for people to jump right in and say, "Oh, this is horrible! I can't believe it; I am so scared!"

Commentary

In scene one of this dilemma, the nurse's thoughts suggest that she is imagining what it must be like to be in this client's situation: *At 33 years old and you're diagnosed with leukemia and have no no idea that it was coming down the line, it has to be terrifying.* In her thoughts, **making generalizations** seems to be a way for her to understand how the client might be reacting to the news that he has leukemia. She imagines how she would react to such news. She draws inferences from the particulars of the client's young age and the suddenness of his diagnosis and then **generalizes** that the news must be terrifying. In this case, **making generalizations** may assist the nurse to further understand the nature of this dilemma, how the client must be feeling, and what to do about it. On the other hand, **making generalizations** could cause the nurse to misinterpret the nature of this dilemma, to misunderstand what this individual client is feeling, and to make inappropriate decisions regarding what to do about it.

Skill in critical thinking should enable us to recognize instances when our thoughts may be influenced by inferences that may or may not be correct and that may stem from our own feelings that we are inadvertently projecting onto our clients.

Thinking Activities

1. Review the nurse's thoughts about scene one. Identify instances where she uses the thinking strategy **making generalizations**.

2. How does **making generalizations** assist the nurse in thinking about this dilemma?

3. Reflect on your own nursing practice. Give examples of instances when you have used **making generalizations** to help you to understand a client situation.

4. Discuss the risks and benefits of **making generalizations** in these examples.

SCENE TWO

The results of the admitting laboratory work on your client are back. His hematocrit is 34.6%, platelet count is 29,000/mm^3, and bone marrow biopsy reveals rods and increased blasts. A disseminated intravascular coagulation screen revealed a prolonged prothrombin time and partial thromboplastin time. Fibrinogen was within normal limits, and fibrin degradation products were increased.

The Nurse's Response

I would be pretty concerned. He definitely has the tendency to bleed here. So I'd automatically put him on bleeding precautions for needle sticks and suppositories. I'd call the doctor to see if he knows about the platelets being only 29,000[/mm^3]. I'd want to see if he wants to give the client some platelets. Depending on the bruises too, if they're still real purple . . . I'd go and mark them with an indelible magic marker to see if he's still bleeding. I can go back a few hours later to see if the bruises are still growing. That's one of those things that I might do or might not do. I have to see the bruises myself.

Commentary

There seems to be a tentativeness in the nurse's thoughts regarding the significance of the client's platelet count of 29,000/mm^3. Normally, the platelet count ranges between 150,000 and 300,000/mm^3, but it is often significantly reduced in conditions such as acute leukemia. It would seem that a drop in platelets to

29,000/mm³ might be very concerning for many nurses. The tentativeness in this nurse's thoughts suggests that she has seen many cases such as this, where patients have a tendency to bleed, but not all cases of low platelet levels (thrombocytopenia) result in bleeding. Thus, her tentativeness implies that experience has taught her that it isn't necessary, and probably not helpful, to panic over this type of laboratory value.

The nurse says she would be *pretty concerned* about this laboratory value. Using the thinking strategy **making predictions**, she anticipates that he might bleed and **chooses** what action to take to try to prevent this from happening: *I'd automatically put him on bleeding precautions.* She then **chooses** an additional action: *I'd call the doctor to see if he knows about the platelets being only 29,000[/mm³].*

SCENE THREE

The day after Joe's admission, when baseline studies have been completed, chemotherapy is started. The doctor's orders are daunorubicin, 60 mg IV piggyback on days 1, 2, and 3; cyclophosphamide, 100 mg IV piggyback on days 1 through 7; and allopurinol, administered daily. The client is also on broad-spectrum antibiotic therapy. It takes six attempts to find a peripheral IV site. Fifteen minutes after you start Joe on his chemotherapy, his call light comes on. You put on a mask and gown and enter his room. You find Joe standing by his bed naked with his gown wrapped around his IV pole and soaked with blood. The chemotherapy solution is draining onto the floor.

The Nurse's Response

BINGO! Six needle sticks to start the IV; this is a big problem. Oncology nurses are pretty good at starting IVs. If I have to stick someone two or three times, then that's not a good sign. If I have to call someone else to try two and three times, then the client has no veins. And we need to get a central line put in. It's one of those situations where I think the risks might outweigh the benefits because this guy is going to be on 3 days of daunorubicin and 7 days of cytoxin. You don't want chemotherapy going through IV sites that are even questionable. You want to be able to get a nice, central IV line into somebody, preferably with a large-gauge catheter that provides a sizable blood return so that you know it's in there. And if I'm going through six needle sticks, then that's not good. I'm going to use up his arms.

Anybody who is on chemotherapy is immediately put on chemotherapy precautions. As a healthy person, you do not want to come in contact with the chemotherapy solution itself. There are guidelines indicating the safe amount of lifetime exposure to chemotherapy for nurses and other caregivers. And that would be important to know about in this client's history. Has he received chemotherapy in the past? Because if he's already received the recommended lifetime dose, or if he's received doses of chemotherapy that has been unsuccessful, then we wouldn't use those again.

Standing in the patient's room, I'd be wondering what happened. I'd have blood everywhere. And it would look like something out of a horror movie. Of course, I'd go over and stop the IV pump and glove up and get my chemo spill kit out. You never want to come in contact with any body fluids from somebody that's been receiving chemotherapy.

Usually, I wouldn't have left the room so soon after starting chemotherapy, although I have. Usually, however, I stick around for a while to see how the client responds. "Is the IV site intact?" "Is it burning?" "Are you having any pain?" After I start a client on chemotherapy, I find that I always stick around the room doing this, that, and the other thing just to keep checking to make sure that the client's okay.

Commentary

BINGO! Six needle sticks to start the IV; this is a big problem. The nurse **recognizes a pattern**. She substantiates her opinion that this is a big problem by **stating** several **propositions**: *If I have to stick someone two or three times, then that's not a good sign. If I have to call someone else to try two and three times, then the client has no veins. . . . And if I'm going through six needle sticks, then that's not good.* She **makes a prediction**: *I'm going to use up his arms.* And she **asserts** several **practice rules**: *You don't want chemotherapy going through IV sites that are even questionable. You want to be able to get a nice, central IV line into somebody, preferably with a large-gauge catheter that provides a sizable blood return so that you know it's in there.*

Responding to the information about starting the client on chemotherapy and then discovering, a few minutes later, that the IV has come out and the chemotherapy is spilling onto the floor, the nurse again **asserts** several **practice rules**: *You never want to come in contact with any body fluids from somebody that's been receiving chemotherapy. . . . After I start a client on chemotherapy, I find that I always stick around the room doing this, that, and the other thing just to keep checking to make sure that the patient's okay.*

◄ **SCENE FOUR**

Finally, the mess is cleaned up. You find a nurse to cover for you so you can take a much needed break. You return to the unit and the nurse says to you, "I took Joe's temperature, and it was 39°C. I gave him 650 mg of acetaminophen, but he's still shaking!"

The Nurse's Response

My first thought with a fever of 39°C would be, has he had blood cultures drawn within the past 48 hours? Usually, we do blood cultures every 48 hours. Somebody who has a low white count can become septic real quick.

And sometimes, even with blood cultures, we are unable to identify the source of the high temperature. So right away I think about obtaining blood cultures and other cultures. I'd call the physician to see what he wants to do.

Commentary

Once again, the nurse **asserts** several **practice rules** (*Usually, we do blood cultures every 48 hours. Somebody who has a low white count can become septic real quick*) as she reasons about what to do about the sudden increase in her client's temperature. She also **searches for information**: *Has he had blood cultures drawn within the past 48 hours?. . . I'd call the physician to see what he wants to do.*

Thinking Activities

1. Think about your practice. Have you ever **recognized a pattern** so clearly that you reacted in a manner similar to this nurse (*BINGO!*)? Describe the circumstances of the situation in which this happened.

2. In responding to this dilemma, the nurse frequently **asserts a practice rule**. Discuss how this way of thinking might assist her reasoning about the case.

3. Discuss how this way of thinking might interfere with her reasoning about the case.

Clinical Dilemma Three

SCENE ONE

It is 8:00 A.M. You are a charge nurse on the unit for the day. The census is high, and a staff nurse has called in sick. You are getting a float nurse from the obstetric unit. You will not be getting home on time because of a meeting you will need to attend when your shift ends. One of the clients that you will be caring for today is John D., who was admitted a few days ago. He is a 40-year-old white man who was diagnosed with human immunodeficiency virus (HIV) 6 years ago. Since then, he has had *Pneumocystis carinii* pneumonia (PCP) twice. His CD4 count is currently less than 50 (mean %). His past history includes seizure disorders, Kaposi's sarcoma, hepatitis B, and oral thrush. He lives with his significant other, has an occasional drink, has smoked one pack of cigarettes per day for 23 years, and has a history of IV drug abuse.

He has a history of cytomegalovirus retinitis and recently had a detached retina repair performed under general anesthesia. Subsequently, he has been experiencing progressive shortness of breath, increased weakness, and lethargy. Before his admission, his shortness of breath had worsened, he had been running a fever up to 39.4°C, and he has had increased confusion, lack of concentration, and emotional lability. His admission diagnosis is probable pneumonia. His chief complaint is increased shortness of breath.

The oral medications that John has been taking at home are phenytoin, 300 mg hS; fluconazole, 100 mg qd; clarithromycin, 500 PO bid; scopolamine, 0.25 mg prn; prednisolone ophthalmic solution, 1 gtt OU tid; lorazepam, 2 mg q4h prn; and hydromorphone 2 to 4 mg q4h prn. He has also been receiving ganciclovir, 150 mg IV qd, and trimethoprim-sulfamethoxazole (Septra), 240 mg IV q6h.

The Nurse's Response

I hate days like this. I mean, it's 7:00 in the morning, and I just know it's going to be one of those days.

His CD4 count would make me real worried. It's obvious he's had a few opportunistic infections. I mean this is where I start getting a feel for how sick a client is and what type of acuity they will be. With his history of retinitis, he'll be on ganciclovir every day for the rest of his life. His CD4 count means that he's probably getting a lot of opportunistic infections, and some of his medications are more prophylactic than anything else. His history is not uncommon. I mean, that's actually not a bad past history. We see patients like this who come in with many diagnoses and pages of history. If I were to guess what his opportunistic infection is, he probably has *Pneumocystis carinii* pneumonia.

Hopefully, he's been worked up in the emergency department, and blood and sputum cultures have been done. We need to start him on IV antibiotics. And if I were thinking that I had to start his IV, then I'd be wondering what his veins would be like, since he was an IV drug user. I'd like to know what his phenytoin level is. The Ativan [lorazepam] would make me wonder, one, what type of IV drugs he's using, or if he's shooting speed. Because, as he withdraws from it, he'll become very lethargic and unarousable. And if he's a heroin user, he'd need to be on methadone or something to control the pain because he'll start developing a lot of pain.

Commentary

From her analysis of the initial information about this client, the nurse is able to **draw conclusions** about his status: *It's obvious he's had a few opportunistic infections. I mean this is where I start getting a feel for how sick a client is and what type of acuity they will be. With his history of retinitis, he'll be on ganciclovir every day for the rest of his life. . . . Some of his medications are more prophylactic than anything else.* According to Crandall and Getchell-Reiter (1993, p. 45), "research on the nature of expertise suggests that exposure to numerous cases enables experts to accumulate knowledge that allows them to judge events in terms of a prototypical case." Since all cases of clients with HIV and acquired immunodeficiency syndrome (AIDS) admitted to this nurse's hospital are treated on the oncology unit, she has no doubt seen numerous cases of clients similar to the one described here. This helps her to *start getting a feel for how sick a client is and what type of acuity they will be.*

She **generates** several **hypotheses:** *His CD4 count means that he's probably getting a lot of opportunistic infections. . . . If I were to guess what his opportunistic infection is, he probably has* Pneumocystis carinii *pneumonia.* Then she **searches for** more **information**: *I'd be wondering what his veins would be like. . . . I'd like to know what his phenytoin level is. The Ativan would make me wonder, one, what type of IV drugs he's using, or if he's shooting speed.*

◀ SCENE TWO

It's 10:00 A.M., and your initial assessment findings on John are temperature, 38.2°C; heart rate, 153 beats per minute; respirations, 30 breaths per minute; blood pressure, 109/63 mm Hg sitting and 93/64 mm Hg standing; and weight, 52 kg.

Your assessment reveals a thin white man, alert and oriented times three; his right pupil is 6 mm and nonreactive to light, and his left pupil is 3 mm and reactive to light; and he is slightly disheveled looking. He is experiencing mild respiratory distress with decreased breath sounds bilaterally and prolonged expiratory wheezes throughout his lung fields. He has gingivitis and thrush. He has active bowel sounds in all four quadrants, and he has 1+ pedal edema bilaterally.

His most recent laboratory data include white cell count, 10,500/mm³; hemoglobin, 9.6 gm/dL; hematocrit, 27.2%; platelets, 102,000/mm³; neutrophils, 74%; lymphocytes, 21%; serum calcium, 8.1 mg/dL; total protein, 5.5 gm/dL; albumin, 2.4 gm/dL; and magnesium, 1.8 mEq/L. His chest x-ray shows bilateral infiltrates.

The Nurse's Response

I wonder if we need to up his IV rate because he's orthostatic [his BP decreases with position changes]. And I'd be a little concerned about a heart rate of 153. I hope he's had blood cultures. And his temperature is 38.2°C. That's kind of borderline and not something I'd be real concerned about. He's hasn't been started on antibiotics yet. I'd be wondering why the antibiotics haven't been started. He's on Septra, right?

I think he's being treated presumptively for PCP. His clinical presentation is consistent with *Pneumocystis carinii* pneumonia. So, if I saw the physician, I would run that by him, maybe ask him what the plan is, what does he think is going on?

Commentary

Given these assessment findings, the nurse **poses** several **questions**: *I wonder if we need to up his IV rate because he's orthostatic. . . . I'd be wondering why the antibiotics haven't been started. He's on Septra, right?* She doesn't seem certain what condition they are treating, what the treatment plan is, and what is going on with this client. Inquisitiveness has been described as an important habit of mind for developing sound critical thinking strategies. This disposition is considered to be particularly important for sound thinking in nursing practice: "Considering that the knowledge base for competent practice continues to expand, a deficit in inquisitiveness would signal a fundamental limitation of one's potential to develop expert knowledge and professional practice ability" (Facione, Facione, & Sanchez, 1994, p. 346). In their text *Asking the Right Questions: A Guide to Critical Thinking*, Browne and Keeley (1994) propose that the "ability to ask and answer critical questions at appropriate times" is essential to critical thinking. In addition, a recent study by Fisher and Fonteyn (1995) revealed that questioning is a thinking strategy that is frequently used by experienced nurses in practice.

Thinking Activities

1. In responding to the information in the first scene of this dilemma, the nurse uses the thinking strategy **searching for information**; in responding to the second scene, she uses the thinking strategy **posing a question**. What do you see as the difference between these two thinking strategies?

2. What do you see as the similarity between these two thinking strategies?

3. What strategies have you used to develop the habit of being inquisitive in your practice?

SCENE THREE

It is now 11:00 A.M. You have John on oxygen at 15 L/min via mask. You have noted that he keeps taking the mask off, subsequently dropping his oxygen saturation from 92% to 87%. He has scattered rhonchi and a persistent hacking cough.

At 12:00 noon, you check in on John. He complains of increased shortness of breath, is becoming increasingly anxious, and is confused. His respiratory rate is up to 40 breaths per minute and is labored, blood pressure is 93/65 mm Hg, heart rate is 140 beats per minute, and temperature is 38°C. You switch him to 100% oxygen via nonrebreather mask, which brings his oxygen saturation up to 90%.

The Nurse's Response

Now I'm getting concerned that he's going into sepsis. He's getting septic. I would have thought of that earlier, that he might be starting to get septic. He has an increased heart rate and decreased blood pressure. That is a major sign right there. And his oxygen saturation is not ideal. An oxygen saturation of 90% on 100% oxygen—I'd be real worried. I mean hopefully the docs would be around. I'd get them in there. What are we doing? What is going on? I'd be concerned. I'd be really worried about him. I think he's getting septic. Somebody's who's had HIV for over 6 years, I'd be wondering about his status. Because he's getting progressively worse. And if something acute happens, are we going to whisk this guy off to the intensive care unit, or is he a no-code and we're going to help him stay comfortable, just provide comfort care? How aggressive are we going to be with this guy? That's the kind of questions I'd start throwing out at people. What should I do with this guy? I don't know.

His respirations are at 40, he has decreased blood pressure—I'd be very concerned. I'd be thinking maybe it's time to get him to the intensive care unit. Sometimes I don't know what's going on, but I just kind of get a gut feeling. Maybe get him on a monitor. If he has a heart rate of 140, then get him on a monitor.

Commentary

In the nurse's thoughts about this scene depicting a marked deterioration in the client's condition, we hear her repeatedly **setting priorities** regarding her concerns about the client: *Now I'm getting concerned that he's going into sepsis. . . . An oxygen saturation of 90% on 100% oxygen—I'd be real worried. . . . I'd be concerned. I'd be really worried about him. . . . Somebody's who's had HIV for over 6 years, I'd be wondering about his status. . . . His respirations are at 40 [breaths per minute], he has decreased blood pressure—I'd be very concerned. I'd be thinking maybe it's time to get him to the intensive care unit. Sometimes I don't know what's going on, but I just kind of get a gut feeling.*

In their study of the cognitive processes used by experienced nurses in making assessments and decisions, Pyles and Stern (1983, p. 54) referred to gut feelings as "the essence of the art of nursing. . . . All of the nurses [in the study] sensed when a patient had taken a turn for the worse, because of a gut feeling. . . . Nurses claimed that when they had those feelings about a patient, most of the time something did happen."

◄ SCENE FOUR

It's now 1:00 P.M. Upon entering John's room, you note his oxygen mask is off and lying on the bed. His oxygen saturation is 77% on room air. His heart rate's 150 beats per minute, and respirations are 44 breaths per minute. Pedal edema has increased to 3+. You listen to his lungs and note bilateral rhonchi. At this time, John is difficult to arouse. John's significant other arrives to visit. On entering the room, he rushes to the bedside and looks very concerned.

The Nurse's Response

Sometimes you don't even have to listen to their lungs; you can hear it when you're standing over their bed. And I imagine if he's breathing 44 times a minute, this might be one of those times. Plus the edema. He's got fluid overload, and I'd probably take his blood pressure too. Because, if he's getting fluid overload, and you call the doctor out, he'll pretty much say furosemide. But if he's got a blood pressure at 90/60, you don't want to give him furosemide because his blood pressure will go a lot lower after the furosemide. Now I'd probably be begging to send him to the [intensive care] unit if he's a full code. Because there's only so much a staff nurse can do outside of ICU. If he keeps progressing along this way, heart rate at 150 and respirations at 44, something's going to give out. The heart can't keep going that fast. Something's going to start giving out.

I imagine he's in fluid overload. I'd cut back on his IV fluids. I'd probably do that without even an order at this point. I think I'd probably have another nurse in the room. At this point, I'd want to get someone in to help me.

If John's significant other [SO] is acting out, it might be a good idea to get him out of the room and with someone who can sit with him and talk to him. Hopefully, someone who has a little bit of an idea about what's going on can sit down and maybe calm him down. I'd tell his SO, "We need to work with John, and we need you to step out of the room for a few minutes."

Hopefully, you can get a client like this to the unit before he codes [has a cardiac arrest]. If we could get an idea of how conservative our treatment is going to be with this man . . . are we going to be very aggressive with him? I have a tendency to think of the patients as my loved ones. If I had someone who was dying and these were the last few weeks of their lives, would they want to be attached to a machine that was breathing for them? Sometimes when you're talking with families about code status you have to ask them that in very nonclinical terms. Do you want a machine breathing for him? Do you want medications making a heart beat? Is this what John would have wanted? If you can get a real clear sense of that, then you can kind of understand what type of treatment to give. If this man is going to continually get worse and wants unaggressive care—he just wants nature to take its course—it's time to cut back on the IV fluids and start him on morphine drip. Get him started on a morphine drip and keep him comfortable because right now he's not comfortable. He's miserable. He's working real hard to breathe. At what point do you stop the antibiotics? Some patients don't want antibiotics stopped. They want everything but the antibiotics stopped, so you can keep giving antibiotics. My own personal feeling is that sometimes prolongs the inevitable. Sometimes, if you get someone on a morphine drip and comfortable and just let nature take its course, they can go much more peacefully. But that's my own personal opinion.

Commentary

In the nurse's initial thoughts about this scene, we see a classic example of **recognizing a pattern**: *Sometimes you don't even have to listen to their lungs; you can hear it when you're standing over their bed. And I imagine if he's breathing 44 times a minute, this might be one of those times. Plus the edema. He's got fluid overload.*

The nurse then **makes** several **predictions**. She predicts that if she calls the doctor to report that the client is in fluid overload, he'll probably order furosemide, which, the nurse **predicts**, will cause his blood pressure to go a lot lower. She'll check the client's blood pressure before calling the doctor so that he'll consider that while determining whether to give the order for furosemide. The nurse also **predicts** that the client's condition is likely to deteriorate: *If he keeps progressing along this way, heart rate at 150 [beats per minute] and respirations at 44 [breaths per minute], something's going to give out. The heart can't keep going that fast. Something's going to start giving out.* In their study of expert nurses' judgment, Jacavone and Dostal (1992, p. 58) report, "It was evident that [these nurse] experts recognized subtle physiologic changes in each patient's response. . . . Prior to acknowledging a significant patient response, the nurse must have a sense of the patient's baseline or continuum of homeostatic changes."

As the nurse continues to think about this client's deteriorating condition, she struggles with the ethical concerns surrounding aggressive treatment of this client in the face of his seemingly inevitable demise. Her thinking includes consideration of the context of this situation, the ominous signs that the client is rapidly deteriorating, his level of comfort (*He's miserable. He's working real hard to breathe.*), as well as her personal feelings about what she would want done in this situation. In her provocative article, "Women and Ethics: A Seeing' Justice," Hepburn (1993) advocates that a component of ethical decision making is to "consider the issue from the perspective of one intimately bound to another by ties of kinship and/or love. . . . What is called for is an ethic which gives due weight to considerations of justice within a setting illuminated by all the information we have at hand," a "seeing," attached justice rather than a blind, detached justice. Benner, Tanner, and Chesla (1996, p. 253) support this perspective: "In the context of generous, knowledgeable, caring practices that are finely tuned by one's own sentient and skilled embodiment, the level of mutual respect and knowledge of the other will allow for more than mere rights and justice."

Thinking Activities

1. The nurse's thoughts about this last scene demonstrate her strong commitment to client advocacy. Discuss how she demonstrates this in her thinking.

2. What are some of the risks involved in putting client advocacy into action in this situation?

3. What are some of the benefits?

4. Think about your own practice. Describe a situation where you felt strongly committed to client advocacy. How did this affect your thinking?

References

Benner, P., Tanner, C., & Chesla, C. (1996). *Expertise in nursing practice: Caring, clinical judgment, and ethics.* New York: Springer.

Browne, M., & Keeley, S. (1994). *Asking the right questions: A guide to critical thinking.* Englewood Cliffs, NJ: Prentice-Hall.

Crandall, B., & Getchell-Reiter, K. (1993). Critical decision method: A technique for eliciting concrete assessment indicators from the intuition of NICU nurses. *Advances in Nursing Science, 16* (1), 42–51.

Facione, N., Facione, P., & Sanchez, C. (1994). Critical thinking disposition as a measure of competent clinical judgment: The development of the California Critical Thinking Disposition Inventory. *Journal of Nursing Education, 33*(8), 345–350.

Fisher, A., & Fonteyn, M. (1995). An exploration of an innovative methodological approach for examining nurses' heuristic use in clinical practice. *Scholarly Inquiry for Nursing Practice, 9*(3), 263–279.

Hepburn, E. (1993). Women and ethics: A "seeing" justice? *Journal of Moral Education, 23*(1), 27–38.

Jacavone, J., & Dostal, M. (1992). A descriptive study of nursing judgment in the assessment and management of cardiac pain. *Advances in Nursing Science, 15*(1), 54–63.

Lipman, M. (1995). Caring as thinking. *Inquiry: Critical Thinking Across the Disciplines, 15*(1), 1–13.

Naylor, M., Munro, B., & Brooten, D. (1991). Measuring the effectiveness of nursing practice. *Clinical Nurse Specialist, 5*(4), 210–215.

Pyles, S., & Stern, P. (1983). Discovery of nursing gestalt in critical care nursing: The importance of the gray gorilla syndrome. *Image: The Journal of Nursing Scholarship, 15*, 51–57.

Waltz, C., & Sylvia, B. (1991). Accountability and outcome measurement: Where do we go from here? *Clinical Nurse Specialist, 5*(4), 202–203.

19 *Clinical Dilemmas in Critical Care Nursing*

The nurse responding to the clinical dilemma presented in this chapter has 16 years of nursing practice experience in medical intensive care. For the last 7 years, she has been the charge nurse of a 13-bed medical intensive care unit (MICU) in a large urban hospital.

Clinical Dilemma One

SCENE ONE

You are the charge nurse in the MICU. Currently, all 13 beds are occupied; you are one of eight registered nurses working the day shift. It is 7:00 A.M. One of your clients is a 78-year-old woman 3 days postoperative status post–partial gastrectomy for gastric ulcer. She is an insulin-dependent diabetic in end-stage liver failure.

Her vital signs at the beginning of the shift are blood pressure (BP), 140/80 mm Hg; temperature, 37.6°C; pulse, 105 beats per minute; respirations, 24 breaths per minute; and oxygen saturation, 93% on 6 L of oxygen per minute by face mask. She was extubated last night after 2 days of stability. Her current laboratory data are hematocrit, 24%; hemoglobin, 8 gm/dl; white blood cells, 10,000/mm³; platelets, 75,000/mm³; glucose, 165 mg/dl; alkaline phosphatase, 295 U/L; and aspartate aminotransferase, 95 U/L.

She is oriented to person only. Her lungs have bilateral crackles on auscultation. She has 2+ lower extremity edema and multiple ecchymoses. She is NPO (nothing by mouth) and has a nasogastric (NG) tube in her right nare, which is connected to low continuous suction. Thirty millimeters of dark drainage has accumulated in the last 3 hours. Her abdomen is firm, and she has no bowel sounds. She has a Foley catheter inserted into her bladder and connected to gravity, which is draining 20 ml of dark amber urine per hour. She has a large primary abdominal dressing with old, marked bloody drainage. There is a 20-gauge IV in her left forearm infusing a solution of dextrose and electrolytes at 60 mL/hr. An 18-gauge IV catheter in her right forearm is locked off at present.

The client received 6 U of regular insulin at 6:00 A.M. Three hours into the shift, at 10 A.M., the client's blood sugar drops to 50 mg/dL, her heart rate increases to 120 beats per minute, her blood pressure drops slightly to 118/60 mm Hg, and she becomes slightly combative, with an increase in confusion.

The Nurse's Response

We don't get a lot of surgical clients in the medical intensive care unit, but I guess we got overflow from the surgical intensive care unit [SICU] on this particular day. We can take care of surgical clients, but it's not our norm; we tend to operate a little differently in MICU. In SICU, they get their clients up and walk them and stuff at 4:00 in the morning. Most of our clients are MIs [patients with myocardial infarctions] or clients that you want to actually let rest or sleep, so that's rather different.

Her surgical problems are not common in our unit. Her abdomen is firm. And what would worry me would be only 30 mL out the NG tube in the last 3 hours, if her abdomen is firm and she's just had bowel surgery. I want to check to make sure the NG tube is working, check for bowel sounds, and determine if she is guarding her abdomen, if that is painful to her.

Her medical problems are common in our unit. Her blood sugar is too low, so we'd get the intern, and give her a bolus of 50% dextrose [D50], and then repeat it, maybe in an hour or two. She's got problems. The blood pressure, what was it before? 140/80 [mm Hg]. Well, it's not really that much less; that's not very critical. I am more worried about her blood sugar, actually. It would depend on what kind of response she had to the low blood sugar. She's only oriented to person.

If she was lethargic and unresponsive, then that would be a worry, but I wouldn't worry if she was still awake, and the rest of her vital signs were okay. Her heart rate is up a little; that's compensating for the little bit of drop in the blood pressure. If she's combative, that could be from her low blood sugar, too. When they find somebody unresponsive in the field, the paramedics automatically give a bolus of 50% dextrose, just to see if the person has low blood sugar, because they could go into a coma from that [the low blood sugar].

A blood sugar of 50 [mg/dL] is rather worrisome; but being in the unit, I can check it, and I can give something right away. I don't have to wait for the intern to write the order. I'd just grab him and push him into the room and say, "We're going to give some D50." What we'd do is give her the D50, and then draw another blood sugar, maybe in a half hour, to see where we are, and then check to see how her mentation and her other vital signs were at that time.

Commentary

While reasoning about this dilemma, the nurse remarks, *We don't get a lot of surgical clients in the medical intensive care unit.* Thus, it may be more difficult for her to reason well about this type of case because, as she explains, *her surgical problems are not common in our unit.* Research has demonstrated that skill in reasoning is specific to an area of expertise, a speciality (Glaser, 1990; Patel, Groen, & Arocha, 1990). Competence in a specialized area of nursing such as MICU does not ensure competence in another (SICU). In the presence of an extensive knowledge base, clinical dilemmas represent familiar, well-structured problems for which there are standard solutions, often associated with established protocols. Thus, the problem of sudden hypoglycemia (a drop in blood sugar to 50 mg/dl), although *worrisome*, can be rather easily resolved without the need for the nurse to do extensive problem solving (*being on the unit, I can check it, and I can give something right away*).

In contrast, the client's surgical problems are less familiar to this nurse and thus are ill structured and without standard solutions or established protocols (*We can take care of surgical clients, but it's not our norm*). When reasoning about these surgical problems (a firm abdomen and only 30 mL of NG output in the last 3 hours), the nurse uses the way of thinking described as **searching for information**: *I want to make sure the NG tube is working, check for bowel sounds, and determine if she is guarding her abdomen, if that is painful to her.* Finding out more information is a way to provide structure to a problem that is ill structured. In his seminal paper "The Structure of Ill-Structured Problems," Herbert Simon (1973, p. 187) emphasized, "There is merit to the claim that much problem solving effort is directed at structuring problems, and only a fraction of it at solving problems once they are structured." This helps explain the nurse's **searching for information** to uncover additional data that will provide more structure to the client's surgical problems and thus provide insight into their resolution.

SCENE TWO

It is now 11:10 A.M. The 10:00 A.M. laboratory results come back with a hematocrit of 21.4%, hemoglobin of 6 gm/dL, and platelets of 58,000/mm^3. The physician has ordered two units of packed red blood cells and six units of platelets. When you start to administer the blood, you discover that the right forearm IV is clotted.

The client's oxygen saturation has dropped to 89% on 6 L of oxygen per minute. Her respirations have increased to 32 breaths per minute, and her abdominal dressing has a new spot of drainage. The resident has left the floor for a code blue (cardiopulmonary resuscitation) on the sixth floor.

The Nurse's Response

Well, she has two IVs, so she's still got one IV left, so one being clotted doesn't worry me right now because she still has an IV site. Her oxygen saturation of

89% on 6 L is a concern because that's pretty low. And she was just extubated last night. Her respirations have increased to 32 [breaths] per minute. They were 24; now they're up a little bit.

Her abdominal dressing has a new spot of drainage. Is it bloody drainage? And her platelets are only 58,000 [/mm³], so they're dropping. Sounds like she's bleeding; what would I do? I'd call the intern or the resident, if they're both off the floor. I'd increase her oxygen. She obviously needs the blood, so I'd start the blood. After I got the blood started, then I would start another IV, in case we needed to give her fluids or administer some other kind of drugs. And I'd wait for the intern or resident to get back.

Her respirations are up. But, to me, it sounds more like she's bleeding. She's in some kind of distress. Her platelets are low, so I know she's at risk to bleed, and I think she needs the blood. We'd be giving her both blood and platelets, so I'd start another IV to give her blood in one site and platelets in another because platelets you can just push in. She could be in failure, too. If she's getting a lot of fluid and getting the blood, and she has crackles already and pitting edema, she is in failure. And we're going to put her into more failure giving her the blood. That's a concern also. But if she needs blood . . .

The other thing would be her blood pressure; what's her pressure? Because that's going to tell me what her volume status is. If she's bleeding, her BP is going to drop. If she's in failure with respiratory distress, she'd be tachycardic. Her respirations are up, and her pressure could be higher too. She's still breathing, right? So I could do a blood gas.

It's hard to tell how the client is from reading this because a lot of what I do is just intuitive. I'd be looking at the client. I wonder, what does she look like? I can't tell by reading this. If I were to walk into her room and she was in respiratory distress, I'd look to see what her color was like, and if she could talk, what her mentation was, and what her vital signs were. All of that would determine what I'd do first.

If she were still awake, and her blood pressure was okay, but she was having a lot of respiratory distress, and she has a history of failure, and she has edema, then I would think she's in failure. We're going to give her blood and put her over the top. We need to address that whole situation. If she's bleeding, and that's the reason for this, then her pressure is going to be low, and her level of consciousness is going to be worse. It kind of depends on what I'd see when I went into her room.

Hopefully, she would have a living will, where she would have expressed her wishes, but most clients don't, unfortunately. She has heart failure, so of course I'm going to wonder about a living will, depending on how bad it is. She's a diabetic and not in real good health. And if there's family members there, then I might want to discuss how aggressive they want to be.

Commentary

In this scene, the nurse identifies a series of client problems: a clotted IV line, leaving only one access; a decrease in oxygen saturation coupled with an increase in respiratory rate; new drainage on the client's abdominal dressing; a decrease in platelets; and the possibility that she's bleeding. Being confronted with all of these problems at once demands skillful and agile reasoning and efficient concentration. Individuals are quite limited in the amount of information that they can concentrate on at one time. The classic work by George Miller (1956) demonstrated that individuals can concentrate on only seven, plus or minus two, bits of information at a time. Miller defined one bit of information as "the amount of information that we need to make a decision between two equally likely alternatives" (p. 83). Subsequent research demonstrated that individuals can increase the amount of information that they can concentrate on at once by using a perceptual ability called "chunking," recognizing a pattern composed of bits of information that fit together in a familiar constellation (Glaser & Chi, 1988). Hence, chunking represents another aspect of the thinking strategy **recognizing a pattern**, which is used frequently by nurses in every area of practice.

In responding to the description of the dilemmas in scene two, the nurse chunks numerous bits of information into two primary problems—bleeding and heart failure—that she is famliar with and knows the interventions usually taken to resolve them. Chunking a great deal of information into these two patterns allows her also to concentrate on the interventions to resolve them, including notifying the intern or resident, increasing the client's oxygen, starting another IV and hanging the blood, doing a blood gas, and discussing with the client's family how aggressive they want to be.

Other thinking strategies that this nurse uses to reason about the client's problems include **generating hypotheses** and **making predictions**. The nurse **generates a hypothesis**: the client is in heart failure [*If she's getting a lot of fluid and getting the blood, and she has crackles already and pitting edema, she is in failure*]. Then, she **makes a prediction**: *And we're going to put her into more failure giving her the blood.* **Making a prediction** helps the nurse to confirm her hypothesis and to mentally prepare and plan for anticipated events.

SCENE THREE

The client becomes difficult to arouse. The resident has reintubated the client because of a continuous drop in her oxygen saturation and is at the bedside. The client's vital signs are blood pressure, 98/58 mm Hg; heart rate, 140 beats per minute; and respirations, 28 breaths per minute. The NG tube output is increasing and is now bright red blood.

The Nurse's Response

I'm wondering, has the surgeon been called? Whoever did the surgery should have been called way back when we first thought that she was bleeding. Her blood pressure is dropping, and her heart rate is up because of that. She still needs blood replacement because she's losing more blood. And they'll end up taking her back to surgery because there's something bleeding in there.

More than likely, we'll start dopamine or Aramine [metaraminol]. A blood pressure of 98/58 is still not that bad. It's bad, it's low for her, and if she is difficult to arouse, it could be her blood gases. Maybe her CO_2 is sky-high; that could be. But ultimately, she needs the volume, the blood. In the meantime, we could be giving her blood and maybe starting her on a drug like dopamine, to see if that brings her BP up. It's going to increase her heart rate, too.

Commentary

The client's condition is continuing to deteriorate. She has to be reintubated, her blood pressure is dropping, and her heart rate is up. The nurse wants something to be done fast: *Has the surgeon been called? . . . She still needs blood replacement. . . . We'll start dopamine or Aramine.* She continues to **make predictions**: *And they'll end up taking her back to surgery. . . . It's [the dopamine] going to increase her heart rate.* And she continues to **generate hypotheses**: *It could be her blood gases. Maybe her CO_2 is sky-high.*

Thinking Activities

1. Think about the various types of client cases that you have encountered in your practice. What types that were the most familiar to you, and what types were the least familiar? List examples of cases in each category.

    Most familiar:

    Least familiar:

2. Describe the similarities among the cases that you've listed as most familiar.

3.   Describe the similarities among the cases that you've listed as least familiar.

4.   Choose one of the cases with which you have indicated you are most familiar. List features of this type of case that fit together to form a pattern.

5.   When you encounter this type of case in practice, do you find that you perceive the case in terms of the pattern you have depicted? How might this assist your thinking?

6.   In your practice, what do you find is most difficult in reasoning about unfamiliar cases? What are strategies that you could use to correct this?

7.   Give examples of how you use the following thinking strategies in your practice.

Generating hypotheses:

Making predictions:

8. What relationship do you see between these thinking strategies?

Clinical Dilemma Two

SCENE ONE

It is 10:30 A.M. The emergency department (ED) has just called to give you a report on an admission they will be sending you at about 11:00 A.M. He is a 62-year-old Russian-speaking man with a long history of chronic obstructive pulmonary disease (COPD). He was brought to the ED for acute shortness of breath that did not respond to albuterol nebulizer treatment (three doses—one in the ambulance, two in the ED). He was a client in the local county hospital for pneumonia/COPD exacerbation 1 month ago. His wife gave a half-filled bottle of amoxicillin-clavulanate (Augmentin) and one mostly filled bottle of prednisone, 5-mg tablets, to the ED nurse. The wife is deaf and used sign language to communicate that her husband wouldn't take his medications. She told the ED nurse that her husband is very confused and fearful since his last episode of illness.

The latest vital signs on the client are BP, 150/92 mm Hg; respiratory rate, 24 breaths per minute; heart rate, 120 beats per minute; and occasional premature atrial contractions (PACs). He can speak only two to three words at a time because of extreme shortness of breath, and he is using his accessory muscles to breathe. His oxygen saturation on room air was 82%, and it is now 86% on 1 L/min via nasal cannula. The ED physician felt that the client should be admitted to the MICU because he's very unstable and requires close monitoring. The client has refused to have any blood drawn for laboratory tests.

The Nurse's Response

If the client's wife is using sign language because she's deaf, then communicating with her and her husband is going to be very difficult because he only speaks Russian and she's deaf. The client needs to take his medication. He's been on steroids forever. It sounds like he's a pretty long-term COPDer, and he probably has pneumonia. He had pneumonia a month ago. And he hasn't been taking his Augmentin or his prednisone, so that's like a double whammy.

His CO_2 is probably a hundred; and you hate to intubate these clients. You do everything you can not to because you never get them off the ventilator. So, we'll call in other respiratory docs, who would follow him anyway, and they'll give him treatments, and morphine, and steroids, and whatever they need to do to try to get him past this without having to tube [intubate] him.

He must have some kind of IV going. I'd have his wife explain to him. Get the doctor in there and explain to them, if he's afraid, that we need to do this; otherwise, he could die. He needs to let us do this.

The client's blood pressure is 150/92, and his respirations are 24. That's pretty good. His heart rate is 120, with PACs. He can only speak two to three words at a time, and he is using his accessory muscles. His oxygen saturation on room air was 82% and now is 86% on 1 L via nc [nasal cannula]. Well, he's probably got pneumonia. And we'll bring him up to the unit, start him on some empirical antibiotics, and do blood gases. But the main thing is getting him to let us stick him to draw labs and blood gases. Usually, these clients get so tired and they're so scared because they can't breathe that, in the end, they'll pretty much just say, "Do whatever you have to do; just help me breathe better." If he absolutely refuses treatment, then what are we going to do?

Commentary

The nurse identifies numerous concerns with regard to this client, including difficulty communicating, not taking his Augmentin and prednisone (*a double whammy*), his fear and anxiety (which are hindering his treatment), difficulty breathing, and low oxygen saturation. Despite these many concerns, she sets a priority regarding one primary concern: *But the main thing is getting him to let us stick him to draw labs and blood gases.* This indicates that she is still **searching for** additional **information** to help her structure the problem. She **generates** several **hypotheses** about what she thinks the problems may be: *His carbon dioxide is probably a hundred. . . . He could die. . . . He's probably got pneumonia.* She seems to **recognize a pattern** of familiar features, and based on her **pattern recognition**, she **makes predictions** about what will be done for the client in the unit: *They'll give him treatments, and morphine, and steroids, and whatever they need to do to try to get him past this without having to tube [intubate] him.* Here again, **making predictions** about the client's treatment helps the nurse anticipate and prepare for that treatment.

◄ **SCENE TWO**

Mr. Leski has arrived from the ER. He has obvious digital cyanosis and circumoral cyanosis too. He is sitting with the back of the gurney straight up, surrounded by pillows, which he leans on heavily. The oxygen saturation monitor registers 84%. He has ceased pushing away staff and does not speak. You quickly slide him over to the bed, with the MICU resident's help, and continue with your assessment.

Lung sounds are almost absent in the bases, with tight inspiratory wheezes and a prolonged expiratory phase with wheezes. Vital signs are blood pressure, 138/92 mm Hg; heart rate, 148 beats per minute and irregular; respirations, 18 breaths per minute; and temperature, 37.8°C tympanic.

The Nurse's Response

Well, he's tachycardic. I would think he'd be breathing a little faster than 18 [breaths] per minute, unless he's getting ready to quit breathing, which he could be. He's got pneumonia. He probably is going to end up needing to be intubated because it sounds like everything they have tried hasn't worked. I would get the resident in there and do blood gases because now he sounds like he's almost unconscious. And he's cyanotic, so he obviously needs more oxygen; his oxygen saturation is only 84[%]. We would probably have the crash cart there already, with everything ready. He's cyanotic; he's kind of unresponsive; he's sounding like he's taken the downhill slide pretty fast.

Commentary

The information provided in this scene causes the nurse to recognize the features of the **pattern** of a client who is rapidly destabilizing: *He's sounding like he's taken the downhill slide pretty fast.* Perkins (1986) describes the mental models that "sit more or less permanently in our minds" (p. 143) as "a repertoire of patterns built up over years [of experience]" (p. 140). This collection of patterns assists experienced nurses in spontaneously recognizing familiar situations in practice, in quickly identifying the problem, predicting what will happen next (*he probably is going to end up needing to be intubated*), and knowing what to do to prepare for action (*we would probably have the crash cart there already, with everything ready*).

Thinking Activities

1. Describe the mental model or pattern that you have of a client who is destabilizing. What features does the model contain?

2. Now, describe a countermodel, or pattern, of a client who is very stable. What features does this model contain?

3. List the features of the pattern of the stable and destabilizing client that you think are the most significant.

   Most significant features of the pattern of the stable client:

   Most significant features of the pattern of the destabilizing client:

4. Describe how the above activities might improve your skill in **recognizing a pattern**.

Clinical Dilemma Three

SCENE ONE

Joshua is a 36-year-old man who's directly admitted to MICU. He is status post–cardiac surgery due to a 1.5 cm tear in his right pericardium. The SICU is full, so you are given this client direct from the operating room (OR). He is estimated to have lost 4 L of blood in all. He is 71 inches in height and weighs 82 kg. He is on a ventilator with the FIO_2 set at 40% and intermittent mandatory ventilation at 12/min. A central line is in place. He has received 2000 mL in total intravenous volume. A unit of packed cells is infusing at a slow rate, and an electrolyte solution is also infusing. A right pleural chest tube is in place and connected to a Pleuravac. He's in semi-Fowler position. His cardiac status is being monitored and shows that his vital signs are generally stable. BP is 100/55 mm Hg, and respiratory rate is 12 breaths per minute on the ventilator. The cardiac monitor shows normal sinus rhythm at 96 beats per minute. His skin appears slightly mottled, and his extremities are cool to touch. There are bilateral pulses present, but with thready quality.

The Nurse's Response

No. We would never take care of a fresh open heart surgery client in MICU. They would go to SICU. If SICU were full, they'd move somebody out. Heart surgery doesn't come to MICU. It wouldn't happen this way. The MICU nurses haven't been trained to take care of fresh open hearts. And although we can float over there, we take care of second-day hearts, but not right from heart surgery. We don't know the equipment, and it wouldn't be safe for the client. What would happen would be that they'd transfer somebody out in order to make room for him.

The clients are usually cold when they come back from the OR because they're on bypass and cooled down in the OR, and they don't warm them up real fast. You don't want to do that. So it takes awhile. I don't know how long. But since this isn't my forte . . .

But his pulses are present, and his blood pressure is okay, and his pulse is okay, so he's getting perfusion down to his extremities, even though they're cool to touch.

Commentary

When asked to reason about a dilemma that the nurse feels she would not ever encounter in her practice, she reacts negatively: *No. We would never take care of a fresh open heart surgery client in MICU. . . . Heart surgery doesn't come to MICU. It wouldn't happen this way.* She goes on to explain: *We don't know the equipment, and it wouldn't be safe for the client.* After these initial explanatory remarks, the nurse then goes on to struggle to reason about the case. Our understanding of how nurses reason in practice can be enhanced by learning what nurses do when trying to reason about unfamiliar cases outside their area of expertise. This nurse tries to identify the features of the typical pattern of a client immediately after open heart surgery: *The clients are usually cold . . . and they don't warm them up real fast.* Then she falters: *So it takes awhile. I don't know how long.* Not knowing means this dilemma represents an ill-structured problem to this nurse, which will make problem solving more difficult.

◀ SCENE TWO

The client's chest tube drains 200 mL of semisanguineous excretions from the right chest. His Foley catheter drains 15 mL/hr. He is alert and oriented times one, recovering from anesthesia, and responsive to loud direct verbalization. The unit of packed red blood cells is completed. He is to receive a second unit of packed cells. His vital signs have suddenly changed. His pulse is 130 beats per minute; respirations are 28 breaths per minute and labored. Joshua grimaces as if in pain. His face appears flushed. Suddenly, you notice traces of blood in the Foley tubing.

The Nurse's Response

Well, I think he's bleeding somewhere. But I would think that if he would be bleeding from postsurgery, that would be dumping out blood into the chest tube, so I'm not sure why he's got blood in his Foley. But his blood pressure is definitely low; SICU has standards post–cardiac surgery. They'd start him on Aramine [metaraminol] right away; they have everything spelled out—they just do it. His blood pressure is low, so start him on Aramine. They'd call a cardiac surgeon and try to figure out where he's bleeding from. I think he is going into shock because his pressure is so low.

You can get blood in your urine from a transfusion reaction. Maybe that's why he has blood in his Foley catheter tubing. We just had a client a couple weeks ago that had a blood transfusion and was hypotensive. That's the first time I've ever really seen that severe a blood transfusion reaction. That's why this kind of threw me. But the blood in the urine . . . usually we see more mild symptoms—elevated temperature and chills, maybe some low back pain. I would stop the blood, and then I'd call the blood bank, and they would check the unit, and then I'd do lab work, send the urine—there's a whole protocol. People can get blood dyscrasias. I mean, people can die from blood transfusion reactions. They get blood dyscrasias that clot their blood in their body, so that's why if it's a reaction that is really severe, it is life-threatening.

He's lost 4 L of blood. We have to give him volume somehow. We'd have to stop that unit and give him volume with the lactated Ringer's or whatever else we have. Albumin or anything to get volume back into him while you're trying to get more blood in the meantime. It might be just that one unit [that caused the reaction], or sometimes they have a real hard time crossmatching people because they've got an antibody. That's very rare. We could just put the next unit of blood on a pump; and there's like 250 to 300 mL in a bag of blood, and we can pump it in 15 to 20 minutes. And sometimes we might have two bags running, if we're just trying to replace the volume with the blood. We'd probably be giving him fluid too, and he's probably going to be on his head [titled into Trendelenburg position]. And a young person like him could tolerate that position. Now you can't always do that with an older person because you might put them into failure. You're kind of walking a thin line here.

Commentary

Although she still sounds unsure about this case, the nurse continues to struggle to reason about it. She does not seem to have a definite explanation for the client's signs and symptoms, so she **generates** several **hypotheses**: he may be bleeding somewhere; he may be having a blood transfusion reaction; he may be going into shock. Despite not knowing the precise cause of his problems, the nurse **makes a prediction** about the plan of action, based on the standard protocol that would be followed in SICU: *They'd start him on Aramine right away. . . . They'd call a cardiac surgeon.*

She also knows what has to be done for this or any patient who appears to be going into shock from bleeding: *We have to give him volume . . . with lactated Ringer's . . . albumin or anything . . . and he's probably going to be on his head [in Trendelenburg position].* In her years of experience with clients in MICU, this nurse has probably seen the **pattern** of hypovolemic shock enough to know intrinsically what needs to be done in this situation. This pattern and its associated interventions evoke a response in her that suggests that she seems to know intuitively what needs to be done. Tanner, Benner, Chesla, and Gordon (1993) describe this type of experiential knowledge as "know-how that allows for the instantaneous recognition of patterns and intuitive responses in expert judgment" (p. 274).

Thinking Activities

1. In your practice, have you found that standard protocols assist you to think about client cases? Give examples of how these protocols have been useful to you in your practice.

2. Do you ever find yourself knowing intuitively what to do in a situation in practice? Give several examples of instances when this has occurred in your practice.

3. What factors contributed to this sense of intuitive knowing?

Clinical Dilemma Four

SCENE ONE

This is your fourth day on, and you are looking forward to 3 days off. A new nurse has just started on the unit who has 1 year's experience on a medical-surgical unit. The day shift is just starting, and you note on the board that patient acuity is high. You also notice a central line placement will take place today at 1:30 P.M. for a patient who is positive for human immunodeficiency virus (HIV) and whose bronchoscopy yesterday confirmed the diagnosis of *Pneumocystis carinii* pneumonia. A resident will be performing the procedure with the staff physician.

The Nurse's Response

Well—so, I have a new nurse. I'd give her somebody who would act as her preceptor. The acuity is high, so who I assigned her to would depend on how long she'd been there. Now, if she was just starting in the unit, but she's had a year of medical-surgical nursing, but she hasn't had any critical care experience, she'd go through like a 6- to 8-week orientation. So if she was new on orientation, she and her preceptor, should have two patients who aren't that sick because I don't want to throw a new orientee right into the fire the first week; otherwise, they're likely to run the other way. They need that time to kind of ease into it a little bit. In other words, I wouldn't take somebody that's new to the unit and give them a really hard assignment if the rest of the patients are really busy, because the nurses might be too busy to help her. So that's probably what I'd do, give her an assignment that's not too overwhelming.

And if the central line placement is scheduled for 1:30 P.M., then it'll probably never happen right at that time. Things never seem to go according to schedule in the unit. It's either that they're putting in a line in an emergency-type situation or, if it's not an emergency, then they do it when they have a spare moment. Unless the physician has a made a commitment to be there at a certain time, then it might happen at 1:30 p.m., or it might not.

And I think that it's kind of risky because the patient's HIV-positive, so we'd be extra careful. But you still have to do the procedure, and you can only be as safe as you can be and wear gloves and goggles and everything you have to do to protect yourself, but the patient still needs a line, so you still have to do it. In other words, if you have a patient who is HIV-positive who needs an IV, and they call down to the unit, and they say can you come start this IV, you can't say no. You still just use your best technique [regarding universal precautions] and hope that you don't stick yourself. But the bottom line is that someone's going to have to get an IV started.

Commentary

The nurse acknowledges that this situation is uncertain and somewhat risky. She is supervising a new nurse working in the unit on a day when there is high patient acuity on the unit. Thus, she factors this information into her plan for patient assignments. She states that she will try not to give the new nurse an assignment that is too hard, so that her assignment is not too overwhelming.

Another concern is the central line placement scheduled for 1:30 P.M.: *It's kind of risky because the patient's HIV-positive . . . but you still have to do the procedure, and you can only be as safe as you can be.*

SCENE TWO

It is now 12:30 P.M. The patient you have assigned to the new nurse is a 65-year old man, Mr. Kirk, who was admitted to the unit with a diagnosis of acute anterior wall myocardial infarction.

His past medical history includes exertional angina for 7 years, adult-onset diabetes for 3 years, and recently diagnosed hypertension. He also has a 45-year history of smoking one to two packs of cigarettes a day. He has complained of continued shortness of breath since coming up from the ER 2 hours ago and is currently receiving 2 L of oxygen per minute via nasal cannula.

As you review his history with the new nurse, you note that the patient looks to be in no acute distress. His vital signs on admission to the unit were as follows: blood pressure, 150/94 mm Hg; heart rate, 112 beats per minute; respirations, 30 breaths per minute; and temperature, 36°C.

The Nurse's Response

First of all, his blood pressure is a little high, and his heart rate is a little high, and his respiratory rate is a little high, so that's a little worrisome. For someone who's had a documented myocardia infarction [MI], he's a little tachycardic. And he's breathing at 30 [breaths] a minute, so he's working hard. He's probably in congestive heart failure, which means he probably needs some diuretics.

If he's a new MI, then my first concern would be to make sure that this nurse was picking up on this and that she felt comfortable. The house staff should get in there. Sometimes a nurse who is new on the unit tends to not be as assertive or aggressive. Most of the nurses who have been there a long time have no problems grabbing the intern or the resident and dragging him in a room if they think something is not quite right. So I'd probably make sure that somebody got in there to see this patient because it sounds like somebody should take a look at him and also check to see if this nurse is comfortable in that situation.

He's got hypertension, and he's presently a little hypertensive; his diastolic is high. And he's a smoker. He's complaining of continued shortness of breath since coming up from the emergency department 2 hours ago and is currently receiving 2 L of oxygen. Well, they should probably do an arterial blood gas. And have they done a chest x-ray? These are all the things I'd ask. Did they do a chest in the emergency department? Have they done a blood gas? If he's been smoking all these years, maybe he's a COPDer [someone with chronic obstructive pulmonary disease].

So if they haven't done those tests in the emergency department, then they need to do them now. We have standing orders for our unit. And depending on how busy the physicians are—if they're tied up with somebody else—I would go ahead and order things and have them write an order later. I'd just tell them, "We got a chest x-ray; you need to write an order."

We have usually two interns and a resident on the unit. And if they're tied up, or if they don't give me any satisfaction as far as coming in to see the patient, then I'll just call the cardiologist. If he wasn't that sick, then we'd probably sit on it for a little while. But if he started to deteriorate, then I'd probably just go get the house staff and tell them, "You need to see him now." If they have a problem with that, then I'll call the cardiologist.

Commentary

In her initial response to the information that she is given in scene two, the nurse uses the thinking strategy **judging the value** to assess the significance of Mr. Kirk's vital signs. She qualifies the meaning of the numerical data regarding the client's vital signs with language that suggests she is interpreting them within the context of a client who has had a documented myocardial infarction. Fonteyn (1991) identifies this tendency to translate quantitative amounts into qualitative ones to be a reflection of a nurse's expertise. She found that experienced nurses do not just accept a particular numerical amount but rather translate numbers into terms such as this nurse used, *a little high*, which is more relevant to the context of the current situation. The attempt to make information context-specific has been previously described by Chi, Glaser, and Farr (1988) and Glaser (1988) as a representational ability associated with expertise within a specific domain.

Elstein (1995) described this thinking strategy as a psychological necessity in the complex clinical environment where care providers need to swiftly and efficiently sift through a great deal of clinical data and try to narrow down the problems before they can begin to try to resolve them.

Here, the nurse uses the thinking strategy **searching for information** to identify the evidence that she will need to confirm or reject her hypotheses. In her attempt to narrow down the client's problems, she looks for the results of two diagnostic tests (*Well, they should probably do an arterial blood gas. And have they done a chest x-ray?*)

◄ **SCENE THREE**

It is now 1:30 P.M. Mr. Kirk suddenly experiences acute shortness of breath. Auscultation of his lungs reveals diffuse crackles. Within 10 minutes, he complains of severe substernal pressure.

His vital signs at this time are as follows: BP, 140/100 mm Hg; heart rate, 126 beats per minute; and respiratory rate, 36 breaths per minute. His nurse, the new RN, has increased the nitroglycerin infusion with no improvement in Mr. Kirk's chest pain. His 12-lead electrocardiogram reveals sinus tachycardia and a new left bundle branch block. As this patient's acuity is increasing, you look around the unit to see if another staff nurse can assist this new nurse. No one is available.

The Nurse's Response

Okay, so he's deteriorating. So if his nurse is not comfortable being in there and there's nobody else to be there, then I would go to his bedside. And the house staff would probably be there too.

The patient probably needs some furosemide. I just tell his physician, "He needs some furosemide, so how much furosemide do you want me to give? Go look at the chest x-ray, and then tell me how much you would like."

So I think the gist of this is that the nurse isn't feeling comfortable being in there, and she's kind of over her head. So if there was nobody else to be there, then I'd be there. But I'd still expect her to be there with me because, even though she feels over her head, it's still a learning experience. There comes a time when you just have to do what you have to do, until either the patient stabilizes, or I might have to switch assignments if there's somebody that's a little bit more stable. It doesn't seem like she should be totally overwhelmed, yet. I don't know, maybe later. But maybe she just needs a little support. I'll let her know that she's doing okay. So, at this point, I'd probably talk to her and say, "How you doing?" and "This is what you need to do."

I'd get the house staff in there, make sure things are moving in the right direction. I probably wouldn't change this nurse's assignment yet because it's not good for her ego and she needs to know that she should be able to take care of this.

It sounds like he was already short of breath. His respiratory rate was already high. He was a little tachycardic.

The nurse needs to be there; it's her patient. The easiest thing for me would be to tell her to go sit in the corner and let me do everything. But that's not a good learning experience for her. So she needs to be there with her patient with somebody supporting her who has more experience, and then she can get through the situation until the patient becomes more stable, and then we'd probably sit down and talk. Now, if she just fell apart, then I'd probably say, "Maybe you just need to go sit down and collect your thoughts for awhile, and we'll talk." But the best thing would be to take care of what's happening here. You don't always have time to go sit and talk about what's happening now because he's crumping.

Commentary

The information given to the nurse in this scene causes her to immediately conclude that the client is deteriorating. This ability to use the thinking strategy described as **drawing conclusions** (*Okay, so he's deteriorating*) depicts a process by which an individual with extensive knowledge and experience in a specific area—domain expertise—uses available information about a case to reach a conclusion based on a limited amount of information (Scott, Clayton, & Gibson, 1991). In this case, the nurse is given the following information: diffuse crackles, severe substernal pressure, BP of 140/100 mm Hg, heart rate of 126 beats per minute, respiratory rate of 30 breaths per minute, and electrocardiogram changes. Rather than evaluating each piece of information individually, she considers all of these data collectively as the basis for **drawing the conclusion** that the client is deteriorating. We do not know, however, whether the nurse's conclusion about this client's status is based on additional assumptions that she is not revealing to us.

When she goes on to reason further about the information in this scene, she makes additional inference statements (in the form of IF–THEN statements, the thinking strategy **stating a proposition**) that tell us the specific condition that initiates her conclusions: *So if his nurse is not comfortable being there . . . then I would go to his bedside. . . . If she just fell apart, then I'd probably say, "Maybe you just need to go sit down and collect your thoughts for awhile, and we'll talk."* IF–THEN statements are commonly used as the basis for building computerized decision support systems. These statements, known as projection rules, are used to represent knowledge in a computer program that can be applied to problem solving (Frenzel, 1987).

SCENE FOUR

At the same time that Mr. Kirk is experiencing the shortness of breath, the physicians have started the central line placement for the patient with *Pneumocystis carinii* pneumonia who is HIV-positive. You are just heading over to bed eight to assist and reassure Mr. Kirk's nurse when you hear one of the physicians inserting the central line yell for assistance, and you see blood gushing out of the patient's left jugular vein. As you approach to assist, you realize you are ungloved. But before you can glove up, the resident attempts to hand you a bloody instrument and shouts for you to apply pressure to the bleeding site.

The Nurse's Response

Well, I'd tell the physician that he could hold onto that instrument. He can apply pressure to the bleeder because he has gloves on and I don't. I'll put on a pair of gloves, and then I'll be glad to take the instrument. In the meantime, he can hold it, and he can also hold pressure because he has two hands.

Where's the nurse assigned to this patient? I don't know where his nurse is, but I'd see if I could offer any assistance. Maybe the patient's nurse stepped out of the room, because we're not always in the room.

I'm just thinking, "Okay, well he's bleeding, so I'll hold pressure on the bleeder, and then he'll stop bleeding. And I'll get this patient's nurse back in the room, so that whole situation should be okay."

Then I'd go back to the other nurse to make sure that patient is all right. I can only be in one place at a time, so sometimes I just have to say, "Listen, I've got this other patient that's crumping down the hall. I need to be down there so, you need to handle things here. There's two doctors and a nurse; you should be fine." In this situation, where somebody is going to hand me something that's bloody, I'd say, "Hang on, let me put on some gloves."

Up in the neck by the carotid arteries, all sorts of things can happen. If it's bleeding that bad, then they'd probably call for a vascular surgeon. So they'd be doing that, and all you can do is remedy the immediate symptoms. We'd give him fluid, and we'd put him in Trendelenburg position and try and replace the fluids he's losing. They might not have blood ready, but we can get random type O blood in an emergency. But more than likely we'd probably just give him normal saline to expand the volume that he's losing while we're getting the vascular surgeon to come repair the big tear that this intern put in his neck!

Commentary

The nurse seems very confident in her response to the information provided in this scene. She states what she would do, and then uses the thinking strategy described as **providing explanations** to justify her response: *He [the physician] can apply pressure to the bleeder because he has gloves on and I don't. . . . More than likely, we'd probably just give him [the client] normal saline to expand the volume that he's losing.* **Providing explanations** for the decisions that she makes seems to help this nurse justify them to herself, moving her reasoning about the case forward.

The nurse also uses the thinking strategy described as **making predictions** in response to the information provided in this scene: *I'll hold pressure on the bleeder, and then he'll stop bleeding. . . . They'd probably call for a vascular surgeon. . . . We'd give him fluid, and we'd put him in Trendelenburg position. . . . We'd probably just give him normal saline . . . while we're getting the vascular surgeon to come repair the big tear that this intern put in his neck!* **Making predictions** helps the nurse anticipate and prepare for the actions that she and other members of the health care team will need to take to correct the situation.

◀ SCENE FIVE

Mr. Kirk continues to complain of severe chest pain and shortness of breath and is becoming increasingly agitated and restless. His skin is cool, ashen, and diaphoretic. His oxygen has been increased to 100%, and his nitroglycerin infusion has been increased by his nurse, with no relief of his pain. You see the nurse's anxiety growing. At this time, Mr. Kirk's systolic blood pressure falls to 40 mm Hg.

The Nurse's Response

Oh dear! I bet this guy is having a big MI. I'd have somebody call the cardiologist. (I hope he has one.) So what I'd want to do is, obviously, turn off the nitroglycerin because his blood pressure is so low. We're going to put him in Trendelenburg position, too, and open up the fluids. Hopefully, he'll have fluids somewhere, some normal saline. It kind of sounds like he's going into cardiogenic shock.

His nurse is probably totally overwhelmed by now, and we're kind of in a pseudo-code situation here, so maybe I'd have her record things so that she's still there getting the experience and seeing what's going on. At this point, the patient is in bad shape, and it's not a time to teach. You don't have time to stop and say, "Okay, his pressure is 40. Now what would you do first?" No. This isn't the time. I can sit down and talk about it later, and hopefully she'll get some of this by watching what's going on.

Commentary

The information that the nurse is given about the client causes her to **generate a hypothesis**: *I bet this guy is having a big MI.* A few sentences later, we discover the basis for this hypothesis: *It kind of sounds like he's going into cardiogenic shock.* The nurse **recognizes this pattern** from the way the client *sounds* in the description provided in this scene. Alfaro-LeFevre (1995) describes **recognizing a pattern** as an important step toward problem identification and toward recognizing what additional data need to be collected to confirm one's hypothesis that a particular problem exists.

In this situation, the nurse describes how she will proceed to carry out certain interventions (turn off the nitroglycerin, put him in Trendelenburg position, open up the fluids). She plans these interventions even though her hypotheses that the client is having an MI and/or is in cardiogenic shock have not yet been confirmed. This method of problem solving seems to contradict the way nurses have traditionally been taught to problem solve, that is, by following the steps in the nursing process in logical order. As Fonteyn and Cooper (1994) have explained, when reasoning in practice nurses frequently do not follow the steps of the nursing process in a linear fashion. For example, they often intervene to assist clients before the etiology (problems) causing their signs and symptoms has been clearly established, or they identify client problems before they have performed a complete assessment.

Thinking Activities

1. Provide some examples of IF–THEN statements that you use when thinking in practice.

2. How do you think that mentally providing an explanation for your reasons for decisions would move your reasoning forward?

3. Give examples of instances in practice when you do not follow the linear steps of the nursing process to reason about a client case.

4. What are the advantages and disadvantages of a nonlinear approach to reasoning?

Clinical Dilemma Five

SCENE ONE

You have just arrived on the MICU to work the day shift (7:00 A.M.–3:30 P.M.) after 3 restful days off. As you walk into the unit, you notice that all but 1 of the 12 beds are occupied. You are then handed a message that indicates that one of the your best nurses for this shift has called in sick.

In addition, you notice that there is a memo on your desk from the VP of nursing indicating two mandatory meetings scheduled for today for all nurse managers.

As you head for the break room to put away your belongings, a code blue [indicating a client in cardiac arrest] on the seventh floor is announced over the loudspeaker.

The Nurse's Response

If somebody is sick, which makes me short to begin with, then the first thing that I will do is call staffing to tell them that I need another nurse. We have a book on the unit that has people that are willing to work extra shifts, so I'll check that and tell staffing to call whoever's willing to work and anybody else, any per diem nurses.

In the meantime, an option might be having one of the night people stay over to have somebody watch the one or two patients that they'd have to watch until things settle down. That would probably be my first concern: staffing the unit for the day.

The memo on my desk from the VP of nursing indicating two meetings would be on the back burner, sorry to say, but there's very little time for me to leave to attend meetings. I only get one management day every 2 weeks, so most of the time, when I'm in the count, my answer is always "If I can make it, I'll make it." If administration really needs for me to be there, then I need to have a day off or a management day because I can't always plan to be somewhere at 1:00 for an hour. So that's like way back there on the list of things to do.

The other thing about the code being called is that the staff from nights is still there until 7:30, so somebody from nights, if they're not too busy, could go to the code. Or somebody from days might be all gung ho and ready to go up there. And if they were, that's fine. Then I'd send them. Because, possibly, if the code were to survive and we get the patient, then that nurse would probably have the patient. So it'd either be somebody from nights or somebody from days. I don't go to the codes. I usually stay in the unit to try to figure out what I'm going to do with the patient if we get them. So that probably means that I'm not only short the one nurse that called in sick, I'll also need another nurse to handle the code patient. So I call staffing again and hope that we can find someone.

Commentary

In this first situation, the nurse has to respond to several management dilemmas: being short-staffed, having to leave the unit to attend a meeting, and determining who from the unit should respond to the code on the seventh floor. The thinking strategy **generating hypotheses** predominates as she reasons about how to resolve these dilemmas.

◀ **SCENE TWO**

It's been a long day, but it's almost over. You were able to call in a replacement for your ill staff member, which resulted in being short-staffed for only 1 hour. The code blue from the seventh floor has taken your last available bed.

This patient is intubated and on a ventilator, making the total number of intubated patients six. You have just walked back onto the unit after your last meeting. You breathe a sigh of relief and look forward to heading home to watch a little television. It is now 5:06 P.M., and as you head for the break room to collect your belongings, you start to feel uneasy and realize that the room around you is shaking and that you are experiencing an earthquake.

Before you can react, the shaking intensifies, and the supply cart in front of you falls violently to the floor, missing you by an inch. You can hear monitors crashing to the floor, and two of the nurses on the evening shift scream. You can barely stand up, and just as you make it to the doorway of the unit, the shaking stops. The electricity has gone off, and the unit is eerily quiet, with all the monitor sounds ceasing.

The Nurse's Response

My first thought is "How are we going to get these patients downstairs and then outside?" That's a lot of ventilated patients. It's very hard to staff the unit with those many patients on the ventilator. It's not only the numbers of patients, but with the number of hours that we can allot in our budget, it's very difficult. It means that we'd probably only be able to have two of the ventilator patients as a one-on-one [one nurse–to–one patient ratio]. Hopefully, there would also be some lighter patients. Some of the patients could walk out of the hospital and downstairs to safety. How are we going to evacuate these patients? We're going to lug them down the stairs.

My first concern would be to make sure that the unit was okay structurally, and then I'd be listening for further instructions, because if there was any damage to the building, we'd have to evacuate. The first thing would be to make sure that all the bedside nurses are okay and that the ventilators are working. If the standby generator were to fail, then all these patients would have to be provided ventilations by a handheld Ambu bag. So that's the first thing I'd worry about with the ventilator patients—I'd want to make sure they're getting their oxygen, which might mean that all the nurses or whoever is around (respiratory therapists would probably be there) would be bagging the patients if needed. We have to triage.

Commentary

Jones and Beck (1996, pp. 70–71) have described the type of vigilant decision making that occurs in management situations: "Vigilant decision making assumes that the individual has gathered the necessary facts, considered the alternatives, weighed competing interests, and finally made a decision that can be defended." "Unfortunately," these authors explain, "vigilant decision making can be maladaptive in situations where split-second decisions are required. . . . [For these situations] a vigilant decision maker will always have a crisis management plan to deal with the unforeseen."

In managing the crisis described in this second scene, the nurse **poses** several **questions**: *How are we going to get these patients downstairs and then outside? How are we going to evacuate these patients?* Another thinking strategy that she frequently uses is **setting priorities** about the major concerns in this situation: *My first thought is. . . . My first concern would be to make sure that the unit was okay structurally, and then I'd be listening for further instructions. . . . The first thing would be to make sure that all the bedside nurses are okay and that the ventilators are working. . . . So that's the first thing I'd worry about with the ventilator patients—I'd want to make sure they're getting their oxygen.* **Setting priorities** helps the nurse to focus on the most pressing concerns in this crisis situation.

◀ SCENE THREE

Ten minutes has passed, and the emergency generator has not come on. You and the evening nurse manager have managed to calm the nurses on duty and, as much as possible, the patients. Without electricity, staff nurses are manually providing respirations with Ambu bags to the intubated patients, and you have checked all the oxygen lines to make sure they have not been compromised, to prevent fire.

The Nurse's Response

This is basically what I was thinking about. The oxygen is the other important thing. All the oxygen lines coming into the unit are what's supplying the ventilators and the Ambu bags. If the oxygen was out due to an earthquake, then we'd just have to bag the patients with room air. We'd have no choice. And the other thing is we wouldn't have a monitor. We rely so much on the monitors to watch the patient's heart, so if we had somebody really unstable, we'd have to be checking their pulse and their blood pressure frequently.

I don't really have any personal experience with earthquakes. We have drills, but everybody knows it's a drill, and I think it would be a different situation if it were the real thing. There's a whole system set up; we have a disaster list. I always feel that no matter what, the first focus is the patient and making sure that they get the care that they're supposed to. And in the unit that I work in, things can happen. We can start out with four patients, and the census can go up. We've had five or six admissions in a day—and I have no more nurses. There's no more bodies, so everybody pitches in, and it's a real cohesive group.

It would depend on how bad the building was or how bad the earthquake. If you have a 95-year-old on a ventilator with pneumonia who's conceivably not going to survive, and you've got a 45-year-old who has had a bad MI, then I would think that the 45-year-old would probably go out first. I wouldn't be making those decisions alone. It would be my boss, who's the director of critical care, and then there's also a medical director of critical care, so it would be several people making those decisions. Each unit would triage their own patients. We have a form that we actually fill out when we have a disaster drill, and they want to know who the patients are, and there's three levels of who's the sickest, from those who are ambulatory, and then middle ones, then finally the real critically ill patients on ventilators or something.

Commentary

Because the nurse doesn't *really have any personal experience with earthquakes*, she intends to follow policy and procedures when making decisions about managing this crisis: *There's a whole system set up. . . . I wouldn't be making those decisions alone. . . . It would be several people making those decisions.*

Thinking Activities

1. Describe a crisis in which you have been involved in your practice.

2. What role did you play in making decisions about how to manage this crisis?

3. Were you comfortable functioning in this role?

4. What did you learn from this experience that would help you in the future?

References

Alfaro-LeFevre, R. (1995). *Critical thinking in nursing: A practical approach.* Philadelphia: Saunders.

Chi, M., Glaser, R., & Farr, M. (Eds.). (1988). *The nature of expertise.* Hillsdale, NJ: Lawrence Erlbaum Associates.

Elstein, A. (1995). Clinical reasoning in medicine. In J. Higgs & M. Jones (Eds.), *Clinical reasoning in the health professions* (pp. 49–59). Oxford, England: Butterworth-Heinemann.

Fonteyn, M. (1991). A descriptive analysis of expert critical care nurses' clinical reasoning. Unpublished doctoral dissertation, University of Texas, Austin.

Fonteyn, M., & Cooper, L. F. (1994). The written nursing process: Is it still useful to nursing education? *Journal of Advanced Nursing, 19,* 315–318.

Frenzel, L. (1987). *Understanding expert systems.* Indianapolis: Howard W. Sams & Company.

Glaser, R. (1988). Thoughts on expertise. In C. Schooler & W. Segaie (Eds.), *Cognitive functioning and social structure over the life course* (pp. 81–94). Norwood, NJ: Ablex.

Glaser, R. (1990, July). Expert knowledge and the thinking process. *Chemtech,* pp. 394–397.

Glaser, R., & Chi, M. (1988). Overview. In M. Chi, R. Glaser, & M. J. Farr (Eds.), *The nature of expertise.* Hillsdale, NJ: Lawrence Erlbaum Associates.

Jones, R., & Beck, S. (1996). *Decision making in nursing.* Albany, NY: Delmar.

Miller, G. (1956). The magic number seven, plus or minus two: Some limits on our capacity for processing information. *Science, 63*(2), 81–97.

Patel, V., Groen, G., & Arocha, J. (1990). Medical expertise as a function of task difficulty. *Memory & Cognition, 18*(4), 394–406.

Perkins, D. (1986). *Knowledge as design.* Hillsdale, NJ: Lawrence Erlbaum Associates.

Scott, A. C., Clayton, J. E., & Gibson, E. L. (1991). *A practical guide to knowledge acquisition.* Menlo Park, CA: Addison-Wesley.

Simon, H. (1973). The structure of ill-structured problems. *Artificial Intelligence, 4,* 181–201.

Tanner, C., Benner, P., Chesla, B., & Gordon, D. (1993). The phenomenon of knowing the patient. *Image: The Journal of Nursing Scholarship, 25,* 273–280.

20 Clinical Dilemmas in Home Health Nursing

The nurse responding to the dilemmas described in this chapter has 6 years of nursing practice experience, 5 of which have been in home health. She currently works full-time in a home health department associated with a large urban hospital.

Clinical Dilemma One

◄ SCENE ONE

It is Thursday at 8:00 A.M. Lucy B. is a 75-year-old woman who is recovering 3 days postoperative after surgical repair of a fractured left hip. She is to be discharged today. During the hospital stay, the client received prophylactic intravenous antibiotics (cefazolin, IV piggyback, 1/gm; D5W, 50 ml) for infection, had one episode of deep venous thrombosis, which is being treated with warfarin, and was diagnosed with osteoporosis. The client's vital signs have been relatively stable, and her latest vital signs were: pulse, 68 beats per minute; blood pressure, 112/72 mm Hg; respiratory rate, 117 breaths per minute; and temperature 36.4°C.

Her husband died 2 years ago, and she has no family in California. She receives money from Social Security, and her insurance is provided by the government. Her living quarters are above street level and accessed by a flight of stairs (15 steps).

Her discharge orders include bed rest with bathroom privileges, regular diet, physical therapy three times a week, and skilled nursing visits three times a week. Medications include multivitamin, PO qd; Os-Cal 500, PO bid; Ensure, 1 can PO tid; and warfarin, 8 mg PO qd.

The patient has made arrangements for a live-in caretaker for the time being. You have set up an appointment to meet the client at her house tomorrow afternoon at 1:00 P.M.

175

The Nurse's Response

Number one, I'm going to definitely see that this client gets an order for physical therapy right away. That's a major concern with a fractured hip. Also of immediate concern is occupational therapy [OT] and social work services because this client is supposed to be on bed rest, and she is alone, there's no family. At this point, I would not even have allowed her to go home unless I can arrange for a 24-hour attendant in place before I admit her to the home health department's service.

I'm also concerned about the warfarin, 8 mg PO qd. I want to know what her hematocrit and hemoglobin are, as well as her white blood cell count, and her prothrombin time [PT] and partial thromboplastin time [PTT]. And I want to make sure there are orders for at least five weekly PT draws at this time.

It doesn't say if there's any family at all. She might have family who are not in California but who might be able to come to stay with her.

IV antibiotics . . . if this was just prophylactic, I'd like to know if she has any infection and what her respiratory status is.

I would do a head-to-toe assessment, check pain, check bowels. I'm concerned that there's no pain medicine ordered for her, not even acetaminophen or ibuprofen. And why is she on Ensure, a nutritional supplement? To me, that means that she possibly is not eating well. She might have had a problem with her oral intake in the hospital. If the client is not taking an adequate number of calories, sometimes they are also not hydrating well, so that's going to be a big concern.

So, the focus on this client, if the admission took place, would be pain control, bowel care, nutrition, and hydration. Those would be my major concerns. And also, getting social work, OT, and physical therapy out to see her immediately.

◀ SCENE TWO

You arrive at Lucy's house to find that there is a steep flight of steps that must be climbed to reach the front door. When you ring the doorbell, you hear a woman yell, "The door is open, come on in." As you enter the house, you notice that the living room is off to the right, with the kitchen directly behind it. Also, there are two rooms down the hall in front of you. There is no carpet; instead, there is only wood flooring.

Your client yells, "I'm in my bedroom! Just go straight down the hall." As you make your way down the hallway, you encounter a rather pungent smell from the kitchen. When you enter Lucy's bedroom, you notice that she is in an old-fashioned bed that is at least 42 inches high. There are dirty clothes all around the bed. Next to the bed you observe a stack of unpaid electric company and telephone bills.

As you begin to interview Lucy, she tells you that the phone has been disconnected and that the electric company is threatening to cut service. Lucy also informs you that she has no clean clothes, including any clean underwear.

The Nurse's Response

I would immediately page the social worker. I would tell them the client's condition is marginal and unsafe; the power might be cut off. And the social worker should ideally be able to get out the next morning. If I had to, if the client was concerned about her power being cut off that day, I would call the power company from the house, explain that I'm a home health nurse, that the client is bedbound, has just gotten out of the hospital, and that we have a social worker that should be working on this case.

Let me see . . . a pungent smell from the kitchen . . . I'd go see what it was. It could be that the client has a psychiatric problem. It might be year-old food in the refrigerator. It could be . . . her dead husband! It could be anything! I would look at everything to find out what's going on. The pungent smell and marginal self-care key me in to possible psych problems. The situation in the home was obviously going on before the client went into the hospital.

The problem with this client is that there's no family that I can contact. One thing I'd be doing when I call the physician is finding out who the heck is responsible for this client. I would maybe go to the neighbors and say, "Do you know this person? Do you know if anyone watches out for her?" I have knocked on neighbors' doors before and said, in cases where someone can't be admitted, "Look, the woman living next to you is in danger. Could you check on her?" And usually my clients have somebody in the world that cares about them, whether it be calling them every hour or checking on them twice a day. There's usually someone that can do that. And they will, especially when I present it as an emergency thing.

It's a real tough one when I really feel the client is unsafe. All I can do, in my capacity as a home health nurse, is contact the right people to get the ball rolling.

SCENE THREE

It is Monday at 9:05 A.M. when you arrive for your second visit to Lucy's house. The caretaker tells you that Lucy suffered a fall last night after having an episode of incontinence of both urine and stool. The caretaker also informs you that the client has been refusing her medications. When you examine the client, you observe a large bruise on the outside of her right thigh and redness on the buttocks. As you begin to question the caretaker about the problem with the medications, Lucy tells you she thinks the caretaker is stealing money and silverware from her. While listening to Lucy, you notice a couple of pills on the floor next to the bed. You recognize them to be the patient's warfarin.

The Nurse's Response

Number one, I'm going to call the physician to tell him that I'm sending this client to the emergency department to have x-rays of her hip. That's the first thing I'm going to do. I can't look at this client and say, "Oh, well, her hip is bruised." She has to have an x-ray today. At this point, I'm not really as concerned about the noncompliance with the meds [medications] as I am about her hip. It could be that her noncompliance with the meds is because she might have broken her hip, and she might be confused. I don't know.

The incontinence of urine and stool is a concern. Was she incontinent before, in the hospital, or is it a new problem?

Right now, to be honest, I'm not too worried about the caretaker stealing money and silverware from her. I'm more worried about her hip. I'm focusing on that hip, and I don't really care about anything else right now because for all I know, she might have broken her hip. This all might be occurring from a fractured hip or from severe pain.

I need to find out why she's being noncompliant with her meds. It could be that she can't swallow them. It could be that the multivitamin or whatever is making her sick to her stomach, and therefore she's not taking anything. If she's just for-getting to take her meds, then I'm going to offer her a Mediset device to hold her pills and help her remember which ones to take when, and I'll teach the care-giver, either this one or a new one, how to use that. And that's the first thing I would do with the noncompliance: find out why she's noncompliant and then take it from there.

Commentary

In response to this clinical dilemma, the nurse frequently uses the thinking strat-egy **setting priorities**. This helps her to focus on the primary concerns regarding the client's treatment plan. For example, the client is taking warfarin, but there is no related laboratory data; the client has recently had hip surgery, but there is no pain medication ordered; the client may not be eating well; she seems confused; she is incontinent of urine and stool; and she may have fractured her hip again when she fell at home. The nurse also uses **setting priorities** to identify those con-cerns that are not as immediate, such as the possibility that the caretaker may be stealing money and silverware from the client; although this concern will need to be looked into later, it is not a primary concern at the moment.

Setting priorities also assists the nurse in deciding on the most essential actions to take first to begin to resolve this dilemma. This includes requesting some con-sultation on the case: a physical therapist, an occupational therapist, a social worker, and a psychiatric nurse. It also includes doing a head-to-toe assessment, helping the client to gain control over her pain, planning for bowel care, and en-suring that the client has adequate nutrition and hydration.

Using the thinking strategy **setting priorities** seems to assist this nurse in fo-cusing on the most pressing concerns for this client and in selecting the essential actions to take to begin to resolve this dilemma.

Another thinking strategy that this nurse uses when reasoning about this dilemma is **generating hypotheses**. Here, **generating hypotheses** is used to speculate about the client's potential problems: she may not be eating or hydrating well; her power might be cut off. **Generating hypotheses** is also used to determine the etiology of possible problems. For example, the nurse guesses that the cause of the pungent smell coming from the client's kitchen might be year-old food in the client's refrigerator, or it might even be her dead husband. The client may be non-compliant with her medications because she has severe pain, because she can't swallow her pills, or because they make her sick to her stomach. Additionally, the nurse uses **generating hypotheses** to speculate about possible solutions to the client's problems. For example, the client is all alone but might have family somewhere else who could come to stay with her, or she might have a neighbor who could check on her. If the client keeps forgetting to take her medications, then maybe using a Mediset and involving the caregiver will help. The thinking strategy **generating hypotheses** seems to provide guidance regarding what additional investigations to make and what direction to take to begin to resolve the problems she has identified.

A third thinking strategy that the nurse uses to reason about this dilemma is **searching for information. Searching for information** helps her remember what information she needs to better understand what is wrong with the client and to assist her in confirming her hypotheses. For example, when the nurse learns that the client was on intravenous antibiotics in the hospital, she **searches for information** that will help confirm one of two competing hypotheses: (1) *if this was just prophylactic* and (2) *I'd like to know if she has any infection, and what her respiratory status is*. This use of **searching for information** may also help the nurse to keep in mind important information that she might otherwise forget or overlook. For example, when the nurse is told that this client is on warfarin, she begins **searching for information** about certain laboratory data that would assist her in determining the effectiveness of this therapy: hematocrit, hemoglobin, PT, and PTT. She also **searches** for an order for at least five weekly PT draws because, as she explains, this laboratory value needs to be monitored closely when a client is on warfarin.

Thinking Activities

1. Review the nurse's response to each scene in this dilemma. What additional examples can you find of her use of the thinking strategies **setting priorities, generating hypotheses**, and **searching for information**?

2. Can you identify any other thinking strategies in the nurse's thoughts about this dilemma? List each additional strategy that you identify, and provide an example of its use from the text.

3. Think about your thinking in practice. Have you used any of the thinking strategies that this nurse uses? If so, provide examples of how you have used these skills to reason about dilemmas that you have encountered in your practice.

Clinical Dilemma Two

SCENE ONE

Mr. W. is a 56-year-old single man who underwent a coronary bypass 2 years ago. He has just been discharged from the hospital following a myocardial infarction (MI). You have been assigned to Mr. W.'s case, and today you are going to visit him to make sure he is complying with his medications and avoiding unnecessary stress. His medications are as follows: digoxin, 0.125 mg bid, and 1 enteric-coated aspirin qd.

When you arrive at his home, Mr. W. tells you he has just returned from a brisk walk and is feeling short of breath. After he sits down to rest, you take his vital signs: pulse, 100 beats per minute; blood pressure, 140/80 mm Hg; respiratory rate, 21 breaths per minute; and temperature, 37.1°C. The client also tells you that he has a hard time sleeping at night because he finds it very difficult to breathe. He is concerned because he is urinating frequently throughout the night.

The Nurse's Response

It sounds like this person might be in congestive heart failure [CHF], or maybe he has pneumonia. First of all, he's finding it difficult to breathe and he's urinating throughout the night. I want to find out if this client has been on diuretics in the past and if possibly that was overlooked when he was discharged. Maybe he should be on Lasix [furosemide] or something.

I'm going to be telling him not to be taking brisk walks. I'm going to give him an OT referral to teach him how to pace his activities. If his pulse is regular, I'm not too concerned about it. I'm more concerned about how his chest sounds and if his heart sounds are distant.

I'm going to tell the client not to take brisk walks, to pace his activities, and to stay in the house. I'm going to call the doctor and tell him the client has been taking brisk walks. I'm going to see if the physician wants to order some furosemide, to diurese the client. I would also ask for some nitroglycerin tablets for prn use. I'm going to find out if the physician maybe wants to see him in the next 2 days, versus the next 2 weeks, for his discharge evaluation visit.

I'm going to see what the client's diet is. If he is on a low-salt diet, what did he learn in the hospital about it? He's had an MI. Has he had chest pain? Sometimes old people urinate a lot at night. Most of my clients who are males urinate at least two or three times a night. I'm going to ask him if he has had his prostate checked. I usually ask my male clients that. But if this is a new thing for him, it's hard for him to breathe, he might have CHF. Or maybe he is having another MI.

SCENE TWO

On your second visit, you find Mr. W. is pale, cool, and clammy to touch. He also has a rash on his trunk. He states that he had a rough night due to the fact that he was up with a headache and repeated episodes of vomiting. He is also worried because he had to increase his aspirin intake due to the pounding headache. His vital signs are: heart rate, 130 beats per minute; blood pressure, 110/60 mm Hg; respiratory rate, 30 breaths per minute; and temperature, 36.4°C.

The Nurse's Response

Hmmm. I don't like this at all. I'm afraid this person is having a bleed. Let me see . . . I'd ask him if he's having any chest pain, ask him if the emesis had any blood in it. I'd be looking to see if he's pallid, and if so, how pale is he? He's not on any blood pressure medicine . . .

I'm going to call the doctor to tell him that I'm suspecting a GI [gastrointestinal] bleed. I'll ask him if I can send the client to the emergency department to be evaluated. And I'd probably stay with the client until the ambulance arrived. I wouldn't want to leave him by himself.

I think this person may be having a cerebral bleed. And the pounding headache could be from hypovolemia. Or it could be an MI; these could be signs of having a heart attack. But, again, I'll ask him if he is having chest pain, any signs of an

MI. Otherwise, I can't tell. But, at this point, I just want the ambulance to get there to evaluate him with a monitor and everything to see what's going on.

I'm wondering, what's the character of his pulse? Is it tachycardia, or is it irregular? What's going on with his heart? I would not call an ambulance unless he was having chest pain. If he's having chest pain, I'm calling an ambulance. If he's talking to me and he doesn't seem like he's in any real distress, he seems okay, he's not having labored breathing. He just said, "God, I have a headache." I'd really check him out because I'm not going to call an ambulance and have an emergency team come in unless I need to. But I am going to stay with him. I'm not leaving.

SCENE THREE

As you continue Mr. W.'s assessment, you note that his lungs have diffuse crackles, and he now has 3+ pitting edema in his lower extremities. He is very anxious. He asks you, "What is going on with me?"

The Nurse's Response

I would tell him that I think he has severe CHF. I would tell him that his heart is a pump, and it's not pumping well. I would try to calm him down a little bit. I would tell him again that we're going to try to diurese him. Probably, his doctor is going to want to admit him for 3+ edema so he could be diuresed intravenously, which is the best way to do this. And, again, I'd probably call the ambulance and stay with him because he's anxious, and I'd try to calm him down.

Commentary

While reasoning about this dilemma, this nurse frequently uses the thinking strategy **generating hypotheses** both to assist her to identify the client's problems (*This person might be in congestive heart failure. . . . I think this person may be having a cerebral bleed*) and to conjecture about possible treatment for problems (*Maybe he should be on Lasix [furosemide]*).

The nurse uses the thinking strategy **searching for information** in an apparent attempt to narrow down both the list of possible problems (*He's had an MI. Has he had chest pain? . . . I'd ask him if the emesis had any blood in it*) and the etiology of problems (*I want to find out if this client has been on diuretics in the past and if possibly that was overlooked when he was discharged. . . . He's not on any blood pressure medicine*) and to identify possible solutions to problems (*I'm going to find out if the physician maybe wants to see him in the next 2 days*).

This nurse also uses the thinking strategy **making choices** to assist her in deciding what to do about the dilemma: *I'm going to call the doctor. . . . I'd really check him out. . . . I'm calling an ambulance. . . . I am going to stay with him. I'm not leaving.* Choosing actions directs the nurse's thinking and thus helps her develop a more organized approach for a plan of action.

Thinking Activities

1. Describe what you see as the relationship among the thinking strategies **generating hypotheses, searching for information**, and **making choices**?

2. Refer back to the nurse's thoughts about this dilemma. What other thinking strategies do you recognize? Describe how their use helps the nurse to reason about this dilemma.

3. Do you see a relationship among the other thinking strategies that you have identified?

Clinical Dilemma Three

SCENE ONE

Mr. A. is a 76-year-old Hispanic man, status post–right-sided cerebral vascular accident (CVA), with a history of hypertension and noncompliance with medications. Discharge medications include nifedipine, 20 mg tid, and furosemide, 80 mg qd. The client is to be sent home by ambulance because he is unable to climb the stairs into his house. Physical therapy will be following him in the home. His strength is good, but his balance is a little bit off after the CVA. Home care follow-up by the RN is recommended once a week and prn due to his history of medication noncompliance.

This is your first visit to the client's home. It is 3 days since the client has been discharged. When you come to the house, you find the client lives with his wife, son, daughter-in-law, and two grandchildren. The carpet has been vacuumed; the stairs and the doorway are well lit. The client is sitting in a chair and appears well groomed.

His vital signs are blood pressure, 122/82 mm Hg; temperature, 37°C; heart rate, 70 beats per minute; and respiratory rate, 20 breaths per minute. You assess the client's mental status and find he is alert and oriented, with no memory changes. The client is slightly aphasic but responsive to verbal stimuli. His pupils are equal and reactive to light, and he has slight weakness in upper and lower extremities.

As you are proceeding with your assessment, his wife asks you, "Why don't they keep my husband in the hospital longer? He is still very weak, and I am afraid that we cannot be with him all the time."

The Nurse's Response

This is a realistic case study. This is really what I see a lot! Usually, when the client has had a CVA, they've been kept in the hospital for a fairly long time compared to for heart attacks and things, and they usually get a little bit of therapy in the hospital before they're sent home. So they have this sense that things are going to progress, which is good.

I'm happy the client is living in a nice house. It's clean, and he's well groomed, and he seems to be okay. I'm glad that he doesn't seem to have a lot of memory deficits or cognitive changes.

The slight weakness . . . I'm going to do a short neuro[logic] assessment on him. I would be checking his eyes, shoulder shrugs, grips, leg strength, etc. I'd watch him ambulate. I would watch him go to the bathroom. One thing I am going to ask him is if he's having any dysphagia, if he's having any problems swallowing, if the family is noticing any drooling. I want to see what his speech is like, if he's slurring his words. I want him to stick his tongue out at me, all that kind of stuff. If he's having any kind of swallowing problems, I'm going to request a speech therapist to evaluate him and to check for cognitive problems with the aphasia because the therapist is really good with that. I would tell the wife (to calm her down) that clients are kept in the hospital shorter stays these days because of economics, etc., but that we're going to take good care of him at home. He's going to have the full service. I'm going to see if she needs help from a home health aide to assist with the personal care of this client. And she'll probably say yes, because she sounds overwhelmed. I'm also going to see if they would like to get an attendant in to care for him, a respite care so they get breaks.

He's on nifedipine and furosemide but is noncompliant with medication. I'm going to find out why. It could be that the furosemide dosage is too high for him to tolerate, and he feels like he's constantly having to urinate, and it's driving him crazy.

Maybe he doesn't need such a high dose. Does he have a history of congestive heart failure to warrant being on such a high dose of furosemide?

The nifedipine is important. It's been ordered for three times a day; maybe we can change the dose so it's only twice a day. Maybe he'd be more compliant with that. Sometimes people are given meds and not told what they're for and how important they are, and they become compliant when I tell them what they're for. Also I'm going to get him a Mediset. I wonder if he's going to be on any kind of anticoagulant therapy because usually clients who have had a CVA are on that.

I would be teaching him and his family the signs and symptoms of a stroke. I would really stress to the family that if this client has any kind of cognitive change or personality change, even if they just have a gut feeling that he's not acting right, they need to call the doctor. Because sometimes strokes are real subtle, and I want to jump on it. So, I'd really be stressing family teaching here.

SCENE TWO

When you return to the client's home for a second visit, there is no change in his home condition. The client is alert and oriented. His vital signs are: blood pressure, 230/90 mm Hg; temperature, 37°C; pulse, 75 beats per minute; and respiratory rate, 20 breaths per minute. The client complains of gastrointestinal upset with medications. His wife says that he does not eat very much and does not take his medications according to the schedule.

The Nurse's Response

A blood pressure of 230/90 [mm Hg] is obviously a real big problem. It could be because he's not taking his nifedipine. It could be that he needs the furosemide as well. I'd also want to know how long it's been since he's been taking his medications, how long this problem with noncompliance has been going on. If he complains of GI upset with his medications, then he can take them with food. There's not a lot we can do about changing the medications. He's got to be on some kind of a blood pressure agent. Maybe his physician will order him a different one, but I can't really offer any more suggestions to him except for taking it with food, etc. He is not eating very much. Again, this might be due to dysphagia. It could be a sign of infection. I'd be trying to find information like: What's going on? Why is he not eating a lot? Does he have an infection? Has he had another stroke?

SCENE THREE

On your third visit to the client's house, his vital signs are: blood pressure, 200/100 mm Hg; temperature, 37.2°C; heart rate, 78 beats per minute; and respiratory rate, 20 breaths per minute. His wife tells you that the client still won't take his medications according to schedule. You notice there is redness at the client's right heel, and it is tender to touch. The client says to you, "Things are getting flustered here. My wife is very forgetful and always nags me. My daughter-in-law doesn't do the cleaning anymore. I'm jailed. I don't take my pills at regular times, but I take the total amount that I'm supposed to." You encourage the client to verbalize his feelings, and he keeps talking about how depressed he is. "I'm a trapped animal. I can't go out."

The Nurse's Response

I can't make another person take their medications. I can teach them why they should take them; I can enlist the family to get them to take them; but ultimately, it's the client's decision whether they take them or not. So, I'd be doing everything I could—constantly stressing that he has to take his medicines, giving him every aid available, trying to teach the family, etc., helping them deal with their frustrations—but ultimately, it's his responsibility to take his medications.

His heel: sounds like a stage one decubitus. I want to see why that's happened. What's he doing to that heel? What's his positioning? I'm going to call physical therapy and also OT to find out if they've been doing anything about the reddened heel or if they have been teaching him any kind of positions. I'd probably put either a Duoderm or a transparent dressing on it and get him to keep that leg up so the pressure is off the heel. And I'd be evaluating him every 3 days at least and teaching the family if the reddened area breaks, if there's actual breakdown, to call me or page me.

The depression is a real concern for me. I'm probably going to ask him if he would be willing to speak to one of the psych nurses, and I'll have one of them do a home evaluation. And also, I'll find out if he has a history of depression, if he's ever been on antidepressants, or anything like that, and if there's anything in the family that's changed as well. Has something happened besides just these little things that could be causing his depression?

And I'd call the doctor about the blood pressure again and report, again, that he's not taking his meds. It doesn't really sound like these are symptoms of the stroke. It sounds like a family issue to me. I'm real concerned about the blood pressure. I'd be asking every visit if he's having any headaches, any visual changes, any muscular skeletal problems, all that kind of stuff. But right now, it seems like something is going on here with the family. So, every visit, I'd be evaluating him for signs of a CVA and also checking with the family to see what they have to say about that.

Commentary

The nurse initially responds to this dilemma by using the thinking strategy **recognizing a pattern**, saying, *This is a realistic case study. This is really what I see a lot!* She then describes the usual pattern of hospital care for a client who has had a CVA and seems to be suggesting that her client fits this pattern. This influences her perception of the type of care that he received before discharge from the hospital. The nurse also **recognizes** another **pattern**, the pattern of living in a nice house and being okay: *The client is living in a nice house. It's clean, . . . and he seems to be okay.* When reasoning about the last scene in this dilemma, the nurse struggles to try to **recognize a pattern** (impending CVA) by putting pieces of data together to see if they fit the pattern of a CVA, thus explaining the cause of the client's hypertension: *I'm real concerned about the blood pressure. I'd be asking every visit if he's having any headaches, any visual changes, any muscular skeletal problems. . . . Every visit, I'd be evaluating him for signs of a CVA.*

Thinking Activities

1. Review the nurse's thoughts about this case. Provide other examples of **recognizing a pattern**. How does its use assist her to reason about the dilemma?

2. Write a list of the thinking strategies that this nurse uses in her home health nursing practice.

3. What similarities do you see in how she reasons about each of the three separate dilemmas?

4. What differences do you see?

5. How would you explain these similarities and differences?

21 *Clinical Dilemmas in Emergency Nursing*

The nurse who thinks aloud in response to these dilemmas has been practicing for over 16 years. For the last 10 years, he has practiced full-time in the emergency department (ED) of a large urban hospital, which is the region's designated trauma center. He is trained in every area of the ED, which includes triage, trauma, medical-surgical, and dispatch. The ED accepts uninsured and homeless as well as insured clients. They frequently admit clients with gunshot and stab wounds and care for both the perpetrators and victims of violence.

Clinical Dilemma One

You are the triage nurse on the evening shift in the ED of a large urban hospital. You have just gotten the report from the previous shift. The waiting room is packed. There is a gunshot wound in the trauma area. There are 13 patients in the medical ward and 5 in the clinic. The following clients arrive at once.

THE FIRST CLIENT

The first client is an irate lawyer with a laceration to his left hand, who demands to be seen immediately or he will "see you in court!"

The Nurse's Response

This sounds like a typical night in the ED. That's an easy one for a county worker. You know, you try to diffuse every situation. And obviously someone, I mean, who has a cut—the patient tends to define the emergency, which is one of the rules. Quite simply, in practicality, when you look at somebody who is a lawyer, who looks like a lawyer, and I would say to him quite honestly, "The wait to be seen for a minor emergency in the TRAUMA center (emphasize that, underline that) is 2 to 3 hours." You say, "Now, if you have insurance you may go to St. Luke's, which is 5 minutes down the road, and you will probably be seen within 10 minutes. Now, if you want to wait and be seen here, we'll be more than happy to see you; however, everybody pays with something. Those people over in the waiting room pay with their time. So if you want to wait and be seen, we'll see you. We'll still bill you, but we'll see you." And usually if you tell people the truth, you tell them the facts and don't lie to them, they go onto another hospital where the emergency department is not as busy. As far as being sued goes, when people threaten to sue me, I always say, "This is my job. This is what I do. I would rather that someone sue me for doing my job right than that I have to show up in court and defend myself when I've done something that I know is wrong." So, that's a groundless threat as far as I'm concerned.

Commentary

In response to the description of this first client, the nurse frequently uses the thinking strategy **asserting a practice rule**. These rules represent maxims, the informal rules that nurses learn from their experience in practice. Examples of these maxims include the following:

You try to diffuse every situation.

The patient tends to define the emergency.

Everybody pays with something. Those people in the waiting room pay with their time.

I would rather that someone sue me for doing my job right than that I have to show up in court and defend myself when I've done something that I know is wrong.

In thinking about this tense situation where, in a waiting room full of acutely ill clients, several of whom seem to be fairly critical, an irate lawyer with a minor injury demands to be seen immediately or he will "see you in court!", the nurse seems confident in how he would respond, and he justifies his response by **asserting** several **practice rules**.

THE SECOND CLIENT

Also waiting to be seen is a diaphoretic and pale 65-year-old woman who has had rectal bleeding since last night, filling the commode four to five different times with bright red blood.

The Nurse's Response

This is pretty straightforward. The golden rule of emergency nursing is that skin signs don't lie. Someone can lie to me and can fake anything, but they can't fake skin signs. Someone who's pale and diaphoretic would be . . . I'd probably take this woman, not to a trauma room, but to the medical ward, give a complete report to the nurse there, express my concerns that this patient is passing bright red blood from her rectum.

So, I'd put this lady on a gurney, and I'd call the intern over and sort of peel back the patient's eye, take a look at her conjunctiva, and say to the intern, "Her hematocrit is going to come back 18[%]."

By doing this, I would be letting the intern know two things: (1) that he needs to order a hematocrit on this patient right away and (2) that it's going to be low. That's a big hint to the intern.

A good nurse would put an IV line in this patient right away. I could tell from looking at the patient that the nurse should put an 18-gauge IV in her and at the same time draw a first hematocrit. Now, the way things work with hematocrits is that they are going drop when you begin giving these patients fluids. Most people who are bleeding—especially someone that's been bleeding during four to five different episodes over the last night (so we're going to figure 12 hours of bleeding)—are probably dry. So, the first hematocrit might come back 26[%] or 27[%], but we'll give a patient like this a liter of fluids in an hour, put it in pretty quickly, and the second hematocrit will be diluted, and it will go down to 18[%]. And the intern would say, "How did you know it would be so low?" And I'd say, "Because I looked in the patient's conjunctiva and I saw that she looked like she'd just walked out of a wax museum, so I knew that she had a hematocrit of less than 20[%]. It's just real simple. If you see one, you'll never miss it." This woman will end up in the ICU [intensive care unit]. If her blood pressure drops in the face of bad skin signs, she would end up in a trauma room and we would take her from there to the ICU.

Commentary

Again, thinking about this second triage client, the nurse uses the thinking strategy **asserting a practice rule** to justify the **priorities** he sets and the **choices** that he **makes** in deciding what to do about this diaphoretic and pale 65-year-old woman who has been having fairly significant rectal bleeding since last night. The nurse seems very confident in his initial response: *This is pretty straightforward. The golden rule of emergency nursing is that skin signs don't lie.* He is so confident in applying this particular **practice rule** that he calls it the golden rule, the sine qua non, of emergency nursing. We also note his confidence in **making a prediction** about how low the client's hematocrit will drop (to less than 20%): *Because I looked in the patient's conjunctiva and I saw that she looked like she'd just walked out of a wax museum, so I knew that she had a hematocrit of less than 20[%]. It's just real simple. If you see one, you'll never miss it.* Facione, Sanchez, Facione, and Gainen (1995) contend that this attitude of self-confidence is an important habit of mind for sound critical thinking.

◄ **THE THIRD CLIENT**

There is also a buff-looking, athletic 21-year-old, clutching a fist over the chest, complaining of "crushing" chest pain radiating down the left arm and jaw.

The Nurse's Response

Boy! To think that a 21-year-old in-shape kind of a guy would say—it didn't say it's a guy, so—if it were a woman it would be even more atypical. But this does not sound like . . . it presents like a heart attack, but it doesn't meet the kind of criteria that I would look for in a heart attack.

However, my first question to this client would be "When did you last smoke crack?" And he might say, "Last night. How did you know?" or "I've been on a 3-day crack binge." Or he might say, "How dare you ask me that question!" to which I'd reply, "Look, pal, look where you are. You're in the county's hospital, all right? I would ask Mother Theresa herself if she came in here, when did she last shoot up and when was her last drink? And don't take offense at that. This is what I do."

Sometimes I can diffuse a situation with a little humor, but I also have to turn around and look them in the eye and say, "I need to know this because you don't fit the typical person who would be having a heart attack. I need to ask you these questions because I'm concerned that you might be having a crack-induced heart attack, and that's very serious. And I would like to save your life."

I would talk to him about risk factors—drugs would be my first one. Second, this is the kind of chest pain presentation that we sometimes see in healthy people with some form of a pneumonia. I'd also ask him if he's been hit recently because he could easily have gotten hit with something like a baseball bat and maybe didn't think anything about it. Now, if he has been hit recently, he could have a couple of things that would cause chest pain. He could have a pneumothorax. He could also be having reflux pain from perineal bleeding. Or, a lot of people complain of shoulder pain when in fact they have a ruptured spleen.

Commentary

Research findings from Pyles and Stern's (1983, p. 54) classic study of the cognitive processes used by experienced nurses revealed a phenomenon that these investigators called "falling out of the pattern." They explain, "The discrepancy between what is and what should be provides the nurse with data necessary in making decisions about whether a patient's condition is improving or deteriorating." We see an example of this phenomenon in the nurse's thoughts about this third client. He is trying to understand why a *21-year-old in-shape kind of a guy* would be exhibiting the classic signs of having a heart attack. This client just doesn't fit the pattern of the typical client who is having a heart attack.

So, the nurse indicates that he would **search** for more **information**, all of which will help him to identify other patterns that look like the pattern of someone who is having a heart attack, but that fit better with a client who is a *21-year-old in-shape kind of a guy*: a crack-induced heart attack, pneumonia, or injury from trauma.

THE FOURTH CLIENT

Another patient in triage is an elderly man brought in by the paramedics, who is intoxicated, unarousable, and lying on a stretcher.

The Nurse's Response

The fact that he is intoxicated does not mean a thing to me at this point. The fact that he is unarousable means something to me. Now there's unarousable, and then there's arousable. We use what we call the mission wake-up call [to determine if someone is unarousable]. You put pressure on the ocular notch, which is very painful, and if the patient jumps up and curses at me and takes a swing at me. . . . Hey, I feel good about that because I then know he is not unarousable. This is not somebody we would put out on the street. He gets medical care.

Commentary

The nurse provides an excellent example of **setting priorities** about what is and what is not a concern in regard to this client. He is not concerned about this client being intoxicated, but he is concerned about him being unarousable. This gives him a focus for further assessment; he will use the *mission wake-up call* to determine if the client really is unarousable: *and if the patient jumps up and curses at me and takes a swing at me. . . . Hey, I feel good about that because I then know he is not unarousable.* Nonetheless, the nurse has already decided on the disposition of this client: *This is not somebody we would put out on the street. He gets medical care.*

THE FIFTH CLIENT

The final client in triage is a 50-year-old woman with occasional headaches of moderate intensity, nausea and vomiting, and gait disturbance. A family member noted a change in her personality, along with confusion. The patient is currently slumped over a chair and staring off in the distance.

The Nurse's Response

This is a pretty easy triage. You have to rule out hypoglycemia and intoxication because this could very easily be intoxication. We get 10 people a day that present like this; half of them are intoxicated. Half the time their families bring them in because they want them to stop drinking. However, as far as I'm concerned, drunk or sober, this is a stroke until proven otherwise. And she wouldn't wait; I would take her back with that report. And I would just simply say to the intern,

"Doc, do you want to order the CAT [computerized axial tomography] scan now or later? You're not going to discharge or admit this woman without a CAT scan, so you might as well order it now because you've got to rule it out." And they'll say, "Okay."

Commentary

Here again, the nurse uses the thinking strategy **setting priorities** to narrow down his focus to what is really the concern with this client: *as far as I'm concerned, drunk or sober, this is a stroke until proven otherwise.* The nurse then **makes a choice** to have this client seen immediately: *And she wouldn't wait; I would take her back [into the treatment area] with that report.* He also **makes** another **choice** to see to it that this client gets a CAT scan. Getting this done is dependent on the intern's order, yet the nurse seems confident that it will be done, and he **asserts the practice rule** (policy): *you've got to rule it out.*

A characteristic of expertise in nursing practice described by Benner, Tanner, and Chesla (1996, p. 167) is the ability to work with and through others for the good of the client: "Having a good clinical grasp, and having interventions and responses linked with that clinical grasp, sets up the possibility for expert nurses to take strong positions with other nurses and physicians to get what they believe the patients need."

Thinking Activities

1. Much of this nurse's thinking seems to be guided by maxims, the informal rules that nurses learn from their experience. Describe the advantages and disadvantages of using maxims to guide your thinking.

2. Think about your own practice. List some of the maxims that guide your thinking in practice.

3. Describe a situation where using maxims has guided your thinking in practice.

4. Describe a situation where using maxims has hindered your thinking in practice.

Clinical Dilemma Two

SCENE ONE

You are assigned to the trauma department on the night shift. It is 2:15 A.M., and there's a lull in the activity, so you are taking a sip of coffee. The dispatcher frantically waves you over to hear a dispatch call regarding an accident that has occurred at a 24-hour construction site. A 25-year-old man has fallen 12 feet and has been impaled by three steel rods, which were being used for concrete reinforcement. Each rod is 6 feet in length, 3 inches in diameter.

The paramedics arrived on the scene to find the patient suspended in a horizontal position 5 feet in the air, skewered on the rods. They used a blowtorch to free the patient from where the rods were attached to the concrete. The patient is alert with stable vital signs.

The Nurse's Response

By the time the paramedics would have called in to us, they would have already carried out their standing orders for this type of trauma. The orders would dictate that they obtain a full set of vital signs, place two large-bore IVs in the patient if possible, stabilize the rods, but not remove them because they could be tamponading off something bad. And this patient would be on full C-spine [cervical spine] precautions, on a backboard.

The paramedics would probably be en route before they even called in to the hospital. At that point, their call to me would be advisory to say, "We're coming in. The man is stable and alert but meets trauma criteria for a 911." Our department has several categories of response for our trauma team; 911 is the highest response, where we send out a hospital-wide page. For 911, in addition to our emergency room doctors, we mobilize the trauma team, which consists of the surgeons who will actually be taking the patient to surgery, as opposed to the emergency room doctors who will stay in the emergency room. The anesthesiologist would also come down to see the patient because he would be going to surgery.

We don't know where these rods are. He may be in need of intubation because people can go bad real fast. The patient won't get anything for pain. Our standing criteria for administering morphine to trauma patients in the field is limited to people who have extremity trauma only. If there's any suspicion of blunt trauma, abdominal trauma, or penetrating trauma, patients do not get pain medication because the surgeons are going to have to evaluate them once they arrive in the ED. In this case, it would be a pretty easy evaluation; he's going to surgery.

Commentary

Given the nature of the extremely unusual life-threatening trauma described in this dilemma, one cannot help but be impressed by the nurse's cool and collected reaction to it. He begins by **making** several **assumptions** about what the paramedics would have done prior to bringing the client in: *They would have already carried out their standing orders for this type of trauma. The orders would dictate that they obtain a full set of vital signs, place two large-bore IVs in the patient if possible, stabilize the rods, but not remove them because they could be tamponading off something bad. And this patient would be on full C-spine precautions, on a backboard.*

Next, he **asserts** numerous **rules** (policy and procedure): *The man is stable and alert but meets trauma criteria for a 911. . . . For 911, in addition to our emergency room doctors, we mobilize the trauma team, which consists of the surgeons who will actually be taking the patient to surgery, as opposed to the emergency room doctors who will stay in the emergency room. The anesthesiologist would also come down to see the patient because he would be going to surgery.* Reviewing the policies and procedures for managing a life-threatening trauma case such as this may contribute to the nurse's ability to remain cool and collected. He seems reassured by the knowledge that he will be assisted by very qualified individuals, that these individuals will have very specific role functions, and that everyone will follow a predictable routine for managing the client.

The nurse also uses the thinking strategy **making predictions** to prepare for what will happen once the client arrives: *He may be in need of intubation because people can go bad real fast. The patient won't get anything for pain. . . . The surgeons are going to have to evaluate them once they arrive in the ED. In this case, it would be a pretty easy evaluation; he's going to surgery.*

SCENE TWO

Twenty minutes later the patient arrives at the hospital.

The Nurse's Response

I know the patient is awake and alert. He's a construction worker; he's kind of a regular guy. If he lives, then he's going to do okay. We feel pretty good about people like this. But motorcycle accidents, we see two or three a day. And we see pedestrian-automobile accidents; we get lots of those. We lead California in pedestrians hit by autos. And boy, a MUNI bus at 20 miles an hour can do a lot of damage. This kind of penetrating stuff . . . if you're alive and you make it to the hospital, you're probably going to survive.

There are some things that do shock you . . . I mean, when people with motorcycle accidents come in and their foot is literally turned 180 degrees pointing the other way, it just gets you in your stomach; but you don't stop what you're doing. You do what you have to do; that's what you're trained to do. It's kind of a reflex that you start doing stuff.

Commentary

Here, the nurse is predicting that the client is probably going to survive and is going to do okay.

SCENE THREE

On arrival, the patient's airway is patent and free from injury, and his respirations are 24 breaths per minute and unlabored. Auscultation of his lungs reveals decreased breath sounds on the right side and clear breath sounds on the left. On a pulse oximeter, his oxygen saturation is 100%. He is in normal sinus rhythm. He has strong radial and pedal pulses bilaterally. His bowel sounds fade out completely for about 15 seconds.

The Nurse's Response

This all sounds pretty normal. He's young, and he is compensating very well. That's good. That's something. It's almost a reflex that whenever I walk in to examine a patient, I feel their feet. Not just to make sure that there is no arterial injury but also because one of the first signs of shock is cold feet. So, I always check their feet.

When I get a report like this, I focus on the rod coming out of the belly; but this guy, penetrating trauma aside, is doing fine. He's immobilized. He's going to need to eventually clear his C-spine to make sure that he doesn't have a neck fracture, and you also can't rule out other lung trauma even if the rod isn't sticking out of there.

But, he's awake now, and he's alert, he's oriented. He probably would not get a CAT scan if he's never been unconscious. Our criteria for CAT scans usually start with unconsciousness. So if he has never been unconscious and he's awake, alert, and oriented now, he probably would not be scanned; but that's something that we would check on.

He's got two big-bore IVs, and the paramedics would have done the first hematocrit in the field, which is sometimes helpful. We would most likely get a second hematocrit right off the bat. We'd probably have to do a groin stick because he has an IV in each arm.

In fact, they would probably put a central line in this guy right away. He's going to the OR (operating room); there's no doubt about it. We're going to get a chest x-ray. That's the first thing. The routine for severe motor vehicle accidents is a C-spine, chest, and pelvis. In his case, he's going to get a chest and pelvis x-ray and then clear the C-spine. He might not even have a C-spine cleared until he goes into the OR because the way that his other injuries are presented makes the likelihood of a C-spine injury minimal, especially if he's now immobilized. He probably has a hemopneumothorax. They would get a chest x-ray, but with this kind of presentation, I would have already had a chest drainage system set up. I would have it set up along with the autotransfuser (with anticoagulant) and assume that he's going to get a chest tube; that's probably a given in this situation. A young guy like this has probably really compensated well for his injuries, so the fact that he says he's okay and that his vital signs are good . . . yet, guys like this can go down the tubes in a minute. They can go from a blood pressure of 130/60 to 80/60 to 60/0 [mm/Hg] in nothing flat when they have a major internal bleed. He needs fluids, he needs another hematocrit, and he needs to be gotten ready for the OR.

Commentary

In the nurse's thoughts about the assessment findings obtained on arrival of the client to the ED, we note his optimism about the client's status through his use of the thinking strategy **drawing conclusions**: *This all sounds pretty normal. He's young, and he is compensating very well. . . . He's awake now, and he's alert, he's oriented. . . . A young guy like this has probably really compensated well for his injuries.* The nurse seems to be **recognizing a pattern** of stability that would account for his optimism about the case.

Yet, the nurse's optimism is tempered by recalling other similar cases that fit a different pattern or that quickly changed into a very different pattern, representing instability and deterioration of status: *Yet, guys like this can go down the tubes in a minute. They can go from a blood pressure of 130/60 to 80/60 to 60/0 [mm Hg] in nothing flat when they have a major internal bleed.* The possibility of this other, ominous pattern emerging seems to trigger the nurse's thinking about the client's immediate needs: *He needs fluids, he needs another hematocrit, and he needs to be gotten ready for the OR.*

◀ **SCENE FOUR**

A secondary assessment revealed no tracheal deviation, neck vein distention, or subcutaneous emphysema.

The Nurse's Response

Man, this guy's lucky. Yeah, he's probably got a pneumo, a hemopneumothorax. First of all, I'm not a doctor, and this is starting to get pretty technical . . . the only way that we're going to see the rods in relationship to the veins and the vessels is if he gets an angiogram.

First of all, the rod in the groin is the worst problem. We don't know where it is, and we're not going to know where it is in the emergency room, but I can tell you what he's going to get. While we're waiting for chest x-rays to be developed, he's going to get a rectal exam. And the report that I want as a nurse from the doctor who does the rectal is, what does his prostate feel like? Is it boggy? Is it high riding? The reason we want to know that is I don't know where that rod went.

He's for sure going to get a Foley catheter, just because of the placement of the rod and the fact that he's going to go to the OR. We want to make sure that he has no blood in the rectum and that he didn't rupture his urethra. The appearance of any blood at the meatus is contraindication for moving the Foley catheter forward. And that's very important to look for, especially when the patient is covered with blood, so that takes a pretty good exam.

So, just from the presentation of the rods, I know that he's going to get a chest tube. They're going to stabilize him, and he's probably going to go for an angiogram, if he's stable. If he's not stable, he'd probably go right to the OR, and then he'd go for an angiogram. They would prefer to send him for an angiogram first in order to get a visualization for that second rod.

Commentary

Predominant in the nurse's thinking about the information presented in this scene are the thinking strategies **setting priorities** and **making predictions**. The nurse uses **setting priorities** to identify which rod is the worst.

Clinical Dilemma Three

You are working in the medical area of the ED on the evening shift. There is one other RN assisting you, one police officer on duty, one resident, and three interns. It's 9 P.M., and there are currently 14 patients. One of your patients is in an incoherent state. He has a 10-year history of IV drug abuse and was diagnosed with hepatitis B 2 weeks ago. He was brought to the hospital by ambulance after he collapsed on the sidewalk outside a liquor store. He had a generalized seizure in the ambulance on the way to the hospital.

The Nurse's Response

This is a very typical patient. We see five or six patients like this every night.

The real question is, why did he have a seizure? Most IV drug abusers will tend to drink, too; it doesn't help their drug abuse, but they will. My first guess as to why he had the seizure is that he's probably in acute alcohol withdrawal. Generally, that is why most of our alcoholic patients have seizures. Our standing rule in the emergency department is to expect that most alcoholics will have all of their withdrawal seizures within roughly a 6-hour period. So, we could expect that this patient would wake up after his seizure. If he doesn't, that's an ominous sign.

The fact that he was found collapsed outside on the sidewalk doesn't necessarily mean that he didn't strike his head, or that he didn't get struck on the head, and that this is a post-traumatic seizure. Although this is a very typical case, it probably requires the greatest amount of nursing judgment. A gunshot wound to the chest does not require an awful lot of nursing judgment; we know what to do with these people. Guys like this patient who could very easily have had an alcoholic seizure but could also very easily be an alcoholic who is having a post-traumatic seizure, and having a major bleed . . . that is very, very difficult to diagnose, especially since we do not routinely do a CAT scan on all of these people. This is the kind of patient who will need an IV and a set of labs [laboratory tests] to rule out the conditions that I mentioned earlier.

This patient wouldn't get Narcan [naloxone] unless he kept seizing. If he was intoxicated and unarousable, we would probably observe him over time. This kind of patient can fall through the cracks. Intoxicated patients usually should wake up over time and become less incoherent. They should eventually know their own name and be able to walk, talk, and get mobilized. If, after 2 or 3 hours of receiving a liter or two of IV fluids, this patient either had continuous seizures or never regained any sense of consciousness, then we would know that something much more serious than alcohol intoxication was wrong.

References

Benner, P., Tanner, C., & Chesla, C. (1996). *Expertise in nursing practice: Caring, clinical judgment, and ethics.* New York: Springer.

Facione, P., Sanchez, C., Facione, N., & Gainen, J. (1995). The disposition toward critical thinking. *JGE: The Journal of General Education, 44*(1), 1–25.

Pyles, S., & Stern, P. (1983). Discovery of nursing gestalt in critical care nursing: The importance of the gray gorilla syndrome. *Image: The Journal of Nursing Scholarship, 15,* 51–57.

22 *Clinical Dilemmas in Pediatric Nursing*

The nurse who responds to the clinical dilemmas described in this chapter has 20 years of nursing practice experience in pediatric nursing. Her current practice is as a nursing supervisor at a large children's hospital in a metropolitan area. She also teaches pediatric nursing to undergraduate students at a private university and conducts research on children who have had head injuries.

Clinical Dilemma One

SCENE ONE

It is 7:00 A.M. You are one of the more experienced RNs on the pediatric unit and have worked there full-time for the last 6 years. The 30-bed unit is full today, although several discharges are anticipated later in the morning. One of the RNs regularly assigned to the unit called in sick at the last minute, and the charge nurse has been unable to find a replacement. You agree to take seven patients today instead of five, which is the usual patient load on the day shift. Four of your patients have respiratory problems (reactive airway disease and pneumonia), one infant has seizure disorders, and you have three surgical recoveries and one burn patient.

The Nurse's Response

I realize that right from the start, since I am the most experienced RN, I will have to prioritize my own assignment to allow time to consult with the other nurses about their caseload as well as time to care for my own clients, since I also have seven patients of my own.

I will start with the clients that are the sickest, organize their care in my mind first, and then try to prioritize which of the patients will need what first. My greatest concern at this point is that I don't seem to have a lot of backup, other than myself, and I think I would probably be looking around at neighboring units or at least try to find out who else is around in the hospital that I myself can call on for consultations.

It looks like the acuity is high in the seven patients that I agreed to take, so I would probably want to know if there are any families around that I can count on to let me know if there is trouble. So, I'd like to prioritize that as well. And, in the meantime, I would be asking the administration if there was a possibility that they could get a replacement for me. I wouldn't like to handle this load for an entire day. Of the seven patients to which I have been assigned or that I assign myself, I would probably like to take one or two of the discharges.

So, if there's a way that I could change the assignment such that, of the seven patients that I would take, one or two of those children would be discharged, then I would feel a lot better about assuming this assignment. The only other question that I would ask myself is, would these discharges take a lot of time? Is there a lot of patient teaching that needs to be done or a lot of respiratory care? I would want to turn over those patients to someone else if they are not going to be discharged very soon. I certainly don't want to add to my burden.

Commentary

As the nurse reflects on her assignment, which she perceives as being quite heavy, she uses the thinking strategy **setting priorities** to plan how she will carry out her assignments the best that she can: *I will have to prioritize my own assignment to allow time to consult with the other nurses about their caseload as well as time to care for my own clients, since I also have seven patients of my own. I will start with the clients that are the sickest, organize their care in my mind first, and then try to prioritize which of the patients will need what first. . . . I would probably want to know if there are any families around that I can count on to let me know if there is trouble. So, I'd like to prioritize that as well.*

When an individual confronts a situation that feels taxing and stressful, and perhaps a little overwhelming, it requires considerable discipline to stop and think and to take time to plan. A more common response to the situation described in this first scene, especially in less experienced nurses, would be to jump right in and get to work, without much thought and without planning or **setting priorities**. Research on cognition (Glaser & Chi, 1988, p. xix) has shown that "at the beginning of a problem-solving episode, experts typically try to understand a problem, whereas novices plunge immediately into attempting to [solve it]."

Thinking Activities

1. Describe how **setting priorities** assists the nurse to plan for client care.

2. Describe a situation in your practice when you did not take the time to reflect or plan, but rather plunged immediately into action. Try to explain your reasons for acting this way.

3. If you were to experience a similar situation in your practice in the future, would you handle it in the same manner? If so, why; if not, why not?

4. What are the advantages and disadvantages of taking the time to reflect, to plan, and to set priorities before acting to resolve a clinical dilemma?

SCENE TWO

In report, you learn that one of your clients, Christy, is a 3½-year-old white girl who was severely burned on her buttocks, lower back, upper thighs, and hands by scalding water. Her father is suspected of causing these injuries and is not allowed to visit. She went to the operating room yesterday for skin grafts. Her mother has been staying in her room since admission. Christy had an uneventful night. Her vital signs are within normal limits. Her pain has been controlled with an IV drip of morphine, 0.75 mg/hr. A new bag is to be hung at 10:00 A.M.

The Nurse's Response

I would really want to know how Christy is doing in terms of her own developmental level. Is this a regular 3½-year-old who's never been sick prior to this? That would impact how I would approach this toddler/preschool child. I would want to know how long ago she was burned, if the burns are new to her, or if these were healing injuries.

I would want to know how much social services has gotten involved in this issue of her father not being able to visit. Is her father really a significant other in her family, or is he just someone who visits on occasion? That would make a lot of difference to me in terms of how many questions I would expect Christy to ask me. I would also have to keep in mind that she's 3½, so she's going to have magical thinking, and she's not going to be able to really verbalize her own needs. At this point, I would be most concerned with her psychosocial needs and her developmental issues and probably, at least from this first report, less concerned about her physiological data.

I'd like to know how much she weighs because I see that there's an IV drip of morphine at 0.75 mg/hr. If she weighs about 30 kg, then that is an appropriate dose of morphine. If her vital signs are within normal limits, then I would suspect that she has pain control. I would want to evaluate that pretty early on to see if she will, in fact, still need the morphine drip at 10:00 or whether we'll be able to titrate that down.

How is her mother handling everything? Are she and the father married? Is she involved in any investigation? When patients have suspicious burns, and the pattern of these burns are defensive . . . burns to the buttocks, lower back, upper thighs, and hands represent a defensive maneuver rather than an accident, where a pot could have been turned [over on the child] and there was hot water spilled, or the client jumped into the tub and then jumped out quickly because it was too hot. The burns that Christy has represent extremely defensive maneuvers. So, no doubt, she was seen by child protective services, who would have investigated the family and, together with the police, would have made some decision about this client.

So, I would be charting exactly what I saw, not my own interpretation with the mother, but things like "mother spent 5 minutes with child." I mean, I would definitely keep it as clean and simple as I could because, in the last analysis, the courts are going to look at that kind of charting as evidence for or against the removal of this child. And one of the problems with removing one child is they tend to want to remove them all because in removing one child, sometimes, if there is abuse, then it would just fall to the next in line, and so the whole family has to be taken into context, really, rather than just this one little girl. And I would probably want to know what the siblings' status was as well.

Commentary

In response to the information provided in this second scene, the nurse searches for a great deal more information than she was given. She would like to know when Christy was burned (are the burns new to her versus healing injuries), where she is developmentally, whether she has ever been sick before, what role her father has played in the family, how her mother is handling everything, how much social services and child protective services are involved in the case, and how much Christy weighs. **Searching for information** in this manner assists the nurse to define and structure the problems associated with this client and thus to better understand them. As was mentioned previously, experts spend a greater amount of time trying to understand a problem than do novices.

Another thinking strategy that helps the nurse to structure the problems embedded in this dilemma is **stating propositions**: *If she weighs about 30 kg, then that is an appropriate dose of morphine. If her vital signs are within normal limits, then I would suspect that she has pain control. . . . If there is abuse, then it would just fall to the next in line.* Groen and Patel (1988, p. 289) explain that the usefulness of propositional thinking "arises from the fact that a given piece of information may have many ideas embedded within it. A propositional representation provides a means of representing these ideas, and the relationships between them in an explicit fashion. In addition, it provides a way of classifying and labeling these ideas. . . . Propositions form manageable units of knowledge representations."

Thinking Activities

1. List several IF–THEN propositions that you have learned from your practice.

2. Describe how these propositions provide a means of representing your ideas and the relationships between them in an explicit fashion.

3. Have you found that the relationships represented by propositions that you listed hold true in every situation in your practice? Explain your response.

SCENE THREE

Between 8:00 and 10:00, the unit gets very busy. You are being pulled in three different directions at once. The charge tells you that she's found a replacement for the RN who called in sick, and she's expected in at 11:00. In your haste to hang the new IV bag, you accidentally set the drip rate at 75.0 mg of morphine instead of 0.75 mg. A few minutes later, you discover that Christy is not breathing, and you initiate resuscitative efforts.

The Nurse's Response

Is that missing a decimal point? Can it be right?

I would immediately give mouth-to-mouth resuscitation. At this point, I would be looking for help, and if I were close enough to be heard, then I would yell for help. If I were close to a phone, then I would dial a code. Whenever help did arrive, I would ask for the crash cart to be brought to me. I would be looking for another IV access line. I would be immediately turning off that morphine and starting something else in that line. I would be prepared to hang something to supersede the shock that, no doubt, is in process, and I would be preparing to reverse the morphine with something that antagonizes morphine, like naloxone.

So, I would be anticipating that right from the start. But at 100 times the dose, I would expect that naloxone probably wouldn't help. I would have to resuscitate the shock and the respiratory depression and only hope to reverse some of it with naloxone, but at this much of a dose, it would be pretty much impossible. It would be hard to imagine this client could be successfully resuscitated at this much of a dose.

If it's only been a short time since the incident occurred, then I would expect that I might be more successful in reversing it.

Commentary

The nurse responds with disbelief to the information that she has given 100 times the prescribed dose of morphine to this child: *Is that missing a decimal point? Can it be right?* After this initial reaction, she wastes no more time but immediately **makes choices** to intervene. Unlike her response to the two previous situations, she does not take time to reflect or to plan in this life-threatening situation. Benner's (1984, p. 110) research described expert nurses' skilled performance in extreme life-threatening emergencies as characterized by "the ability to grasp the problem quickly, to intervene appropriately, and to assess and mobilize the help available."

SCENE FOUR

The client is immediately resuscitated with no apparent complications. Her physician is aware of the error.

The Nurse's Response

I wonder how I could have possibly hung 100 times the dose of morphine. I would go back to look at my mathematical calculation. I wonder if I should have taken on so much responsibility, a seven-patient assignment, five of whom were pretty high acuity. I wonder why I didn't ask someone else to watch my clients while I took the time to investigate the exact morphine dose for someone Christy's size and to check my IV setup.

I would go back and reconstruct the events to find out if this was something that I could have prevented, if it was my error, or if something else could have caused it—a machine error, the wrong dose was sent up by the pharmacy. I would try to go away somewhere to try to reconstruct the events; I would sign out my clients to somebody. I would suspect I would be blaming myself, and rightly so to have hung that amount of morphine. I should have known better.

Commentary

In her reflections on this unfortunate incident, the nurse manifests several of the dispositions toward critical thinking that were identified by the American Philosophical Association's Delphi study (Facione, Sanchez, Facione, & Gainen, 1995, pp. 7–8), including truth seeking, inquisitiveness, systematicity, and analyticity. Truth seeking is defined as "being eager to seek the best knowledge in a given context, courageous about asking questions, and honest and objective about pursuing inquiry even if the findings do not support one's self-interests or one's preconceived opinions." Inquisitiveness is defined as "one's intellectual curiosity and one's desire for learning even when the application of the knowledge is not readily apparent." Systematicity is defined as "being organized and diligent in inquiry." And analyticity is defined as "prizing the application of reasoning and the use of evidence to resolve problems, anticipating potential conceptual or practical difficulties, and consistently being alert to the need to intervene."

The nurse's thoughts reveal her struggle to determine the cause of this significant error: *I wonder how I could have possibly hung 100 times the dose of morphine.* She **provides** several possible **explanations**: she made a mathematical error; she had too many clients, too much responsibility; she should have taken more time to calculate the morphine dose and check the IV setup; maybe there was a machine error; or maybe the pharmacy sent up the wrong dose. In the end, she suspects she would be blaming herself *and rightly so to have hung that amount of morphine. I should have known better.* Kassirer and Kopelman (1990, p. 47) state, "When we are wrong, we must be willing to admit that we have erred; we need to rethink. . . . Our responsibility for the patient has a long history and distinguished origin."

The nurse indicates her desire to *go away somewhere to try to reconstruct the events.* Newell (1994, p. 79) described the importance of this type of reflection in our professional lives: "Reflection seems to allow us to examine covert processes in professional life, in much the same way as psychoanalysis claimed to do for personal life during the early years of this century. . . . Reflection touches a need within the professional to make sense of her situation."

Thinking Activities

1. Evaluate the nurse's reaction to the realization that she made a medication error that could have cost her client her life.

2. Despite the seriousness of this error, the nurse's thinking about the situation indicates her possession of several valuable critical thinking dispositions. How do you explain this paradox?

3. How does **providing explanations** help the nurse to understand the meaning of this incident?

4. How will the nurse's intention to *go away somewhere to try to reconstruct the events* be helpful to the nurse?

5. Describe a situation in your practice when you were involved in an incident similar to the one described in this situation.

6. What was your response during and after the situation occurred?

7. What similarities and differences are there between the manner in which you coped with that situation and the manner in which this nurse coped?

Clinical Dilemma Two

SCENE ONE

It is 11:00 on a fairly quiet day on the pediatric unit; you have six clients. Everything is going quite well until you are told that you are getting an admission from the emergency department (ED), a 6-month-old girl with an undetermined seizure disorder. The child arrived in the ED via ambulance while having a seizure. Her symptoms are nystagmus, hypertonic spasms, and coughs with seizures.

The Nurse's Response

I'm expecting that the ED is going to send me this patient prior to the diagnosis being confirmed, so all I will know is that this child has a seizure disorder. I would want to know if this child had any prior history of seizures. Is the patient on a seizure medication? Has the child had a fever? This would rule in the possibility of fever seizures. If the answer to these questions is no, then I know I have a situation in which it's unlikely this child is going to get well fast.

So, with a child with nystagmus, hypertonicity, coughing spasms, and seizures, I would want to put this patient close to the nurses' station where she could be watched by people at the desk. I would probably want to order an apnea and bradycardia monitor for this patient. I certainly would want to follow the oxygen saturation. I would set up suction at the bedside and set up an Ambu bag and mask, to be ready to ventilate this child, should she need it. And I would ask how frequent the seizures are because that would determine whether I would accept or refuse the patient.

Afterward, the physician will come to the ward and order these things, but if I'm going to be taking this patient from the ED, then I'm not going to wait for orders to tell me what I need. I want to have these things prepared so that I can monitor and care for this patient until the physician gets there. At my level of experience, it is expected that I would take care of these things prior to someone writing the order because I certainly know that they would be needed for this kind of patient. And I would definitely have a lot of control over whether this patient would come to my unit or go to the intensive care unit, and I would base it on how frequent the seizures had been. That would make a big difference on whether I would say I'd take the admission.

Commentary

In her response to the situation described in this first scene, the nurse demonstrates the disposition toward critical thinking described as critical thinking self-confidence: trusting in the soundness of one's reasoned judgments and in the ability to lead others in the rational resolution of problems (Facione, Sanchez, Facione, & Gainen 1995). She feels confident enough in her own judgment not to wait for the doctor's orders to initiate the actions that she deems necessary to care for the client when she first arrives from the ED. Findings from Benner, Tanner, and Chesla's (1996, p. 287) study of expertise in nursing practice indicate that "expert practice . . . is characterized by the tacit acceptance of responsibility for much of medical decision making."

SCENE TWO

After admission to your unit, the client, E. A., is diagnosed by the neurologist as having infantile spasms. She is put on oxygen therapy and begun on antibiotic therapy. A complete blood count (CBC) with differential is drawn, and a portable chest x-ray is done on the unit. An intravenous infusion of 5% dextrose in half-normal saline to run at 40 mL/hr is begun.

The history and physical examination reveal the following: She was a term infant delivered via cesarean section. She is a fraternal twin, and her sister has no health problems. E. A. showed signs and symptoms of pneumonia 2 days ago. She is currently living with her mother and the other twin.

Her vital signs are temperature, 37.5°C; heart rate, 110 beats per minute; and respirations, 32 breaths per minute. Her lungs are clear. A neurologic assessment shows decreased muscle tone.

The Nurse's Response

I think that they're probably trying to rule out some sort of sepsis or meningitis. The diagnostic tests would certainly help bring the picture of pneumonia into place. The IV ordered is a very common solution for an infant. I don't know the baby's weight, and I would want to know the weight to see if that was an appropriate IV rate in mL per kilogram.

Her temperature is a little bit elevated. It doesn't tell me whether it was ancillary or rectal or tympanic, so I'd want to check on the source for that temperature. A heart rate of 110 [beats per minute] is a little on the high side for a 6-month-old infant, but still okay. The respiratory rate is within normal range.

Right from the start, I know that she's gone from a hypertonic state to a state where she has decreased tone and decreased reflexes; that tells me that they've either given her medication to stop the tonicity or she's deteriorating. I'd want to check to see if any medication had been given between the hypertonicity and the loss of reflexes or the decreasing reflexes.

I would want to know why she was delivered via C-section [cesarean section]. Did the mom only have the section because they were twins, or was it fetal distress?

We do not know where the father is in the picture, but it looks like there's some extended family support. Other than the temperature—which I would need to know the source of the temperature to find out if that was somewhat normal—the patient is in pretty stable condition with these vital signs. I would want to check on the weight to make sure that 40 [mL]/hr is appropriate, because knowing what I know about her neurological condition, I certainly wouldn't want to overload her and risk increasing her intracranial pressure.

I would really want to know what medication had been given in the ED. I would also want to look at her fontanelle to see if it were bulging, considering this is an issue with pneumonia. I would also worry about an insidious meningitis. I would certainly want to get the results of the lab work as soon as I could. I'd like to know her CBC before starting the antibiotic.

I would have expected her to be lethargic and kind of spacey, but I'm not so sure I would expect decreased tone.

As I'm doing things, I would explain to the mom what I was doing. But I would get my house in order, as they say, first. I'm always of the opinion that prevention is the best cure, so I would want to make sure that I have all the physiological things tied down before I spoke to the mom. I would say something to the mom like, "It's going to take me a few minutes to orient myself to your daughter and to check her over; as soon as I'm finished, I'll sit down to talk with you." In the meantime, I would try to verbalize what I'm doing at the time. "I'm checking her IV right now," etc., so I would allay some of her fears. I wouldn't remain silent, but I wouldn't take the time to spend with the mom until I was assured that things were plugged in correctly and the doses were right and the patient was in a safe situation; then I'd feel like I could make a little bit more time for the mom.

Commentary

This is another situation where much of the nurse's thinking focuses on **searching** for additional **information**: *I'd want to check to see if any medication had been given between the hypertonicity and the loss of reflexes or the decreasing reflexes. I would want to know why she was delivered via C-section. Did the mom only have the section because they were twins, or was it fetal distress? We do not know where the father is in the picture. . . . I would really want to know what medication had been given in the ED. I would also want to look at her fontanelle to see if it were bulging. . . . I would certainly want to get the results of the lab work as soon as I could. I'd like to know her CBC before starting the antibiotic.* Barrows and Pickell (1991, p. 70) explain that "with almost any presenting patient problem, the clinician will need more information than is available at the outset."

Although the nurse states that she would need to be sure that her client is settled in and safe before she spent time talking to the mom, she indicates, *In the meantime, I would try to verbalize what I'm doing at the time. "I'm checking her IV right now," etc., so I would allay some of her fears.* This indicates that the nurse recognizes that caring and concern can be expressed to clients and their families in many ways. No doubt the client's safety and well-being are as much a priority for the mom as they are for the nurse, so we can assume that just allowing her to remain in the room and to listen to the nurse explain what she is doing would be comforting to the mom.

Thinking Activities

1. Describe strategies that you use in your practice to communicate caring and concern for your clients and their families.

2. Do you ever talk aloud or think aloud while you are assessing or caring for your clients?

3. What would be the advantages and disadvantages of this approach?

SCENE THREE

You find out that your client's seizures were successfully arrested in the ED with one dose of IV diazepam. The neurologist takes the mother aside and explains the pathophysiology of infantile spasms, which are characterized by intermittent seizures worsened by acute illness or upset. Infantile spasm seizures are difficult to control with medications, and the life expectancy with this diagnosis is about 3 years. The doctor leaves the room to find you to ask if you can put aside your other duties to help E. A.'s mother. You enter the room to find the mother standing over her sleeping infant and crying.

The Nurse's Response

I'm going to need some time with this mom because the physician has basically left this in my hands. I would probably let the mom cry for awhile. I think that's real appropriate. This is an infant who's not going to be so aware that her mom is upset and crying. I think it's appropriate that mom express her emotions. I would try to make some sort of physical contact with her, just put my hand on her shoulder or come closer somehow to let her know I was there.

And I would try to read her nonverbal cues to see when she'd be ready for me to say something, but I would let her have her time. I would do all the different things that need to be done, and then I would say to her, "Do you need some time alone or do you want to talk to me? Is there something that we can talk with about?" I'd let the mom direct that. I don't think it's my purview to demand a discussion when I've got all of these patients to watch. If the mom said she wanted to talk, I would organize my morning so that I could return to that mom at a specific time when I could get someone to watch the rest of my patients so that I wouldn't need to worry about them.

If I couldn't get someone else to keep an eye on my other patients for a little while, then I would call the social worker, and I would ask that person to speak with the mom. This is not something that's going to be resolved in 5 minutes. But I think that having support at this really dramatic time, if nothing else but to let the mom know that we're thinking of her in this time, is important. That is often enough to make mom begin to trust us.

My concerns would be that she would be grieving over the loss of this infant at a time when she would be experiencing joy about the sibling, which is tough when you have twins and one is sick and one is well. There will always be that guilt that comes from these mixed feelings. So, I would try to hook the mom up with someone who would understand the feelings of mothers with twins. I'm presuming the other twin is normal.

Commentary

In her thoughts about how to help the mom, the nurse demonstrates a sensitivity regarding not only the mother's feelings but also those of the young client. She will let the mom cry for a while, assuming that her 6-month-old infant will not be *so aware that her mom is upset and crying*. The nurse says that she will try to come close to the mom *to let her know I was there . . . but I would let her have her time*. These actions exemplify many of the characteristics that Barry (1996, p. 55) attributes to a healer: "a gentleness of spirit, compassion for others, respect for the dignity of others, respect for the choices of the other, and mindfulness of the potential of the healing act to release the healing energies of the other."

Clinical Dilemma Three

◀ SCENE ONE

Oscar, a 9-month-old Hispanic boy, was admitted to the pediatric unit at 3:00 in the morning for observation. Oscar is a severe asthmatic and had been running a rectal temperature of 38°C for the last 24 hours. His patients were worried because their pediatrician had told them that a fever is often the first sign of a respiratory infection. The parents felt incapable of dealing with another severe asthma attack, so they brought Oscar in.

At report the following morning, the night nurse tells you that Oscar is listless and irritable, refusing food, and he has vomited once. The nurse reports that at 5:30 in the morning, Oscar's rectal temperature was 36°C. His only medication is acetaminophen (Tylenol) to keep the fever down. The night nurse has neglected to give Oscar his last dose. When you take his morning vital signs, you find he has a rectal temperature of 39°C.

The Nurse's Response

I would jump on his temperature. At a temperature of 39°C, this child is already going to be tachycardic, his respiratory rate's going to be up, and his metabolic rate will be high. Given his asthmatic history, he won't be able to manage the work of breathing very well, so I would jump on this temperature. At 39°C, I'd probably want to use something that's cooling, like wet cloths under the axilla. I certainly wouldn't put a wet cloth on the child's entire body because I wouldn't want him to start shivering and therefore increase his metabolism even further. But I'd use some mechanical means to lower the temperature at the same time I was giving him his Tylenol.

I would want to monitor his sensorium. He's 9 months old, so he should still have an anterior fontanelle open. I would feel that. I'd want to know what his normal behavior is because the nurse said that he is a little bit listless and irritable.

And I would ask the mom what his baseline behavior was. Is this typical of him when he's hospitalized or when he's with strangers? If she said, "No, that's not typical," I would wonder if he's on any medications that would cause irritability and vomiting. Many medications that are given for asthma cause those two things, so I'd want to find out about the medications that he takes at home.

This could also be a sign of a decreasing sensorium; I would be really concerned about his mental status. The fever could be the reason for his irritability as well, and could certainly be the reason for his vomiting. But I would want to rule out the most serious things, and I'd be working on the fever while I was ruling things out.

Research regarding febrile seizures shows that it's not so much how high the temperature is, but how fast it went in that trajectory. Some children can seize at 38°C if their temperature went from normal to 38°C in one really fell swoop, versus a slow incremental increase. A fever of 39°C in a 9-month-old asthmatic child is not all that high. It's high for an adult, but it's not all that high for a child.

Commentary

The nurse's initial thoughts about this dilemma demonstrate the use of two thinking strategies simultaneously: **making choices** (*I would jump on his temperature. . . . I'd use some mechanical means to lower the temperature at the same time I was giving him his Tylenol*) and **making predictions** (*At a temperature of 39°C, this child is already going to be tachycardic, his respiratory rate's going to be up, and his metabolic rate will be high. Given his asthmatic history, he won't be able to manage the work of breathing very well*).

A second sequence of thoughts depicts the association of two other thinking strategies: **searching for information** (*I'd want to know what his normal behavior is*) and **providing explanations** (*because the nurse said that he is a little bit listless and irritable*). Another example of this association can be seen in the following text: *I would wonder if he's on any medications that would cause irritability and vomiting. Many medications that are given for asthma cause those two things, so I'd want to find out about the medications that he takes at home.*

Thinking Activities

1. In what way does the simultaneous use of the thinking strategies **making choices** and **making predictions** help the nurse to reason about the information presented in this dilemma?

2. In what way does the simultaneous use of the thinking strategies **searching for information** and **providing explanations** help the nurse to reason about the information presented in this dilemma?

References

Barrows, H., & Pickell, G. (1991). *Developing clinical problem-solving skills: A guide to more effective diagnosis and treatment.* New York: Norton Medical Books.

Barry, P. (1996). *Psychosocial nursing: Care of physically ill patients and their families.* Philadelphia: Lippincott.

Benner, P. (1984). *From novice to expert. Excellence and Power in clinical nursing practice.* Menlo Park, CA: Addison-Wesley.

Benner, P., Tanner, C., & Chesla, C. (1996). *Expertise in nursing practice: Caring, clinical judgment, and ethics.* New York: Springer.

Facione, P., Sanchez, C., Facione, N., & Gainen, J. (1995). The disposition toward critical thinking. *JGE: The Journal of General Education, 44*(1), 1–25.

Glaser, R., & Chi, M. (1988). Overview. In M. Chi, R. Glaser, & M. Farr (Eds.), *The nature of expertise.* Hillsdale, NJ: Lawrence Erlbaum Associates.

Groen, G., & Patel, V. (1988). The relationship between comprehension and reasoning in medical expertise. In M. Chi, R. Glaser, & M. Farr (Eds.), *The nature of expertise* (pp. 287–310). Hillsdale, NJ: Lawrence Erlbaum Associates.

Kassirer, J., & Kopelman, R. (1990). Lest we become smug. *Hospital Practice, 25,* 33–47.

Newell, R. (1994). Reflection: Art, science or pseudo-science. *Nurse Education Today, 14,* 79–81.

23 *Clinical Dilemmas in Cardiovascular Nursing*

The nurse responding to the clinical dilemmas in this chapter has 11 years of experience in nursing practice. For the past 7 years, she has practiced full-time on a telemetry unit in a nonprofit urban Catholic hospital.

Clinical Dilemma One

SCENE ONE

You are a nurse on a telemetry unit. Your shift is from 7:00 A.M. to 3:30 P.M. You have been assigned to eight patients today. One of them is Mrs. Whitney, who was admitted to your unit from the emergency department 2 days ago at 6:30 A.M.

Mrs. Allison Whitney is a 58-year-old woman recently diagnosed with coronary artery disease. She was admitted to the hospital for severe chest pain that she perceived to be a heart attack. This occurred while she was moving furniture. Her serum lipid level is 299 mg/dL (less than 200–220 mg/dL is normal). She's been smoking since the age of 16. She has a history of hypertension, has type II diabetes, and is obese. All the medications that she takes at home are in a brown paper bag in her room.

At 7:30 A.M., after you receive report on your clients, you make rounds to check on them. Mrs. Whitney is on bed rest. You go through her paper bag of medications with her to find out what she has been taking. She is taking nifedipine, 60 mg bid; glipizide, 10 mg before morning and evening meals; albuterol (Ventolin), 1 to 2 inhalations q4–6h; lovastatin, 30 mg bid; and nitroglycerin, sublingually prn for chest pain. Mrs. Whitney said she stopped taking the nitroglycerin because it gives her a headache.

An electrocardiogram (EKG) performed during an anginal episode showed an ST depression. Her chest x-ray was normal because no heart failure was present.

Treadmill stress test showed angina occurring with activity more vigorous than normal ambulation. Radionuclide studies showed adequate cardiac profusion and ventricular muscle activity when the patient is at rest. Coronary arteriography via cardiac catheterization showed a lesion in the coronary artery that is 70% occluded. Serum enzymes ruled out that she had a myocardial infarction (MI).

The Nurse's Response

She was recently diagnosed with a coronary artery disease, so I know she already has that problem. If I know she has coronary artery disease and that she has come in with chest pain, then I'd wonder if it's true cardiac pain versus perhaps GI [gastrointestinal] pain. And a lot of times women tend to be underdiagnosed for chest pain with an MI. But she already has a lot of risk factors here: smoking, high cholesterol, hypertension, diabetes, and obesity—almost all the risk factors that you can have. One thing she doesn't seem to have as a risk factor is heredity, which is probably the biggest one when it comes down to it. But she has every other risk factor, so chances are this is chest pain caused by a myocardial ischemia. The chest pain was precipitated by moving furniture and a lot of activity. So, I'd probably believe that it was some kind of true cardiac event, just because of all the risk factors she has.

It's good that it's been ruled out that she had a myocardial infarction, although I'm thinking with all this stuff going on, she's definitely prone to them in the future. Let's see . . . her cholesterol is 299 [mg/dL], which is very high. The EKG showed ST depression. A lot of times there is ST depression from angina or cardiac pain, although you might see a little different portrayal if it was an actual MI. Chest x-ray is normal, which probably is to be expected without any other symptoms. Her treadmill result is probably what was expected also. She has increased chest pain with anything more than normal ambulation. Her cardiac cath[eterization] showed a lesion in one of her coronary arteries causing 70% blockage. It didn't mention which coronary artery, but that's definitely a significant amount of occlusion in there.

So at this point, what should we be doing to keep her comfortable to decrease the anginal periods? She's already on bed rest. I'd want to maintain a calm environment, decrease the noise, keep her comfortable. She may or may not be on oxygen at this point. If she's still having angina, then she's probably on oxygen. If she's not, then it might just be that prn oxygen is all right for now.

So, she's on the monitor. She's already had some ST depression. I want to keep watching her monitor to make sure that there aren't any more changes.

She brought her medicines in a brown paper bag. She's on lovastatin, and she's not taking the nitroglycerin because it gives her a headache. Patients usually don't take nitroglycerin routinely, unless they're having chest pain. She's on a Ventolin inhaler, so chances are she has a history of chronic obstructive pulmonary disease.

Sometimes people can be having pain that they say is around the rib cage or chest area, and it's actually pulmonary in origin. But because of all the other things that they found, it's most likely that this client's pain is cardiac this time.

Commentary

In thinking about the initial information about the client that is provided in scene one, the nurse uses the thinking strategy **judging the value** (*Her cholesterol is 299, which is very high. . . . That's definitely a significant amount of occlusion in there [one of her coronary arteries]*) to identify the most significant data that would support the hypothesis that her chest pain is true cardiac pain (*I'd probably believe that it was some kind of true cardiac event, just because of all the risk factors she has*) versus the competing hypothesis (*perhaps GI pain* or *actually pulmonary in origin*). *But,* she concludes, *because of all the other things that they found, it's most likely that this client's pain is cardiac this time.* Kassirer and Kopelman (1991, p. 33) remind us that "in general, working diagnoses are highly likely and parsimonious. They explain all principal clinical findings and are coherent, in the sense of causal and physiological relations. They survive the test that no competing diagnostic hypotheses are plausible. Such hypotheses usually produce valid predictions, both of test results and of the patient's future clinical course."

In this situation, the primary diagnostic hypothesis guides the nurse's decisions about therapeutic intervention: *I'd want to maintain a calm environment, decrease the noise, keep her comfortable. . . . I want to keep watching her monitor to make sure that there aren't any more changes.*

Thinking Activities

1. In their text *Learning Clinical Reasoning*, Kassirer and Kopelman (1991) stress the importance of diagnostic verification when reasoning in clinical practice. They describe several criteria that are useful in verifying a hypothesis:

   a. Adequacy—the hypothesis accounts for all of the clinical findings.

   b. Parsimonious—the hypothesis accounts for the simplest possible explanation of all the findings.

    c. Likelihood—the hypothesis with the highest probability is the most credible.

Using these criteria, evaluate the nurse's primary diagnostic hypothesis that the client's chest pain is cardiac in origin.

2. Use the same criteria to evaluate the nurse's competing hypothesis that the chest pain is GI pain or pulmonary in origin.

3. Describe how you could use these criteria to verify the hypotheses that you generate in your practice.

SCENE TWO

It is 10:00 A.M., and Mrs. Whitney's call light comes on at the nurses' station. You find her in her bathroom, where she was trying to sneak a cigarette. She fell and is on the bathroom floor. She says she felt a squeezing tightness in her chest and then felt really dizzy.

The Nurse's Response

Well, I wonder if she has any psychiatric history. I'd put the cigarette out and flush it down the toilet. She's on the floor. I'd ask her how she fell. Did she just slide down?

She feels a squeezing tightness . . . she's fallen, and I have to assess did she hurt herself, as well as assess how bad the anginal pain is right now. I really don't know whether my first instinct would be to pull her up; who knows what else she's injured during the fall? I'd get some help, have someone call the medical intern to come up to assess her. I'd like to know what her oxygen saturation is.

Meanwhile, I'm in there with her, and I'm assessing her chest tightness. If she appears okay and she indicates she feels fine to get up, then I'll probably get her up and get her back to bed.

A squeezing tightness in her chest . . . I want to assess how strong her chest pain is. Usually, for cardiac pain, I ask my clients to rate its severity on a 0 to 10 scale. I'll ask her to describe it more—if it's radiating down the arm. Or a lot of times people get it in the jaw. Does she have shortness of breath with it? I'd check her vital signs. Assuming she's still on the monitor, I'd check her monitor. I'd want to get another EKG to see if she's had any changes since this episode. There's usually standing orders for an EKG when the client has chest pain. Because we already know that she came out positive on her stress test. She had an occlusion. We're already pretty sure it's anginal pain.

A lot of times if I'm not sure it's really cardiac pain, then I might call the doctor to ask if he wants an EKG to be done before I give nitroglycerin. In this case, it's pretty much been established in this patient already, so usually there will be a prn order for nitroglycerin. So I would give her some nitroglycerin, make sure she gets some oxygen, use 2 to 3 liters, and make sure that she's stable. If the pain did not go away for 20 to 30 minutes, and it stayed at a high level, 7 to 9, and did not get better with nitroglycerin, then I'd have to wonder if she was actually experiencing a myocardial infarction.

If so, then I ought to start thinking about getting her down to the intensive care unit [ICU]. It has been found that just giving a crushed aspirin to someone suspected of having an MI will decrease their risk of mortality. Just one aspirin—it's amazing what it can do. It really lessens the severity of an MI. When they get someone who is having an MI down to the ICU, they may start them on an IV drip of nitroglycerin, or heparin, or both.

Commentary

The nurse reacts to the news that her client has fallen in the bathroom and has chest pain by **searching for information**: *I'd ask her how she fell. Did she just slide down? . . . I'd like to know what her oxygen saturation is. . . . I want to assess how strong her chest pain is. . . . I'll ask her to describe it more—if it's radiating down the arm. Or a lot* *of times people get it in the jaw. Does she have shortness of breath with it? I'd check her vital signs. Assuming she's still on the monitor, I'd check her monitor. I'd want to get another EKG to see if she's had any changes since this episode.* In their text *Asking the Right Questions: A Guide to Critical Thinking*, Browne and Keeley (1994) describe the process of asking critical questions as "panning-for-gold." They contend that searching for additional information is an essential component of critical thinking because it moves us toward interpretations, identifying patterns, and making inferences. Facione, Facione, and Sanchez (1994, p. 346) have identified inquisitiveness as a critical thinking disposition that is essential to nursing practice: "Considering that the knowledge base for competent nursing practice continues to expand, a deficit in inquisitiveness would signal a fundamental limitation of one's potential to develop expert knowledge and clinical practice ability."

Searching for information to determine what happened to cause the client to fall and to confirm the etiology of the client's chest pain does not deter the nurse from **making choices** for action, even in the face of uncertainty: *Meanwhile, I'm in there with her, and I'm assessing her chest tightness. If she appears okay and she indicates she feels fine to get up, then I'll probably get her up and get her back to bed. . . . I would give her some nitroglycerin, make sure she gets some oxygen, use 2 to 3 liters, and make sure that she's stable.* Results from a descriptive study of nursing judgment in assessing and managing cardiac pain (Jacavone and Dostal, 1992, p. 57) revealed that the more experienced nurses "were willing to administer nitroglycerin aggressively in a situation where there was doubt concerning the cardiac versus noncardiac origin of the pain. Data revealed that a sense of urgency is pervasive in the treatment of cardiac pain. . . . Experts rule in the possibility of an ischemic process, rather than rule it out [based on] the fundamental concept of myocardial salvage."

Thinking Activities

1. Describe a situation in your practice when you had to quickly respond to an unexpected occurrence similar to that described in scene two. Was the thinking strategy **searching for information** useful to you in that situation? Explain why or why not.

2. Was the thinking strategy **making choices** useful to you in that situation? Explain why or why not.

3. Do you recall what additional thinking strategies facilitated your judgment in that situation?

Clinical Dilemma Two

SCENE ONE

G. C. is a 47-year-old, unmarried, white man, who is vice president of Tandem Computers. During a 1:00 P.M. meeting, he felt persistent chest pain but dismissed the discomfort as indigestion from the big lunch he had earlier at L'Escargot. He sent his secretary to Walgreens on California Street to buy some Pepto-Bismol while he continued to close a contract deal with IBM Computers. G. C. became increasingly nauseated and vomited. He became weak, his skin became dusky in appearance, and his lips were blue. In an anxious voice, he complained of crushing chest pain, "almost like I can't breathe." The pain radiated to his left arm, and he was extremely short of breath and eventually collapsed. He was immediately rushed to the emergency department (ED) of your hospital.

The Nurse's Response

He's 47 years old and the vice president of Tandem Computers. A lot of men start to develop coronary artery disease in their 40s. In women, it doesn't tend to show up until their late 50s or early 60s. One reason is that estrogen is thought to protect females until they are postmenopausal. If he's the vice president of a big computer company, then that's stress right there.

It sounds like he had a big lunch at a very nice French restaurant. If he usually lunches at these places, then imagine what he's eating. He thought it was indigestion. Well, right away I think he's having a heart attack. Not only was he having some chest pain, but also he was anxious and dusky in appearance. His lips were blue, indicative of poor perfusion throughout his system. He had crushing chest pain, was extremely short of breath, and collapsed. At first thought, I would suspect that he is experiencing a heart attack. Okay, so he goes to the ED.

Commentary

When reasoning about the information presented in this first scene, the nurse uses the thinking strategy **forming relationships** (*He's 47 years old and the vice president of Tandem Computers. . . . It sounds like he had a big lunch at a very nice French restaurant. If he usually lunches at these places, then imagine what he's eating. . . . Not only was he having some chest pain, but also he was anxious and dusky in appearance. His lips were blue, indicative of poor perfusion throughout his system. He had crushing chest pain, was extremely short of breath, and collapsed*) to **generate a hypothesis** (*Well, right away I think he's having a heart attack. . . . I would suspect that he is experiencing a heart attack.*)

SCENE TWO

In the emergency department, his vitals are heart rate, 120 beats per minute; respiratory rate, 32 breaths per minute; blood pressure (BP), 90/50 mm Hg; and temperature, 38.0°C. Immediate treatment includes oxygen at 4 L/min via nasal cannula and nitroglycerin IV drip titrated at 5 μg/min, to be increased by 5 μg q3–5min × 3. EKG shows elevation of ST segment and inversion of T wave in the precordial leads and frequent premature ventricular contractions (PVCs). Laboratory work indicates potassium level, 6.0 mEq/L; creatine kinase (MB), 13 mg/24 hr; lactate dehydrogenase (LDH), within normal limits; aspartate aminotransferase, 45 U/L; and glucose, 300 mg/dl.

The Nurse's Response

Okay, he has a lot of a changes going on, including EKG changes. If there is ST elevation and T wave inversion, then there's definitely ischemia going on. He's having frequent PVCs. His potassium level is 6 mEq/L, so it's very high. Glucose is 300 [mg/dl], which is high. Is he diabetic? This man probably had a humongous carbohydrate lunch. His CPK [creatine kinase] is okay; LDH is okay. He received nitroglycerin. Okay, let's go on a little bit.

SCENE THREE

There are a total of nine high-acuity patients, and each nurse has three. It is 7:50 A.M., and you just finished hearing report. You have been assigned to three patients, one of whom is to be transferred today to another floor; the other two need to be prepared for various procedures such as cardiac catheterization this morning, and both patients verbalized anxiety about their test procedures last night.

All three of your patients have 8:00 A.M. medications. As you finish checking the charts for any new orders on your patients, G. C. is brought to your unit from the ED with no prior notice; ED claims to have informed your unit about the transfer.

Your supervisor has assigned G. C. to you, since one of your patients will be transferred later this morning. You try to find out what is going on with G. C. and notice that his admitting orders cannot be located (ED does not have them). No one seems to know much about the patient's history, but laboratory values, EKG information, and the treatment carried out while the client was in the ED are recorded in the chart. Because you are distracted trying to find out what is going on with the patient, you are late distributing your 8:00 A.M. medications.

You hear the alarm from one of your client's cardiac monitor and see that he is in ventricular tachycardia at 180 beats per minute. At the same time, another of your clients screams from his bed saying, "I think I'm going to have a bowel movement!" At 8:30 A.M., patient transport is scheduled to arrive on the unit to transport both of these clients to the cardiac catheterization laboratory for cardiac catheterization and arteriography.

The Nurse's Response

Why did I come to work today? Why me? How many hours until 3:00? These are all things that I'd be thinking at that time.

Let's see. First of all, there's a lot of things going on. I'm going to need a little help. I'll go to the charge nurse to let her know what's going on. She will probably see what I'm going through written all over my face. I'll ask for some help.

The bowel movement . . . okay, if the bed catches it, I'll clean it up later. I can't take care of everything at once. The charge nurse and I need to get together.

The patient with Vtach [ventricular tachycardia] would be first because he could have a cardiac arrest. I have to take care of that first. I'll call the cardiologist immediately about the ventricular tachycardia.

The patient from the ED is okay for a couple minutes in the hall while I get the patient with Vtach taken care of. Then I can get this new admission settled in, maintain his oxygen, take his vital signs. Let's see. Cath[eterization] lab would probably start calling for my two patients at this point.

As far as 8:00 meds . . . well, sorry, but it's not going to hurt someone to wait for their meds. Yeah, there's some things I have to let go. I have learned what things I can let go. I have learned how to prioritize, and I've learned what things could wait a little bit.

The cardiologist should be in the house because he's scheduled to do the cardiac cath on this person who is having Vtach, so I'm taking it for granted that he's on his way up to see the patient. He might have to end up starting some meds on him. Chances are he will try to stabilize him and get him down to the cath lab immediately or tell the surgeons to prepare an OR [operating room] room in case he has to go for an emergency bypass surgery.

Let's see. I really hope that there's a nursing assistant on the unit that I can delegate to a little bit, to have them clean up the patient who had the bowel movement. I'll call the cath lab to explain what's happening and that I'm trying to get the patient down to them as soon as possible.

Commentary

Benner's (1984, p. 149) earlier classic work examining clinical nursing practice demonstrated that "experienced nurses learn to organize, plan, and coordinate multiple patient needs and requests and to reshuffle their priorities in the midst of constant patient changes." The nurse's response to the description in scene three, where everything seems to be happening at once, provides an exemplar of the ability to coordinate and meet multiple client needs and requests and to set priorities. Fisher and Fonteyn's (1994) study of nursing expertise revealed that two important dimensions of nurses' expertise were (1) their ability to adapt and adjust to clinical circumstances and (2) their capacity to manage competing demands and data in complex, risky clinical situations.

As would seem appropriate in the chaotic situation described in this scene, the nurse frequently uses the thinking strategy **setting priorities**: *The patient with Vtach would be first because he could have a cardiac arrest. I have to take care of that first. . . . The patient from the ED is okay for a couple minutes in the hall while I get the patient with Vtach taken care of. Then I can get this new admission settled in, maintain his oxygen, take his vital signs.* In her text *Critical Thinking in Nursing*, Alfaro-LeFevre (1995) identified **setting priorities** as an important critical thinking strategy for nursing practice. Rubenfeld and Scheffer (1995, p. 170) concur: "Nurses set priorities during many aspects of care, but it is particularly important in planning."

Another thinking strategy that the nurse uses to reason about the information in this scene is **making predictions**: *I'm going to need a little help. . . . Cath lab would probably start calling for my two patients at this point. . . . I'm taking it for granted that he's [the cardiologist] on his way up to see the patient. He might have to end up starting some meds on him. Chances are he will try to stabilize him and get him down to the cath lab immediately or tell the surgeons to prepare an OR room in case he has to go for an emergency bypass surgery.* **Making predictions** in this hectic, multifaceted situation will help the nurse to prepare for the events that are most likely to follow.

Thinking Activities

1. Think about your practice. Evaluate your ability to cope with multiple activities happening at once. Support your evaluation with one or two examples from your practice.

2. What strategies do you use to cope with hectic, multifaceted situations in your practice?

3. Describe how **setting priorities** assists nurses to manage chaotic situations in clinical practice.

4. Describe how **making predictions** assists nurses to manage chaotic situations in clinical practice.

◀ **SCENE FOUR**

Your initial assessment of G. C. reveals that his vital signs are: heart rate, 110 beats per minute; respiratory rate, 27 breaths per minute; BP, 100/65 mm Hg; and temperature 38.0°C. He is weak, his voice is barely audible, he is oriented times one, his skin is cool to touch, his nail beds are slightly cyanotic, apical pulse is distant, heart rhythm is irregular, he has weak radial pulses, his capillary refill time is 3 seconds, peripheral pulses in his lower extremities are weak, he has bilateral edema of his lower extremities of 2 to 3+, he has fine crackles scattered throughout his lung fields and diminished breath sounds bilaterally at the bases, his oxygen saturation is 95% on oxygen at 6 L/min, and a heplock is in place in the vein of his left wrist.

At 8:45 A.M., you reach the physician by phone and are given verbal orders: total bed rest; 6 L/min of oxygen to keep saturation above 97%; sublingual nitro glycerin, 1/150 grain, 1 tablet q5min × 3 prn for chest pain, then notify physician if no relief; morphine, 4 mg qh IV prn for pain; furosemide (Lasix), 80 mg IV stat and bid; indwelling Foley catheter; D5W, 20 mL/hr IV; regular insulin, 25 U SQ now; and digoxin, 0.25 mg PO qd (A.M.), hold if pulse is less than 60 beats per minute.

The Nurse's Response

So, basically, his vital signs are a little bit better than when he was in the ED. He's having some changes in his level of consciousness, perhaps doesn't know he's in the hospital, and so on.

I think that this man belongs in the medical intensive care unit, not on the telemetry unit, because his tissue perfusion is lousy. He's blue. He has a weak, thready, irregular pulse and rales scattered throughout. He could be going into pulmonary edema. He has rapid, shallow breathing.

Yeah, he probably needs to be in the intensive care unit. All these presenting signs and symptoms are very serious. Not only will he take up so much of my time, but also we don't have certain medications and certain medication drips that he might need; we aren't equipped to provide the one-on-one attention that he needs. So, for these reasons, I believe that this patient belongs in intensive care. Sometimes I might have to have a little argument with the doctor, the house staff, interns, but I get a feel pretty quickly that what I think is right.

He better have a Heparin-lock IV in with all this stuff going on. That's just one of the things I know to do, and I don't wait for a doctor's order. He might be in a real life-threatening situation. It looks like it's pretty close to that now, and I'd darn well better have some kind of venous access so I can be prepared to administer medications. I can get the order later. And hopefully, that's not an issue because in an emergency situation, it's going to slide.

And I'm to keep the oxygen saturation at greater than 97%. Usually if it's greater than 93% or above, I'm pretty happy. At 6 L[/min] of oxygen via nasal cannula, and he already has scattered crackles throughout, I'm wondering whether he's going to need a mask if they'd really want to keep his saturation that high. If I can get it to 93% or above, they should be pretty happy.

He has morphine, 4 mg, ordered every hour. If he's having frequent chest pain, we would want to give morphine a lot more frequently than that. It can be given every few minutes in certain emergency situations. And if he was requiring morphine very frequently, then that's a good reason to send him down to the intensive care for treatment. He has Lasix, 80 mg, ordered IV bid. That's good because it will help get rid of some of that extra fluid on board. He has rales and 2 to 3+ edema.

This man's in no condition to feel like messing with the urinal when he can't get out of bed, so a Foley catheter is a good idea. He has an order for regular insulin, 25 U SQ now. With that glucose of 500 mg, I would think the physician would order frequent blood sugar checks, to make sure his level comes down.

He has digoxin ordered qd, 0.25 mg PO, and hold if pulse is less than 60 [beats per minute]. If the physician feels like the digoxin is really needed, then most likely at least the first dose will be given IV. A lot of cardiologists feel that digoxin doesn't have as strong an effect on the heart rate as we've all learned. And usually if it's [pulse] in the 50s, we still go ahead and give the digoxin. If it's lower than 50, then I start to worry. If it's less than 60 and I don't know the doctor, then I'm going to ask. But once I start to know the cardiologist, they always say even if the pulse is 58 or 56, give it. I've learned that digoxin isn't held that often for a pulse less than 60 anymore. We usually give it if the pulse is at least in the 50s. It's absolutely appropriate to order no extra visitors. The lab that is ordered is to assess all the data that is needed to rule out MIs and just to get an even better picture of what the patient is doing.

Commentary

In response to the information presented in scene four, the nurse frequently uses the thinking strategy **drawing conclusions**: *He's having some changes in his level of consciousness. . . . I think that this man belongs in the medical intensive care unit, not on the telemetry unit, because his tissue perfusion is lousy. . . . He probably needs to be in the intensive care unit. All these presenting signs and symptoms are very serious.* She **provides explanations** for why she thinks that this client needs to be in the intensive care unit: *Not only will he take up so much of my time, but also we don't have certain medications and certain medication drips that he might need; we aren't equipped to provide the one-on-one attention that he needs. So, for these reasons, I believe that this patient belongs in intensive care.*

Ennis (1996) explains that the ability to give understandable reasons in support of statements is essential to sound critical thinking, and Paul (1993) proposes that good reasoners assert claims only when they have sufficient evidence to back them up. **Providing explanations** was identified as a critical thinking cognitive skill by the expert consensus (Delphi) study of critical thinking conducted by the American Philosophical Association (1990), and **drawing conclusions** was identified as an important critical thinking subskill in the same study.

◄ **SCENE FIVE**

At 10:00 A.M., G. C. experiences chest pain and labored breathing. His vitals are heart rate, 117 beats per minute; respiratory rate, 30 breaths per minute; BP, 100/65 mm Hg; and temperature, 38°C. His oxygen saturation has remained stable at 97% to 98% most of the morning but dips to the low 90s with exertion. He is oriented times three now.

The Nurse's Response

This is not too much different from the way he first presented when he arrived on the unit. His pulse is a little bit faster. He's being well saturated. It's good he's on bed rest because even with a little bit of exertion, his oxygen saturation really drops. So his lungs are really compromised. He probably has a lot of fluid in his lungs. Not only are we giving Lasix now, but he's also on oxygen. He needs to be on daily weights, have frequent assessments, frequent checks of his edema, and so on.

SCENE SIX

It is the end of your shift now, and you inform the nurse in report that throughout your shift G. C. has remained relatively stable with occasional PVCs and complaints of chest pain. You inform the nurse that the physician has been notified of this information. You go home knowing that you will return to care for G. C. tomorrow.

The Nurse's Response

It's about time for another blood sugar check, especially with the initial glucose having been high. He is still having chest pain off and on. He sounds a little more stable, but he's definitely not really stable. We need to watch his oxygen saturation. If he goes into some kind of pulmonary crisis or has more chest pain . . . he still needs a lot of attention.

Commentary

In response to this last scene, the nurse seems to be continuing to think about this case even as she is getting ready to leave for the day, and we can imagine her thinking about this client (whom she knows she'll return to care for tomorrow) during the time between when she leaves the unit and when she returns the next morning. In his classic text *The Reflective Practitioner*, Schön (1983) describes the importance of reflecting on action, thinking about and reviewing our actions afterward. Indeed, he says, this type of reflection assists practitioners to develop and improve the art of their practice.

Thinking Activities

1. Describe how **drawing conclusions** assists your reasoning in practice.

2. Do you frequently **provide explanations** for your statements or actions in practice? Support your response with one or two examples from your practice.

3. Describe a situation from your practice when you reflected on your actions after they had occurred.

4. What effect does reflecting on action have on your practice?

References

Alfaro-LeFevre, R. (1995). *Critical thinking in nursing: A practical approach.* Philadelphia: Saunders.

American Philosophical Association. (1990). *Critical thinking: A statement of expert consensus for purposes of educational assessment and instruction. The Delphi Report: Research findings and recommendations prepared for the committee on pre-college philosophy.* (ERIC Document Reproduction Service No. ED 315 423.)

Benner, P. (1984). *From novice to expert: Excellence and power in clinical nursing practice.* Menlo Park, CA: Addison-Wesley.

Browne, M., & Keeley, S. (1994). *Asking the right questions: A guide to critical thinking.* Englewood Cliffs, NJ: Prentice-Hall.

Ennis, R. (1996). *Critical thinking.* Upper Saddle River, NJ: Prentice Hall.

Facione, N., Facione, P., & Sanchez, C. (1994). Critical thinking disposition as a measure of competent clinical judgment: The development of the California Critical Thinking Disposition Inventory. *Journal of Nursing Education, 33*(8), 345–350.

Fisher, A., & Fonteyn, M. (1994). The nature of nursing expertise. In S. Grobe & E. Pluyter-Wenting (Eds.), *Nursing informatics: An international overview for nursing in a technological era* (pp. 331–335). Holland: Elsevier Science B. V.

Jacavone, J., & Dostal, M. (1992). A descriptive study of nursing judgment in the assessment and management of cardiac pain. *Advances in Nursing Science, 15*(1), 54–63.

Kassirer, J., & Kopelman, R. (1991). *Learning clinical reasoning.* Baltimore: Williams & Wilkins.

Paul, R. (1993). *Critical thinking: How to prepare students for a rapidly changing world.* Santa Rosa, CA: Foundation for Critical Thinking.

Rubenfeld, M., & Scheffer, B. (1995). *Critical thinking in nursing: An interactive approach.* Philadelphia: Lippincott.

Schön, D. (1983). *The reflective practitioner: How professionals think in action.* New York: Harper Books.

24 *Clinical Dilemmas in Psychiatric Nursing*

The nurse responding to the clinical dilemma in this chapter has been in nursing practice for 17 years, almost all of which have been spent in psychiatric nursing. For the past 5 years, he has worked full-time on the human immunodeficiency virus (HIV) psychiatry unit in a large urban hospital.

Clinical Dilemma One

SCENE ONE

At 7:15 A.M. Michael J. is transferred to your unit. You're in the middle of taking report from the night shift; you are working the day shift. A nurse from psychiatric emergency service (PES) calls to give you report on Michael J. At the same time, the transporter brings him to the unit.

The Nurse's Response

Well, my first thought is, who approved this transfer in the middle of a shift change at 7:00 in the morning? Because if there is a critical incident about to occur, you're not going to have the manpower to handle it. And it's notorious that they schlep people up to you, and they don't tell you about them—things like, "Oh, his Po_2 is 68 [mm Hg], and he's a little cyanotic, but we want him up there anyway because we don't want the patient in the PES right now." And I think a PES transfer is a hot potato, and I need some time to handle it appropriately.

So, I would call someone from the night shift in PES, who is still technically on duty, and tell the charge nurse I refuse to accept the transfer right now. What are they doing approving a transfer? This is still her problem. It's not mine. I have to take report. Until I finish report, I am not responsible for these clients. I think somewhere in the Nurse Practice Act it may say that a nurse can refuse to accept responsibility for an unsafe situation. If I feel like I'm being handed an unsafe situation during shift change, there are some legal technicalities regarding my refusal to accept it. I wouldn't say I'd run up the flagpole that far, but if I'm handed a mess, I don't have to own it. As soon as I step out of report and onto the floor, I now own the mess.

So the first thing is I would turn it back to the charge nurse who accepted this transfer and tell her she needs to admit this patient. I guess that's the most of it. The transport is bringing him, and the nurse is calling me to report; well, why is the nurse calling me to report when the patient's on the way? The nurse calls report to prepare me to accept the patient. It's not like an after-the-fact thing. They want to tell me something about the patient to help me to take care of him. They don't do that after the client arrives, like, "Oh, by the way, he's paranoid about bald people with beards" [this nurse is bald and has a beard]. Little things like that are helpful. I mean we get this all the time coming up from PES. They neglect to tell me really important stuff about clients until I find out just happenstance that the client has a central line in place that's clotted off, and I now have a mess on my hands. I had a patient come up recently who had massive abdominal surgeries and consequently had some very extensive scarring, and the nurse in PES didn't tell me about that. When the client stepped off the gurney and I noticed that his tummy was not like normal, I thought this is news.

Let me read through this again [reads]: "Transferred to your unit. You're in the middle of taking report from the night shift. A nurse from PES calls to give report."

Well, if I've got a nurse on the phone telling me about this guy and I have the guy already up on my unit, then obviously the first thing I need to do is take care of the guy, not the nurse. So, the first thing I would do, assuming I'm going to have to bite this bullet, is to go out and take a look at this client and say, "Hi, how are you? Are you going to be okay for 10 minutes? Can I put you in a bed and leave you?" And the guy may be fine, or he may be climbing off the walls, or he may be overmedicated, or he may be undermedicated. I don't know anything about him yet because nobody's told me.
How sick is this guy? It may be appropriate for me to drop everything and go get some vital signs on this guy, put him into a bed, and then watch him closely. When in doubt, take care of the client; you can always take care of the charts later; you can always take care of the nurse later. I would like to have a talk with the staff in PES after the fact to see who approved this. [I'd tell them,] "Don't do that to us. This is not a good thing."

Commentary

This nurse sounds angry and frustrated over the news that he is getting a new admission from PES right now, when he has just come on duty and is not even finished getting report: *Well, my first thought is, who approved this transfer in the middle of a shift change at 7:00 in the morning?* In response, he **provides an explanation** for his feelings: *Because if there is a critical incident about to occur, you're not going to have the manpower to handle it. And it's notorious that they schlep people up to you and they don't tell you about them—things like, "Oh, his PO₂ is 68 [mm Hg], and he's a little cyanotic, but we want him up there anyway because we don't want the patient in the PES right now." And I think a PES transfer is a hot potato, and I need some time to handle it appropriately.*

He **makes choices** about how he'd handle this situation: *So, I would call the night shift, who is still technically on duty, and tell the charge nurse I refuse to accept the transfer right now. . . . The first thing is I would turn it back to the charge nurse who accepted this transfer and tell her she needs to admit this patient.* To justify these choices, the nurse **asserts** several **practice rules**: *Until I finish report, I am not responsible for these clients. . . . If I'm handed a mess, I don't have to own it. As soon as I step out of report and onto the floor, I now own the mess. . . . The nurse calls to report to prepare me to accept the patient. It's not like an after-the-fact thing. They want to tell me something about the patient to help me to take care of him. They don't do that after the client arrives.*

Although it is somewhat unsettling to hear this nurse's initial thoughts that are laden with sarcasm and hostility, we must remember that these are just thoughts; they do not necessarily reflect what the nurse would do or say in a situation like this. When confronted with a stressful and frustrating situation in practice, it often is helpful to ruminate as this nurse does until one can settle down enough to view the situation more objectively and to respond to it less emotionally. Feltovich, Spiro, and Coulson's (1989, p. 117) study of clinical reasoning revealed that the problems encountered in practice "can be ill-structured: they can be highly variable in their application, requiring tailoring to context, recognition of numerous exceptions, the ability to deal with substantial gray areas, and so on." Thus, another purpose that the nurse's ruminating seems to serve is to help him to understand the nature of the problem embedded in this situation, to convert an ill-structured problem into a well-structured one.

Halfway through the nurse's response to this situation, there is evidence that the nurse has come to understand the nature of the problem and that he has converted it from an ill-structured to a more well-structured problem: *Well, if I've got a nurse on the phone telling me about this guy and I have the guy already up on my unit, then obviously the first thing I need to do is take care of the guy, not the nurse. So, the first thing I would do, assuming I'm going to have to bite this bullet, is to go out and take a look at this client and say, "Hi, how are you? Are you going to be okay for 10 minutes? Can I put you in a bed and leave you?"* The nurse has thus determined that the more important problem is *not the nurse*, but rather *the guy already up on my unit*.

He indicates that he does not as yet have enough information about the client to know what is wrong with him: *I don't know anything about him yet because nobody's told me.* In response to not knowing, the nurse **generates** a series of speculative **hypotheses**: *And the guy may be fine, or he may be climbing off the walls, or he may be overmedicated, or he may be undermedicated.* Findings from studies of clinicians in practice suggest that the clinical reasoning process is characterized by "a highly efficient hypothetico-deductive process . . . the process begins with attention to initial cues which lead to the rapid generation of a few select hypotheses, on average five in a single workup" (Patel, Evans, & Kaufman, 1989, p. 260).

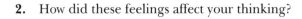

Thinking Activities

1. Describe a situation in your practice when you felt frustrated and angry.

2. How did these feelings affect your thinking?

3. What coping strategies did you use in this situation?

4. Were there similarities between your way of coping and that of this nurse?

SCENE TWO

You receive this information in report from the PES nurse. The client is Michael J., a 24-year-old white man who was brought into the PES by two police officers. He had been found walking down the middle of Market Street waving a knife in his hand and screaming at motorists and pedestrians.

On arrival to the PES, Michael is agitated and angry. He says, "Don't anybody touch me! I've had enough of this!" One of the police officers informed the emergency nurse that in Michael's rage he shouted out that he is an AIDS (acquired immunodeficiency syndrome) victim.

The Nurse's Response

This is not implausible. So far this is not unusual. My first thought is that this data may or may not be grossly distorted. We get people coming in, and what you see is not what you get, or what you hear is not quite what actually happened. Police officers are frequently not the most adept in doing psychiatric assessments on patients running down Market Street with knives. Their job is to get this person off the streets, and if that means going to the psychiatric emergency department, they'll do that.

But they're not very sophisticated practitioners, so they may have missed the boat entirely. This guy may have been running down Market Street with a knife for a reason. There may have been somebody after him, literally. And maybe he needed to defend himself. Maybe he just blew out of an apartment where there was a robbery going on. Who knows? I can't automatically assume that he's crazy at this point. Maybe there's something going on that made it necessary to do this. Now we all tend to think that this type of behavior would be indicative of paranoid thought disorder. Well that might be true, but it might not be true. I mean, you have to leave that doubt in your mind that maybe everything you're hearing about this guy is total baloney. After the fact, we may find out that his roommate is on speed and had just come home with a handgun, and the appropriate behavior for this client was to go out of the apartment screaming and waving a knife.

We still don't know much about this guy. I would just take this information and sort of file it in my head. And when I first meet a client like this, I usually say something like, "How are you?" I might not flat out be confronting him about shouting out that he's an AIDS victim. This is a human being, and he's probably not having a good day. And in our work we often forget that these are people who are frequently doing the best they can with a situation that's actually not very good.

I don't know what has been going on. Maybe he's been on a speed run for 5 days and he has finally topped out and become paranoid, and he needs to be here on the psychiatric unit, in which case he may assault me. I mean, he's giving me a message: Don't touch me. I would say, "Michael, I'm not going to touch you." I'd reassure him. If he's not out of control, I don't need to do anything except say, "Okay. Why don't you sit there. Let's talk."

I don't know what being an "AIDS victim" means. And I don't think, if he's there yelling at me, that he's about to have a circulatory collapse. So I'm not too worried, immediately, about his medical situation. In a little bit, I'd like to take his temperature; but if he doesn't want me to touch him, that's okay. If he can scream, he's not dying, immediately. So, I'm not going to get too concerned about his medical condition right off the bat.

But somewhere down the pike I would say, "There's some data indicating you may have some involvement with the HIV virus. What do you know about that?" And let him tell me. A lot of the people in this city know a lot about their HIV disease, and they can tell you a lot about it. People who are not in a gay white male population may not have access to the information that other people do, and they may not understand that very much.

Maybe being an AIDS victim means that his roommate has AIDS or his wife has AIDS or that he's been perceived as a person with AIDS and is being treated that way. Who knows? So I would file some of this away.

I start with basic safety. That's where I would begin, and because I'm a psychiatric nurse and this guy's been dragged in by the police, I would be most concerned with psychiatric safety: Is he going to hit me, or is he going to hit somebody else? Those are the basics. Is anybody going to get hurt in the next 2 minutes? Once you're beyond that, then this other information can be dealt with.

Some of these clients have been admitted here before, so we have medical records on them floating around somewhere. Sometimes, when a client comes in with handfuls of AZT [zidovudine], you kind of know that HIV is somehow involved. And sometimes you don't know. We've had some people who just had paranoid thought disorders, and their paranoia had crystallized around the delusion of having AIDS. In which case, having them on an HIV-focused floor is frequently helpful because the staff can provide them with information.

We can tell them, "You're HIV-negative. Your T-cell count is this. The notion that you have AIDS is not grounded in fact." At the same time, for a client with a delusion about AIDS to be around people with AIDS can be very provocative for them; it's a hard call. People with AIDS don't necessarily look this way or that; that's my point. He could have a whole wide range of symptoms. The clients at this hospital and in this city are pretty clear about telling you if they are HIV-positive because the level of consciousness in the community is so high. That's probably not true of a couple specific zip codes nearby. And if you drive out of the city a little ways, you'll find that most people would probably hide the fact that they are HIV-positive. Anyhow, I would stick with basic safety, his safety, my safety, our safety.

An axis one diagnosis is your major psychiatric illnesses—your psychoses, your major depressions. Axis two, such as paranoid thought disorder, are your personality disorders: people who are not very nice, but not psychotically not nice. So axis two is personality disorders, and one rarely should get admitted because they're having a personality problem, unless they have private insurance and it's a private hospital and the hospital wants to get the money. But still, it's a weak diagnosis for admission into an acute care psychiatric unit. An adjustment disorder with disturbance of emotions basically is saying, "Something bad happened, and you're not handling it well." It's called human nature.

Commentary

The nurse seems quite skeptical about the information that he receives in report about this client: *My first thought is that this data may or may not be grossly distorted. . . . They may have missed the boat entirely. . . . You have to leave that doubt in your mind that maybe everything you're hearing about this guy is total baloney. . . . We still don't know much about this guy. I would just take this information and sort of file it in my head. . . . I don't know what has been going on. . . . I don't know what being an "AIDS victim" means.* This type of skepticism is indicative of the critical thinking disposition that Facione, Sanchez, Facione, and Gainen (1995, p. 6) call open-mindedness, which they define as "being tolerant of divergent views and sensitive to the possibility of one's own bias." Similarly, Paul (1993, p. 535) describes this characteristic as intellectual humility, which he defines as "awareness of the limits of one's knowledge, including sensitivity to bias and prejudice in, and limitations of one's viewpoint. Intellectual humility is based on the recognition that no one should claim more than he or she actually knows. It implies insight into the strengths and weaknesses of the logical foundations of one's beliefs."

The nurse's thinking about the information provided in this scene reveals frequent use of the thinking strategy **asserting a practice rule**: *And when I first meet a client like this I usually say something like, "How are you?" . . . And in our work we often forget that these are people who are frequently doing the best they can with a situation that's actually not very good. . . . I start with basic safety. . . . Is he going to hit me, or is he going to hit somebody else? Those are the basics. . . . People with AIDS don't necessarily look this way or that. . . . An adjustment disorder with disturbance of emotions basically is saying, "something bad happened, and you're not handling it well." It's called human nature.*

Johnson (1988, pp. 212–213) reminds us that "in decision making under uncertainty no single correct procedure exists . . . experts report that they use complex configural rules." The informal rules that guide nurses' thinking arise from their experiences in practice; they discover what are "the basics," what approaches work best in certain situations, how clients with a particular diagnosis such as AIDS do and don't look, and so on.

Thinking Activities

1. How does the disposition described as open-mindedness or intellectual humility guide the nurse's thinking about this case?

2. What strategies could you use to develop and to improve your use of this disposition in your practice?

3. How does **asserting a practice rule** influence this nurse's thinking?

SCENE THREE

You've been assigned as Michael's nurse. Admit orders are as follows: transfer to the AIDS psychiatric unit; diagnosis—adjustment disorder with disturbance of emotions and conduct; give 2 mg of lorazepam (Ativan) prn for agitation; vital signs every 4 hours.

At 8:00 A.M., your admission assessment shows that his vital signs are: temperature, 37°C; respiratory rate, 18 breaths per minute; heart rate, 82 beats per minute; and blood pressure, 128/80 mm Hg. There are cutaneous lesions indicative of Kaposi's sarcoma on his chest and face. There are superficial cuts and bruises on his hands and arms. He has a strong body odor.

The client states that he is homeless and has been on the streets for 2 months. He also drinks frequently.

The Nurse's Response

On our unit, an order for vital signs every 4 hours would tell me that this guy's a little unstable medically, or that we don't know what's going on, or that he may be going through detoxification, in addition to whatever else is going on.

His vital signs are not bad. He has lesions indicative of Kaposi's sarcoma on his chest and face. Okay, the plot thickens. This does tell me a few things. First of all, the guy's not apparently in acute detox, although we all know now that the primary symptom of acute alcohol withdrawal, the number one symptom, is anxiety.

By the time you get to vital sign changes, you have a problem. I don't let them get to vital sign changes. I medicate them early. Librium never hurt anybody! Really. A lot of people detox without sedation all over hospitals in this city and in every city in America for no reason, and they are not better people for having gotten sick detoxing. So there's no reason not to make them comfortable; it's inhumane not to. The staff frequently have adverse feelings about people with drug and alcohol problems. That's the staff's problem, not the client's problem. And if the client's care is compromised because of the staff's feelings about him, then we've done something wrong.

This client has Kaposi's sarcoma [KS]. Now that tells me that he's got a full-blown AIDS diagnosis on paper. That doesn't necessarily mean he's very sick. We know now that KS is actually a separate disease. It's a separate organism from HIV, and it just tends to have the same transmission routes. There are a few people around with KS who don't have HIV. By and large, though, people with KS do have HIV. The KS and HIV organisms have the same routes of transmission. They occur in the same risk groups.

It used to be, and still is on paper, that KS gives that client a full-blown AIDS diagnosis. That has no relationship to life expectancy. A diagnosis of KS with organ involvement may not actually have any bearing on how the patient's feeling and doing. It's not pretty, but it's not medically dangerous. So, it just tells me a little about this client. It tells me he was probably infected with HIV relatively early because KS is actually not around much anymore. For some reason it dropped out. It's not as virulent an organism as HIV is, and we rarely see any new cases with KS. It does still occur in HIV-positive clients, but it used to be that everybody got KS, and that's no longer the case. So he probably had his HIV infection for 10 or 15 years. He got infected early in the epidemic.

Was he intoxicated? Has he been in fights? Has he been on the streets? Is he so out there that he can't take care of himself? I would just sort of file some of this information away. And I always start worrying about detox. He doesn't smell nice. Okay, does he have a residence? People who live on the streets don't tend to smell nice. It's not that they don't want to, it's just that they can't bathe.

Yes, this actually is not unrealistic. Since I know that he's been screaming, "Don't touch me," and he has been drinking a lot, and he doesn't look well, and I have a lorazepam order for agitation, I would use my nursing judgment and give it, knowing that actually lorazepam will help him if he's going to go into the deep detox. It's not the greatest choice, but when it's all you have, you give it. And then you say to the physician, "Oh, he was agitated." But he is agitated because he's detoxing.

So he's been on the streets; then we can no longer say, "Oh, he doesn't want to bathe, he has a depressive disorder." No. He doesn't bathe because he

doesn't have access to water. And he's got cuts and bruises. Well, he's probably been stumbling around in some sort of intoxicated state and maybe the
problem we have on our hands here is delirium tremens [DTs]. He may be a
guy with schizophrenia and AIDS and DTs, but the problem we have on our
hands is the DTs. And if we don't treat that, he's not going to get to enjoy any of
his other problems.

And I wonder what day of the month it is, too, because the client population at
our hospital get their social security and welfare checks on the first of the
months, and that's when they go on their speed and alcohol runs. They tend to
come into the hospital in an acute detox on day 3, 4, and 5 of the month. Very
rarely can they afford a speed run at the end of the month. If he comes in at the
end of the month because he's been on a speed run, then somebody's been buy-
ing it for him.

Commentary

The nurse's thoughts about this case consistently reveal caring and compassion, especially in his thoughts about information given in scene three. These sentiments
are manifested by such thoughts as *there's no reason not to make them comfortable; it's
inhumane not to. The staff frequently have adverse feelings about people with drug and alcohol problems. That's the staff's problem, not the client's problem. And if the client's care is
compromised because of the staff's feelings about him, then we've done something wrong. . . .
And he doesn't smell nice. Okay, does he have a residence? People who live on the streets don't
tend to smell nice. It's not that they don't want to, it's just that they can't bathe.* According
to Watson (1988), the most basic and essential factor associated with professional
caring is a humanistic and altruistic system of value. This nurse's thoughts are indicative of this system of value.

Additional evidence is demonstrated by his thoughts in response to an earlier
scene: *This is a human being, and he's probably not having a good day. And in our work
we often forget that these are people who are frequently doing the best they can with a situation that's actually not very good.* Sellman (1996, p. 44) reminds us, "There is a tendency to consider questions of morality as those life and death questions such as
euthanasia and abortion. However, nurses are subject to much more mundane aspects of morality." This nurse's thoughts seem to be guided by the system of ideas
of right and wrong reflective of the type of morality associated with a practice that
adheres to altruistic and humanitarian values. Lipman (1995, p. 12) contends that
"caring has ample credentials as a cognitive enterprise, even though it consists of
low visibility mental acts like screening, inferring and defining. . . . Without caring,
higher-order thinking is devoid of a values component." Benner, Tanner, and
Chesla's (1996, p. 234) study of expertise in nursing practice revealed that it is
characterized by "the embodied skilled know-how of relating to others in ways that
are respectful and support their concerns."

Thinking Activities

1. How does this nurse's sense of morality influence his thinking about this dilemma?

2. Describe a situation in your practice that required the type of caring thinking that was described by Lipman (1995).

3. How did your sense of morality influence your thinking about this situation?

SCENE FOUR

You are called out of Michael's room to receive another admission from the PES. At 10:00 A.M., you return to Michael's room to find him at the window banging on the window and screaming. You attempt to calm him down and to give him an oral dose of lorazepam, but he screams, "No. I refuse to be poisoned."

The Nurse's Response

What time did I leave the room? That's what I'm thinking. Why has this client been left alone for 2 hours? He's an acute client who just rolled in from the PES; hasn't anybody peeked in on him in 2 hours?

So, he's getting worse, and he's banging and screaming; we're about to hit unsafe. Banging and screaming on windows is one step away from banging and screaming on his nurse, so it's time to do something. Now back here when I got the medication orders and it said give 2 mg of Ativan prn for agitation, I would like it to have had the order say PO/IM because I would like to give this client some Ativan IM.

But this is realistic. Clients come up to our unit with orders like this, no IM backup, and you're just stuck. We had a guy come in recently from jail, direct from jail to us, with no IM orders. He was a big, menacing, weird guy, and he had no IM orders. I was not happy.

He says, "No, I refuse to be poisoned." I would say, "Hey, could you stop banging on the window and screaming?" Maybe he can. Who knows? I would like to know what he thinks is going on around here. I'd say, "Michael? What's going on here?" People think you need to use a special approach with psychiatric patients. They're actually human beings. You just ask them what's going on. Now then, what you get in response may or may not be problematic. If he says, "There are radios in my teeth," you have a new problem. But if he says, "I had a really bad night and it was scary, and I'm hearing voices telling me to hurt people." I mean, he may just be so tortured that what he needs is some tender loving care and some physical space. Or he may be banging on the window because nobody's come to talk to him for 2 hours and he wants to know what's going on. Banging on the window may be appropriate behavior given his situation; maybe not. So he says, "No I refuse to be poisoned," and I would say, "Okay, we're not going to poison you." And I would just wait and see. Maybe he'd like to talk.

If he were an imminent danger to himself or others, then I would have the right to give him medications against his will. And if this behavior persisted and he was out of control, then I would go get four or five other staff, or security, and we would grab him, and take him to a seclusion room, and put him in restraints, and give him an IM, which may be less harmful than him breaking the glass and then slashing his neck with a broken piece of it.

But, yeah, danger to self, danger to others, imminent harm. I wouldn't just do that because he's having a bad day or that I'm having a bad day. In a perfect world, what I'd do is, if he's banging on that window, I would sit over by the door so I could get out if I needed to, and I'd say, "Michael, could you stop banging for a minute and tell me what's going on?" And then just sit. Sit for awhile. But if he lunges at me, then I'm out the door. So I sit near the door. I don't let him get between me and the door.

There's a lot of questions about this young man for which I don't have answers. I would say that what I have on my hands here is an acute detox with whatever else involvement may or may not be present. He may have HIV involvement in his brain; he may not. He's got KS. In this day and time, when a client presents with KS, I would assume that he's had HIV on board for probably, not definitely, but probably 10 years. Because KS is no longer currently a real prominent symptom of HIV. But it was 5 or 6 or 8 years ago. And it was only gay men, by and large, that got KS, but it's dropped out of the subgroup. IV drug users, for some reason, didn't get KS. Transfusion AIDS people did not get KS, so it's a transmission route problem.

So, I would wonder, how advanced is his HIV? And how bad has it been? And how many friends of his have died? There are a lot of questions here. But as far as acute psychiatric care goes, we need to treat this guy's detox situation. We need to provide him with some reassurance. I shouldn't leave him alone for 2 hours. And I need to provide him with some safety. And if that means I manhandle him right now, that may be a better option than him hurting himself. If he did that, then not only do I have the same situation on my hands—which is to get him into a safe environment, whether that be seclusion or restraints—but I also have to treat his self-inflicted injuries and then complete an incident report about why I didn't provide some safety measures for an acutely agitated patient brought up from the ED [emergency department] with an alcohol problem.

Yeah. Get safety established. And it may be that he would feel very reassured when he's in restraints and he is no longer capable of being out of control. And I can sit near him, but not too close. So I sit near him. I let him stay over there, and I sit by the door. I do this a lot in my practice because being in restraints is very frightening for clients, and when I'm standing and looming over the client and he's pinned down in restraints, it's very imposing. So what I would do is to go sit on the floor about 4 feet away from him, so I'm not so imposing. I'd just sit over there for a little while. Sometimes they want to talk. I'd say, "Are you okay? What happened?" Show I care. This guy may be really sick, and he may need some help. Who knows? But I'd continue to establish some safety, and that includes medical safety, for him.

This could be a drug reaction. We see this stuff a lot. Clients with HIV who have been at home with horrible diarrhea; it's not an unusual event. They take Lomotil (diphenoxylate-atropine); it's not an unusual event. They have tons of it at home; it's not an unusual event. If someone takes enough of that stuff, then they get atropine psychosis. Maybe he had diarrhea at home and all of this came from taking too much Lomotil. It's not impossible that could be the case. And what I would do is to hold him on the unit for 3 days, switch him to tincture of opium or to Imodium [loperamide] for a few days, and see if he clears. Maybe he's a nice young man who has diarrhea. I mean it could be nothing more than that.

I'd say I see 10 or 15 cases like this a month. Clients with HIV, back 8 or 9 or 10 years ago, got pneumonia and died. They were coughing one day and dead the next. And that's no longer the case. These people are now around long enough to develop psychiatric symptoms and end up in PES. In the past, the medical treatment was so inexact that the people expired before the symptoms described in this dilemma could happen.

My goal in this situation would be that by the end of the shift, nobody gets hit. That would be nice. And that the client doesn't hurt himself. The client counts as a somebody. I would also like to see his physiological parameters stay stable—at the end of the shift, that he's not febrile, and that his vitals are still okay, and that he has achieved some level of psychiatric comfort, that this guy is not as tortured and terrified and paranoid 8 hours after meeting his nurse, that somehow he's a little better.

Maybe he needs to be snubbed a little bit. If this guy's been on speed for 3 or 4 days, he needs to crash, so maybe a desirable end point is sleep. He may be asleep for a day or two and should not be having me in there messing with him, saying, "Oh, tell me about your mother." I should get him his medications, make sure he's safe, and let him crash. So maybe the desirable end point is some measure of comfort for him, including physiologic comfort, meaning his vitals are stable. And I would like to have, at the end of the 8 hours at least, some more data that tells me what's going on here. Let's get a blood toxicology screen; let's get some lab work drawn.

It could be just be an overdose of atropine. I'd call his roommate and say, "Would you mind looking in his medicine cabinet and tell me if there's any like empty vials in a garbage can in the bathroom?" Maybe he just really wolfed down a whole bunch of Lomotil. Or if I find out he's been complaining of really bad headaches for about a week, I'll start thinking about toxic psychosis, *Cryptococcus* meningitis, HIV stuff. Maybe he just has a headache! But, when I hear symptoms and I see a few mental status changes, I start looking for a fit.

Commentary

Despite the rather extreme behavior that is exhibited by this client, the nurse's thoughts reflect a calm, matter-of-fact attitude. He would simply ask the client, *Could you stop banging on the window and screaming?* He goes on to indicate that he would take the same approach with this client that he would with any other human being: *You just ask them what's going on.* Many of the **choices** that this nurse **makes** about how he would respond to this situation centers around his plan to spend time in the client's presence: *I can sit near him, but not too close. So I sit near him. I let him stay over there, and I sit by the door. I do this a lot in my practice because being in restraints is very frightening for clients, and when I'm standing and looming over the client and he's pinned down in restraints, it's very imposing. So what I would do is to go sit on the floor about 4 feet away from him, so I'm not so imposing. I'd just sit over there for a little while. Sometimes they want to talk. I'd say, "Are you okay? What happened?" Show I care.*

Benner, Tanner, and Chesla's (1996, p. 165) research illustrates that "expert practice is constituted by a caring relationship with the patient and guided by the patient's responses. These [expert] nurses take for granted that their work is located in relationship [including] the skill of being [with the client]." Nurses in a study of clinical decision making (Jenks, 1993, p. 401) "expressed a strong need to establish personal relationships with patients to facilitate clinical decision making." Spending time with this client who is agitated, as this nurse indicates he would do, helps him to establish a relationship with the client, which may facilitate the nurse's subsequent decision making.

The nurse also indicates that he doesn't have enough information about the client to really understand the meaning of his behavior: *There's a lot of questions about this young man for which I don't have answers.* Because he does not yet have enough information to identify the etiology of the client's disruptive behavior, the nurse **generates** several **hypotheses**: *[He may be in] acute detox . . . whatever else involvement may or may not be present. He may have HIV involvement in his brain; he may not. . . . This guy may be really sick, and he may need some help. Who knows? . . . This could be a drug reaction. . . . Maybe he had diarrhea at home and all of this came from taking too much Lomotil. It's not impossible that could be the case. . . . Maybe he's a nice young man who has diarrhea.* In their text *Learning Clinical Reasoning*, Kassirer and Kopelman (1991, p. 7) identify this type of hypothesis generation as the first step in diagnosis: "[Clinicians] formulate hypotheses at first contact, and continue to evoke new hypotheses as long as [they] fail to satisfy themselves that they have the right answer. . . . Quite likely, only a small number of hypotheses remain active at any given time. . . . Many hypotheses must be quite evanescent as others take their place, although discarded hypotheses can and do re-emerge at a later stage in the process." In the nurse's thoughts about the dilemma described here, several hypotheses to explain the client's behavior reemerge at later stages of his reasoning: that he may be going through detoxification or that he may be experiencing a paranoid psychosis.

The nurse identifies what he believes are the important outcome goals in this situation, regardless of the cause of the client's behavior: *My goal in this situation would be that by the end of the shift, nobody gets hit. That would be nice. And that the client doesn't hurt himself. The client counts as a somebody. I would also like to see his physiological parameters stay stable—at the end of the shift, that he's not febrile, and that his vitals are still okay, and that he has achieved some level of psychiatric comfort, that this guy is not as tortured and terrified and paranoid 8 hours after meeting his nurse, that somehow he's a little better.*

Naylor, Munro, and Brooten (1991, p. 212) propose that "through the process of linking outcomes to nursing practices, [nurses] will more clearly define those health outcomes that they are in the best position to influence." The outcomes that this nurse identifies as important are all within his realm of influence. Moreover, this nurse's outcome goals set the direction for care, identify the criteria for evaluation of the outcomes, are patient focused, are measurable, and include a time frame, all of which are important components of goal statements in nursing practice (Rubenfeld & Scheffer, 1995).

Thinking Activities

1. Describe a situation from your practice when spending time with a client helped facilitate subsequent decision making.

2. Which of the various hypotheses generated by this nurse do you believe he thinks provides the most likely explanation for the client's disruptive behavior. Justify your response.

3. Think about your practice; how does identifying outcome goals help your thinking about a client case?

4. Review the nurse's thoughts about scene four; provide several examples of his thoughts that reflect caring and compassion.

Clinical Dilemma Two

SCENE ONE

You are responsible for six clients on the AIDS psychiatric unit. Your shift ends at 3:00 P.M. At 1:30 P.M., the phlebotomist comes to take blood from each of the two clients in room 103. When she enters their room, the client in bed one says to her, "Take my blood first; that guy has AIDS." The phlebotomist replies, "I understand," and then proceeds to draw blood from the client in bed one. When she finishes, she approaches the client in bed two, who refuses to allow her to take his blood saying, "I could sue you for discrimination."

The Nurse's Response

Does this phlebotomist speak English? She's just validated somebody's goofball thoughts about AIDS. Please don't do that. She's not operating on accurate information. I would have said, "Honey! You've missed the boat! The client is not at risk for getting HIV from having his blood drawn after you've just drawn blood from someone with AIDS." Just the facts please. If I were in her situation, then I would not have said, "I understand." Yet, this is not far from what actually happens sometimes.

What I should do before my shift is over, but after this event is over, is call the supervisor of the laboratory department and say, "You need to provide some counseling and/or some in-service education for your phlebotomists. If your phlebotomists are going to provide services to psychiatric patients, then they need to learn how to do it appropriately. And if they can't do it correctly, then they shouldn't do it at all." Maybe the psychiatric nurses should be the ones to draw the blood on the psychiatric units. I could also take the phlebotomist aside and say, "You know, that wasn't a helpful way to handle that situation."

I'm going to have a problem here. As soon as I cross disciplinary lines, I have a problem. I now have a nurse criticizing a phlebotomist. I have a problem. But if I'm going to be a nurse, then I'm going to have to deal with other disciplines and recognize the issues around that. Nurses have a lot of disciplinary issues amongst themselves—so do the other services—so I need to do it comfortably. And I won't call the head of the hospital, but I will call the director of the laboratory and say, "You know, there's a problem here, and we need to look out for this."

If her practice is that poor, she has a problem. Maybe down the pike I can work with that, but so far it's not my problem. Now, if when I walk into the room I find two agitated psychiatric patients because of this goofball phlebotomist, then I have a problem. The clients will need prn sedation or whatever. But right now, it is not a nursing problem. I would go in afterwards if I heard this rigmarole and say to the client in bed two, "You have the right to not have your blood drawn. It may not be helpful to your treatment, but you have the right to refuse." I have often told my clients, "You have the right to ruin your life. It's your life."

But in this case, I would say, "I need to correct some information that seems to have been given out in this room. Letting someone draw your blood has no effect on your viral illnesses. They're separate issues." So, I may have to come in after the fact. And maybe I could walk into the room to do my assessment and say, "What do you guys know about AIDS?" or "Do you know how HIV is transmitted? What are the risk factors?" I need to find out what they know. They may have the most hair-brained ideas, or maybe they've seen somebody draw blood from two different clients using the same needle. It happens. It happens in America. It happens in this city. So I'd find out what they need to know. I'm there to provide some education. And we provide education around safe sex and HIV transmission to the craziest people in this city, including giving them condoms and telling them about the needle exchange program. They may be psychotic, but they can still get AIDS, and it won't help them if they get sick. So maybe there's a place here for me to provide these psychiatric clients with AIDS education, because they're obviously worried about it.

Commentary

As this nurse indicates, resolving interdisciplinary dilemmas requires a certain finesse. Yet, the nurse expresses his determination to follow through with steps to correct both the phlebotomist's and the client's misconceptions about transmission of the AIDS virus. Through this determination, the nurse demonstrates the critical thinking disposition truth seeking, "being eager to seek the best knowledge in a given context, courageous about asking questions, and honest and objective about pursuing inquiry even if the findings do not support one's self-interests" (Facione, Facione, & Sanchez, 1994, p. 346).

Besides **making choices** for resolving the dilemma regarding the inappropriate behavior of the phlebotomist, the nurse also **makes choices** regarding how to assist the two clients involved: *I would go in afterwards . . . and say to the client in bed two, "You have the right to not have your blood drawn. It may not be helpful to your treatment, but you have the right to refuse." . . . I would say, "I need to correct some information that seems to have been given out in this room. Letting someone draw your blood has no effect on your viral illnesses. They're separate issues." . . . Maybe I could walk into the room to do my assessment and say, "What do you guys know about AIDS?" or "Do you know how HIV is transmitted? What are the risk factors?" I need to find out what they know.* These are very appropriate choices, since client education is obviously needed in this situation, and as this nurse indicates, *We provide education around safe sex and HIV transmission to the craziest people in this city.*

Thinking Activities

1. Describe a situation in your practice when you were involved in an interdisciplinary dilemma. How did you handle this situation?

2. To what degree do you possess the critical thinking disposition truth seeking? Provide evidence that you possess this disposition.

3. How is your thinking in practice influenced by this critical thinking disposition?

4. Evaluate the choices that this nurse makes to resolve this dilemma.

> **SCENE TWO**

Christopher P., the client in bed two, is a 32-year-old bisexual black man who tested positive for HIV 8 months ago and has told his friends about his HIV-positive diagnosis.

He was admitted to the unit 3 days ago with a diagnosis of borderline personality disorder and depression. He recently lost a close friend to AIDS. Christopher's physical status has just begun to deteriorate. He has lost 10 pounds (4.5 kg) within the last 2 months. He is chronically fatigued and has just started to experience night sweats.

Christopher approaches you as you are making your 2:00 P.M. rounds and tells you there's no way around it, he's suing the hospital.

The Nurse's Response

So, now he's suing the hospital because he's been discriminated against because the phlebotomist said, "Okay, I understand." Well, that's not a real strong reason for a lawsuit. This guy is angry and wants to engage me around something that's probably not what he's really angry about, "I'm going to sue you because the phlebotomist said this to my roommate"; I don't think so. So he's going to sue the hospital. So I have a client who's mad at THE SYSTEM. That could be any system. And bisexual black males with AIDS tend to have a lot of systems with which to be angry. So he wants to talk to me about something; well, enough has happened to him in the recent past that he should have plenty to talk about.

He lost a close friend to AIDS. Hmmm. Well, I'm a very here and now kind of nurse. I would like to sit down with this client, assuming that I have the time, and say, "How are you?" and not say, "You're doing okay, aren't you?" which tells him, "Don't tell me if you're not." "You're not suicidal, are you?"—that's telling him, "Don't tell me if you are." So I'd just say, "Hi, how are you?" and see what happens. He may want to talk about all of this stuff, or he may not want to talk about all of this stuff. I need to be aware of what these clients are avoiding, which is just as important as being aware of what they want to talk about.

This client has had a lot happen to him, and it may be that he's not yet ready to talk about what it's like to be a black bisexual male or what it is like to be a 32-year-old with HIV and to be losing weight and having night sweats. He's depressed. He may not be ready to talk about that. So he may want to talk about how awful it is that he's being treated this way at this hospital. I may need to sit there and listen to that for awhile, recognizing that it's only part of what he's angry about. He's got all this stuff built up that I may never get to the bottom of. And, frankly, I probably shouldn't even forage into it, but I should be aware that it's there because if he wants to sue me because of this flimflam thing that happened half an hour ago, I just wonder what we're really talking about.

Borderline personality disorders have a lot of qualities that make them very unpleasant in psychiatric settings. One of the things they frequently do is try to engage people and yet distance themselves from people at the same time. This makes it very hard to know how to present yourself to them because you get this approach, avoid, approach, avoid, all happening simultaneously. And it's very easy to respond to the avoidance and not recognize the need for closeness, or to let them get too close until they feel that they need to reject you. They do this stuff all the time. And my job is to present the same attitude to them whether they are being incredibly loving and caring or just the opposite.

Yeah, clients with borderline personality disorders do that. So there's a lot going on here. Maybe the issue is just about the inappropriate response from the phlebotomist; I can help with that. But if the issue is about his feelings about being part of a minority, who is also part of a sexual minority class, and who has a slow-acting, deadly virus, these issues may be more than I as a nurse in this setting can resolve. And if that's what I feel is coming at me, then I need to say something like, "This is important. You need to talk to your therapist about this, so take it up in your session tomorrow."

Knowing my role boundaries is really important here. I'm also not going to go beating the phlebotomist with a rolling pin. That's their supervisor's job. Know your own role boundaries. It's a very fine art to kindly keep someone at a distance, and it's something I have not perfected, even today. One of the things that's helpful to do with a client like this is to point out to them the pattern they're exhibiting by saying, "You know, it seems that some days you want to be very close to me and other days you really want to get away from me. Can we work out some way to find a midpoint?" You have to know he probably can't, but you try anyway.

I have to remember that these are people, and I forget that a lot. These are not diagnostic categories; these are humans. This guy's not having a good day. This is the second time I've said that. And it's just important for me to remember that. It's not just that he's trying to ruin my shift, you know. This is his life, and I'm part of that right now, and I can either be helpful or neutral or detrimental. And probably the worst thing I could do would be to remain neutral. I mean, I believe I am not actually going to harm anyone through one interaction. But I see a lot of people who meet these criteria. And I have learned a lot, and I'm learning a lot now, about how to do a diagnostic workup for major depressive symptoms against the backdrop of HIV disease. For me, AIDS has changed psychiatry because all rules we've been able to rely on are becoming unreliable. All the rules don't apply when you have a 32-year-old who will probably not see 35 and who has probably seen most of his friends die in a manner that is not very nice.

For example, rating scales to determine how much stress is in someone's life don't work anymore. Those rating scales ask things like "Has a friend near you had a fatal illness recently?" A friend? Well, you know, as a bisexual or gay male in San Francisco, "a friend" does not begin to describe what the last 10 years have been like. Or if you're a nurse and you are asked on those rating scales, "Have you had a patient with a fatal illness recently?" and you work on an HIV unit, those questions don't apply. The AIDS epidemic is changing psychiatry because it's changing people's lives. This client's life is not what the textbooks used to suggest. This client has had to deal with developmental issues that are more appropriate for people who are 60, 70, and 80 years old. These issues come crashing down on what may be a rather immature 32-year-old with a drug problem, and he's not ready to cope with them. There's a lot going on there. I have to be careful, again, about what issues I go into because I may not help him if I get lost in an issue that isn't really the important one.

Commentary

In thinking about how he would respond to the client, the nurse **asserts** several **practice rules**: *Well, I'm a very here and now kind of nurse. . . . I need to be aware of what these clients are avoiding, which is just as important as being aware of what they want to talk about. . . . My job is present the same attitude to them whether they are being incredibly loving and caring or just the opposite. . . . These are not diagnostic categories; these are humans.* Research has demonstrated that as individuals gain experience within a specific area (which, in this case, is psychiatric nursing practice), they develop a repertoire of rules that guide their thinking and decision making. Groen and Patel's (1988) study of reasoning in medical practice indicates that a clinician's expertise resides in the rules that he or she develops and that it is these rules that allow clinicians to frame (structure) the problems they encounter in practice, which then facilitates their resolution, since a well-structured problem has standard solutions that are generally agreed upon within a specified community of problem solvers (Voss & Post, 1988).

The nurse's response to the information given in scene two is indicative of his perception that the issues that are really bothering the client involve much more than just his anger with the phlebotomist: *So I have a client who's mad at THE SYSTEM. That could be any system. And bisexual black males with AIDS tend to have a lot of systems with which to be angry. So he wants to talk to me about something; well, enough has happened to him in the recent past that he should have plenty to talk about. . . . This client has had a lot happen to him, and it may be that he's not yet ready to talk about what it's like to be a black bisexual male or what it is like to be a 32-year-old with HIV and to be losing weight and having night sweats. He's depressed. He may not be ready to talk about that. So he may want to talk about how awful it is that he's being treated this way at this hospital. I may need to sit there and listen to that for awhile, recognizing that it's only part of what he's angry about.*

According to Jenny and Logan (1992, p. 255), nurses come to know their clients by acquiring and using their clinical knowledge and applying it to each unique client situation: "The ability of the nurse to identify needs for care involves various kinds of knowing, including knowing something about the person to enable need determination and knowing what could be done to improve the situation." In this situation, the nurse senses that the client has a lot on his mind that is making him angry; the nurse also acknowledges that the client may not yet be ready to talk about all of the things that are making him angry: *I may need to sit there and listen to that for awhile, recognizing that it's only part of what he's angry about.* This response will help the nurse to get to know the client better, leading to a greater understanding of him as a unique human being, something that the nurse indicates is really important in his practice: *I have to remember that these are people, and I forget that a lot. These are not diagnostic categories; these are humans. This guy's not having a good day. This is the second time I've said that. And it's just important for me to remember that. It's not just that he's trying to ruin my shift, you know. This is his life and I'm part of that right now, and I can either be helpful or neutral or detrimental.* Jenny and Logan (1992) propose that getting to know the client facilitates clinical judgment about his or her clinical status and facilitates decision making about the most therapeutic approaches and actions.

Thinking Activities

1. Describe the approaches that you use to get to know the clients in your practice.

2. How does knowing your clients facilitate your clinical judgment?

3. How does knowing your clients facilitate your therapeutic approaches and actions?

4. This is the second time that this nurse has reminded himself that *these are humans. This guy's not having a good day.* What do you think is the significance of his repeating these thoughts?

References

Benner, P., Tunner, C., & Chesla, C. (1996). *Expertise in nursing practice. Caring, clinical judgment and ethics.* New York: Springer Publishing Co.

Facione, N., Facione, P., & Sanchez, C. (1994). *Journal of Nursing Education, 33*(8), 345–350.

Facione, P., Sanchez, C., Facione, N., & Gainen, J. (1995). The disposition toward critical thinking. *JGE: The Journal of General Education, 44*(1), 1–25.

Feltovich, P., Spiro, R., & Coulson, R. (1989). The nature of conceptual understanding in biomedicine: The deep structure of complex ideas and the development of misconceptions (pp. 113–172). In D. Evans and V. Patel (Eds.), *Cognitive science in medicine: Biomedical modeling.* Cambridge, MA: MIT Press.

Groen, G., & Patel, V. (1988). The relationship between comprehension and reasoning in medical expertise. In M. Chi, R. Glaser, & M. Farr (Eds.), *The nature of expertise* (pp. 287–310). Hillsdale, NJ: Lawrence Erlbaum Associates.

Jenks, J. (1993). The pattern of personal knowing in nurse clinical decision making. *Journal of Nursing Education, 32*(9), 399–405.

Jenny, J., & Logan, J. (1992). Knowing the patient: One aspect of clinical knowledge. *IMAGE: Journal of Nursing Scholarship, 24*(4), 254–258.

Johnson, E. (1988). Expertise and decision under uncertainty: Performance and process. In M. Chi, R. Glaser, & M. J. Farr (Eds.), *The nature of expertise* (pp. 209–228). Hillsdale, NJ: Lawrence Erlbaum Assoc.

Kassirer, J., & Kopelman, R. (1991). *Learning clinical reasoning.* Baltimore: Williams & Wilkins.

Lipman, M. (1995). Caring as thinking. *Inquiry, 15*(1), 1–13.

Naylor, M., Munro, B., & Brooten, D. (1991). Measuring the effectiveness of nursing practice. *Clinical Nurse Specialist, 5*(4), 210–215.

Patel, V., Evans, D., & Kaufman, D. (1989). A cognitive framework for doctor-patient interaction. In D. Evans and V. Patel (Eds.), *Cognitive science in medicine: Biomedical modeling* (pp. 258–312). Cambridge, MA: MIT Press.

Paul, R. (1993). *Critical thinking: How to prepare students for a rapidly changing world.* Santa Rosa, CA: Foundation for Critical Thinking.

Rubenfeld, M. G., & Scheffs, B. (1995). *Critical Thinking in Nursing. An interactive approach.* Philadelphia: J.B. Lippincott.

Sellman, D. (1996). Why teach ethics to nurses? *Nursing Education Today, 16,* 44–48.

Voss, J., & Post, T. (1988). On the solving of ill-structured problems. In M. Chi, R. Glaser, & M. Farr (Eds.), *The nature of expertise* (pp. 261–286). Hillsdale, NJ: Lawrence Erlbaum Associates.

Watson, J. (1988). *Human science and human care.* New York: National League of Nursing.

25 Clinical Dilemmas in Case Management

The nurse responding to the clinical dilemmas in this chapter has 24 years of nursing practice experience. She has her master of science in psychiatric nursing. For the last 6 years, she has worked full-time as a case manager with the crisis resolution team of the psychiatric emergency service (PES) at a large urban county hospital. PES is a locked unit that consists of one large dayroom with lounge chairs that convert to daybeds for sleeping, four seclusion rooms, and several small interview rooms. Clients waiting for admission to one of the six psychiatric units in the hospital or to a residential treatment center may have to be held in PES for up to 3 days, until a bed on a unit or a space in a residential center opens up. The crisis resolution team consists of four psychiatric technicians, a social worker, a MFCC, and two clinical nurse specialists who function as case managers. Almost without exception, the clients who are seen by the crisis resolution team are indigent. Most are homeless and have a history of drug and alcohol abuse and of chronic mental illness, usually some type of psychosis.

Clinical Dilemma One

SCENE ONE

It is 8:00 A.M. You are a clinical nurse specialist who is a case manager on the crisis resolution team of the PES. You have been in this role for 6 years and before that have functioned as a clinical nurse specialist on an inpatient psychiatric unit. Your shift started at 7:00 A.M. with report, where you learned that the census in PES has risen to 20 overnight. There are currently 15 patients sleeping in the dayroom area, and 5 others are restrained, 4 in seclusion rooms and 1 on a gurney in an interview room.

From report, you learn that one of your patients, Larry, has come in during the night. Larry was brought in by the police for attacking his mother with a butcher knife in her kitchen. He has been living on the streets for the past 6 months after his mother refused to have him back in her home. According to report, Larry had gone to the mother's house late last night seeking money. When she refused, he attacked her. Her screams alerted a neighbor, who called 911.

The Nurse's Response

When I hear that there are 20 patients in the PES, the first thought I have is, what does my schedule look like for the day in terms of my returning clients? And I'm really just trying to figure out how I can help the PES staff. So that's one of my first thoughts: can I clear my schedule?

So, okay, I know I have one case I'm going to see immediately. I wonder if Larry has taken his med[ication]s lately. There's a real problem here, probably because Larry's mother gets his check because he won't let us set him up with a social worker who could arrange for someone other than his mother to hold his money for him. And I just have to figure out how to get him to do that or how to get his mom to let him do it.

How old is Larry? I think that the main problem with Larry getting violent with his mom is the fact that his mother does get his money, and it really causes a very bad situation. What she probably tries to do is to send it out to him. One of the major reasons that a family member ends up getting attacked is because of the money issue. And I'm always rather surprised that no matter how psychotic somebody seems to be, they still seem to know their money situation quite well.

The crisis resolution team can only assist with crisis management for 30 days, although we can extend to 60 days. We get our patients straight from the PES or the inpatient units, and our primary goal is to connect them to ongoing treatment in the community. And Larry would be a really good case because Larry is probably somebody who continuously uses PES, probably gets into altercations with mom or family or gets in trouble on the street when he's been out there doing whatever, and he's brought into the PES and never really manages to get to a clinic. A lot of the patients that I see are very recidivistic.

Larry probably has a history of violence and tends to go after his family the most often. I don't know if he has ever attacked anybody in the hospital—other staff or clients.

Commentary

In response to learning that there are 20 clients in PES, the nurse's *first thought* is *how I can help the PES staff. . . . Can I clear my schedule?* She **recognizes a pattern** of high acuity and immediately thinks about how she can help; she doesn't have to wait to be asked. This sense of esprit de corps, a common spirit of enthusiasm and devotion among members of a group, is impressive, especially in light of the fact that helping out the PES staff is above and beyond the expectations of this nurse's role as a member of the crisis resolution team.

On hearing the description of Larry's behavior, attacking his mother with a butcher knife, apparently because she wouldn't give him any money, she does not focus on this bizarre, inappropriate behavior but rather focuses on what she suspects is the most likely cause of this behavior: a money issue. She suspects that *Larry's mother gets his check . . . and it really causes a bad situation.* **Generating a hypothesis** to explain the client's bizarre behavior provides a focus for problem resolution that may then eliminate the undesirable behavior.

Thinking Activities

1. Evaluate the esprit de corps attitude demonstrated by this nurse. What might be the positive consequences of this type of attitude? What might be the negative consequences of this type of attitude?

2. Describe a situation in your practice where you experienced this sense of esprit de corps. What were the positive and negative consequences of your feeling that way in this particular situation?

3. What did you learn from that experience?

◢ SCENE TWO

Larry is a chronic paranoid schizophrenic with a long history of poly-substance abuse. He is a 32-year-old single white man who is homeless and who has a criminal history involving assaults and disorderly conduct. He consistently stops taking his haloperidol when out of the hospital. He has an extensive history of hospitalizations from age 18. Larry has been your patient for the last 2 months, following his most recent inpatient hospitalization.

Currently, Larry is in one of the seclusion rooms in four-point restraints. He received 5 mg of haloperidol and 100 mg of diphenhydramine IM during the night.

The Nurse's Response

Automatically, the thing I think about with somebody who has a criminal history of assault and disorderly conduct is a clinic that is called The Center for Special Problems. So I'll work on getting him there, since my job is to get patients into another setting and get them hooked up into treatment.

If he's typical of many of my clients, then he probably threw his haloperidol in the trash can as soon as he walked out the last time he was here. Larry probably doesn't particularly like the haloperidol because it makes him stiff, and that's painful, so he tosses it.

So I've had trouble getting him clustered. Clustering is a new system in mental health services that requires that every patient go through a particular point of entry to get services. And it's very difficult to get patients into the system through clustering, so I'm probably having trouble getting Larry into the system. He's got a long history. He's very recidivistic. He's been in and out of the hospital. I'm going to go back and go through his chart to determine if he has ever assaulted people in PES or in the hospital. I'm going to assess his assaultive history, primarily because if I have to sell him to a clinic [get them to take him] or if I have to sell him to a residential program, then they'll want to know about his assault history, so I really have to get down to the facts. So I will go through all of his clinical records.

I would sit down and talk to Larry and say, "Okay, what's going on? You don't want take the haloperidol?" Many clients will say, "They make me stiff. I don't like them." Sometimes when clients are on antianxiety medications such as benzodiazepine, they have movements that are really ugly looking. It makes other people stare at them, and they don't want that. Some clients develop a blank face, or they look strange when they walk. They walk with a shuffle, and it's horrible. It feels bad. They don't want to do it, and I wouldn't either. If I were a psychotic patient, I probably wouldn't take these medications either if they caused these side effects. So I would work with the client to try to figure out what dose would be the most beneficial with the least side effects.

I think that part of working with any client is to assess why they're not taking their medications. I ask myself, "What does it mean not to take the medications?" Most of us wouldn't be faithful in taking medications if we had to take them day after day after day after day. And I try to get my clients to talk about that, and I try to work with them on it.

The other issue here is that many clinics and a lot of places won't take people who are doing drugs. I mean, if you're a psychiatric patient, or if you're doing drugs, you won't get care in a clinic. For somebody like Larry, this placement center for special problems works with people who are violent—that's one of their specialties. There are a lot of patients that I cannot hook up with services, so what I do instead is to provide brief therapy to them myself for 8 weeks because I can extend the 30 days of coverage to up to 60 days, and that's what I do. And then if they need me again, they call me up, and I reopen their case. I have cases that I've reopened several times.

Larry is homeless. I don't know that much about his assault history except that he assaults his mother, he's been arrested for assault, and he's been in jail. I would like to try to find housing for him. Most of my patients are homeless, and much of what I do is just try to find housing for them. And the first thing I think about with somebody who's pretty ill, which he is, is some kind of residential treatment program. Sometimes, if the patient is likable, the staff at the treatment center will let them come through two times, but then they're out. And a drug problem is really one of the hardest things that I deal with; a patient who is dual-diagnosed, has some kind of psychiatric disorder plus substance abuse, closes a lot of doors.

I've had staff at these placement centers say to me, "No, not another crack user. We won't take him. We already have seven patients here who are crack users, and we won't take another one." So then I'm stuck with somebody to shelter who's a chronic paranoid schizophrenic and therefore is not going to make it in a homeless shelter. The homeless shelters around the city are disgusting! They're really bad. There's drug deals going on in them. There are these rooms filled with cots, and if you're paranoid, it would be pretty horrible to be in there around all these people who are trying to sleep in one room. I couldn't sleep in that way at all, and I'm not schizophrenic.

Commentary

After getting additional information about the client, the nurse **generates** another working **hypothesis** to explain his violent behavior: he may become violent because he stops taking his medication, and he probably stops taking his medication because he doesn't like the side effects that it causes. She recognizes that the unpleasant side effects of the haloperidol are a legitimate concern; she expresses empathy (identification with and understanding of another's situation, feelings, and motives) for what it must be like to experience these unpleasant side effects and for what it must be like to have to take this medication *day after day after day.* Barry (1996, p. 15) contends that empathy "is an essential quality in a helping relationship." In this instance, the nurse's empathy gives her additional insight and understanding regarding the nature of Larry's problems, including the reason why he may not be willing to take his medication on a regular basis.

As she considers how to manage his case, the nurse already anticipates (**predicts**) she'll have difficulty getting Larry placed (a process that she refers to as *selling him*) in a residential program: *a patient who is dual-diagnosed, has some kind of psychiatric disorder plus substance abuse, closes a lot of doors.* As she considers the consequences of not being able to place her client in a residential program (*so then I'm stuck with somebody to shelter who's a chronic paranoid schizophrenic and therefore is not going to make it in a homeless shelter*), she again expresses empathy: *There are these rooms filled with cots, and if you're paranoid, it would be pretty horrible to be in there around all these people who are trying to sleep in one room. I couldn't sleep in that way at all, and I'm not schizophrenic.*

Thinking Activities

1. After getting additional information about the case, the nurse **generates** a second working **hypothesis** to explain Larry's violent behavior. How does this influence her reasoning about the case?

2. How are the nurse's feelings of empathy helpful in her reasoning about the case?

3. Describe a situation from your practice when your feelings of empathy toward a client influenced your reasoning about the case?

4. How does **making predictions** about finding a placement for Larry after his discharge from PES influence her reasoning about the case?

SCENE THREE

It is 8:15 A.M., and you enter the seclusion room to assess Larry's status. As you enter, you discover that his left hand has been let out of the restraints so he could eat breakfast. His breakfast remains on the tray uneaten. You notice that he is mumbling to himself, looks preoccupied, and laughs occasionally to himself. He is unable or unwilling to make eye contact with you. As you begin your formal mental status examination he screams, "You're trying to hurt me. Take this poison out of here!"

You start to attempt to reassure Larry, and he very quickly throws the breakfast tray in your direction. It just misses you, but the food goes everywhere.

The Nurse's Response

I'm walking in, and he's looking very preoccupied. He's mumbling to himself. He's obviously in his own little world. He received 5 mg of haloperidol and 100 mg of diphenhydramine IM during the night. I would guess that this person probably needs more meds or that the haloperidol is at too low a dose for him to deal with his paranoid delusions. He's telling me now that he thinks that people are trying to poison him. If he doesn't seem to have any sense of even who I am, then I might try to reinforce that I'm his case manager. Since I've worked with him, I'd try to get him to look at me to see if that would help him to recognize me. But I think the big problem is that he probably needs some more medication and maybe some more time in seclusion, just to settle down. I would probably go check to see if I could get the doctor to order more medication for him and then give the medication some time to work.

Many of the patients who come into PES are in handcuffs or are put straight into restraints. Many times what the nurses do is to try to get the client to say that he won't harm anybody, that he is in control. The staff will attempt to keep him from having to be restrained; they'll first try just putting him in a seclusion room without restraints. They might lock the door to the seclusion room, have the patient sit on the bed and just stay there until he can calm down, until he can get himself together. And if he can't, then he'll be put into restraints.

I think you have to think of the person's dignity. The staff try to work with the patient around things. A lot of trays do end up against the wall. But at the same time, you want to maintain the client's dignity. You want to try to give him a chance to show that he's getting himself together.

I would stand at the foot of his bed or to the side. I would not get near his free hand. Part of what I do is deal with people who still might be internally preoccupied. I try to get them to talk to me so they can move away from that internal focus, or I see if they can focus during my initial assessment of them.

After years of practice, I just don't think that much about walking into a room with someone who is violent. So he throws things at me. Okay. I'm not sure what was going through his mind just then, why he threw his tray. He asked me to leave, to get out of there and leave him alone; I didn't move fast enough, so he threw the tray at me. That's kind of provocative. Yeah, it's assaultive, but again, I wouldn't get that upset about it. I'd probably walk outside and start laughing or something like that. He didn't hit me or anything, and I just don't know what's going on inside a person's head, so what I would do is, later on, try to assess what was going on, when he's more settled down.

I've had a history with this guy for 2 months, so that should mean something. I would assume that he's not even seeing me, recognizing who I am, but is seeing something else, whatever that might be. I'm not sure that I would judge this as a definite assault or as just acting out because he's frustrated.

Commentary

The nurse's reaction to this situation may surprise many of us: *He asked me to leave, to get out of there and leave him alone; I didn't move fast enough, so he threw his tray at me. That's rather provocative. Yeah, it's assaultive, but again, I wouldn't get that upset about it. I'd probably walk outside and start laughing or something like that. He didn't hit me or anything.* The nurse attributes her calm response to extensive experience with disturbed, violent clients: *After years of practice, I just don't think that much about walking into a room with someone who is violent. So he throws things at me.* The nurse seems to be able to focus on her client's rather than her own concerns, to rise above any fear or anger that she might be feeling to focus instead on what the client is feeling: *I'm not sure what was going through his mind just then, why he threw his tray.* Despite his threatening behavior, she expresses her intent to maintain her client's dignity: *I think you have to think of the person's dignity. The staff try to work with the patient around things. A lot of trays do end up against the wall. But at the same time, you want to try to maintain the client's dignity. You want to try to give him a chance to show that he's getting himself together.* A study of the caring experiences of experienced nurses (Walters, 1995, p. 495) revealed the importance of preserving the client's dignity: "There is also a recognition of the potential for the patient to lose his/her dignity and be treated in a dehumanizing way. Because of the involvement that the nurse has with the patients and their families and friends, it is possible for the nurse to act as a patient advocate. The nurse can bring knowledge and important information about the personhood of the patient to the decision-making process."

Thinking Activities

1. What is your evaluation of the appropriateness of the nurse's response to being told that the client threw his tray at her?

2. How does focusing on the client's dignity affect the nurse's perception of this incident?

3. Describe a situation in your practice when you felt threatened by a client. What was your reaction to feeling threatened?

4. Do you think that your reaction to threatening situations in your practice will change *after years of practice*, as it has for this nurse? Why or why not?

5. What are the advantages and disadvantages of focusing on the client's rather than your own concerns in a threatening situation?

Clinical Dilemma Two

◀ SCENE ONE

It's 9:00 A.M. You have a series of appointments scheduled with your clients who are coming to the PES to see you. You are reviewing the records of the clients you expect to see this morning.

Your first client is Molly. She has an appointment at 9:30 A.M., but she's been unreliable with her appointments, so you aren't sure she'll show up. Molly is a 37-year-old woman who was diagnosed with schizophrenia approximately 20 years ago. Since then, she has been hospitalized several times in acute care psychiatric facilities. During her last hospitalization, she received a diagnosis of borderline personality disorder. She has an 8-year-old daughter and is currently jobless. Over the years, she has held several part-time jobs as a waitress or dishwasher in local restaurants, but her disruptive behavior has escalated in the last 3 months, and she has been unable to find work. Additionally, she and her daughter were recently evicted from their apartment in the Tenderloin district.

The Nurse's Response

Just because a person is homeless doesn't mean they don't care about what happens. It's often because they're homeless and they're getting pushed around from one place to another that they come in late for their appointments, but most of my homeless clients do keep their appointments.

Let's give this client a chance. If a client wants treatment, they will come back for an appointment. If they don't come back, then they don't want treatment. Mine's a totally voluntary program. I have people who show up 2 hours late, or maybe I give them a 9:00 A.M. appointment, and they show up at 7:00 P.M. It's okay, no big deal.

Since Molly often shows up late, I think that I might have time to go through an evaluation and maybe to attend a meeting in PES; I still have other patients to see.

Several thoughts come to me about this case. First of all, people with a diagnosis of schizophrenia very rarely marry. And since she's had some kind of relationship with a man—I'm making a judgment here—she's not married, but she says she has a daughter, so maybe she isn't schizophrenic. And she has held some jobs, which is also rather interesting. I don't see many people who are schizophrenic holding jobs. She's been working recently, which to me indicates that she is able to keep it together enough to work.

I'm trying to figure out what she might have done to get evicted from the apartment. I'm not sure I had that history. But usually clients get evicted because they've been dancing in the halls and screaming and yelling in the middle of the night or banging on their neighbor's doors, etc. I'm also surprised that she still has her daughter with her; that's not common, at least with a lot of the patients that I see. Often, a family member will take the client's children because they don't think that the client is capable of caring for them. But this client has done very well because she manages to hold some kind of a job; she has her daughter with her; and, until recently, she had an apartment in the Tenderloin. I'm concerned about why she's not coming in for appointments. If she can hold a job, that would indicate to me that she's pretty reliable on some level. So I'm not sure why she's not coming in for her appointment.

Commentary

The nurse **recognizes a lack of fit** with the typical **pattern** of schizophrenia: *First of all, people with a diagnosis of schizophrenia very rarely marry. And since she's had some kind of relationship with a man—I'm making a judgment here—she's not married, but she says she has a daughter, so maybe she isn't schizophrenic. And she has held some jobs, which is also rather interesting. I don't see many people who are schizophrenic holding jobs.* This lack of fit raises her suspicion that perhaps Molly has been misdiagnosed. If not, then she is at least able to function at a higher level than many of the schizophrenics that the nurse sees in her practice.

The nurse learns that Molly has been unreliable in keeping appointments with her. This the nurse also **recognizes** as a **lack of fit** with the **pattern** of reliability that Molly is exhibiting in other aspects of her life: *I'm concerned about why she's not coming in for appointments. If she can hold a job, that would indicate to me that she's pretty reliable on some level. So I'm not sure why she's not coming in for her appointment.*

SCENE TWO

Molly arrives at 9:50 A.M. and begins telling you what's been going on since her last visit with you in PES 2 weeks ago. She and her daughter, Marie, had been living in her friend's car until that was stolen. Since then, they've been living at various shelters around the city. Her daughter is in and out of foster care homes. She attends school occasionally but is rarely at the same school for more than a few weeks in a row. At 8 years old, she cannot read or write.

In addition to Molly's psychiatric problems, you notice a medical problem has developed; she has a large weeping ulcer on her swollen left ankle. She says she doesn't remember when her ankle got sore. You notice that she also has multiple scars, abrasions, and bruises. Her feet are callused and cracked. Her blood pressure is 160/98 mm Hg. Her heart rate is 104 beats per minute, her respiratory rate is 28 breaths per minute, and she refuses to have her temperature taken.

The Nurse's Response

It's good that Molly arrived for her appointment at 9:50 A.M. It's disgusting when people like her are out there homeless and someone steals from them. So many of the homeless have been victimized. Everything they have disappears within a few days sometimes; it's awful. Her car was stolen, which is her home. Probably everything that was in it was stolen too, clothes and so on. They've been living in various shelters around the city. Usually women have a better chance of getting into shelters, especially women with children. They can get into shelters for longer periods of time than the men. I'm trying to find out if she's checked out these sanctuaries because they can usually stay up to 3 months if they behave themselves.

Okay, so the daughter does get pulled away from her at times. I guess there are some times when she has probably been too sick or something to care for her daughter, and the daughter is then put in a home, and when the client gets better, she gets her daughter back. Again, I'm really impressed by that.

By whom was her daughter taken away? Where was she taken? Did the client get to see her while she was away? I'd want to know more history about that. When you're moving from place to place, it's very difficult for a child to stay in school. I have this thing about trying to keep mothers or parents and children together, and sometimes I find myself really opposed to the legal issues such as just because a woman gets admitted for psychiatric problems, they take the child away. I have a problem with that.

I don't have any problems with foster homes, but many times the authorities take the child away forever, or it's very difficult for the client to get their child back. And for some clients that's appropriate. A lot of psychiatric clients have had children removed from them. Molly's not a drug user. I don't believe Molly's doing anything harmful to the poor child. It's really an ethical dilemma, but the problem is there's no place in the city that takes a mother and a child except the Salvation Army shelter. So there's no other choice. There's no residential treatment program around that will take a mother and their child. And I think it's a crime because some of these mothers are very good with their kids. They're a little crazy, but they love their children.

It sounds like Molly has provided pretty well in the past. And then she's been hospitalized. But, if a mother had diabetes, then would they take the child away? That's how I think about it. It's the same thing. It's a chronic illness. I have very strong feelings about the importance of children remaining with their mothers.

In regards to the ulcer on her leg, I would have the nurse practitioner who works in PES look at it. We'll probably find out that, since the car's been stolen, Molly has been walking most of the day. Because the shelters basically want you out in the morning. And she's probably just been walking and walking, so her feet are a mess. She has dependent edema and probably has bugs, and her scratching has caused an abrasion and an ulcer. The scars, abrasions, and bruises might indicate that she's been beaten up somewhere along the line. That's quite possible out there on the streets. And she's probably not able to bathe because she doesn't have a place to bathe.

Sometimes the doctor or the nurse practitioner will say, "I want you to go home and soak your feet, then put your feet up, keep them elevated." Those kind of instructions are a joke for these homeless clients. If that happened, I'd respond by saying, "What is going on? This person is walking; this is how she survives." In that case, we may end up having to put her in the hospital if the ulcer is bad enough and requires antibiotics. Where will her daughter go if the client's in the hospital?

It looks as if we probably will need some kind of child crisis team to come in to see Molly and to find out how to help her with her daughter during hospitalization. I would think the daughter is just terrified that her mom is going to be taken away, that they're going to be separated. If I were able to do family therapy with them, I could probably get them to a point where Marie would go to school regularly and they would feel safe, but at this point the mother is not capable of dealing with this type of therapy.

Commentary

The nurse exhibits a strong sense of the ethical issues embedded in the information provided in this second scene, including the victimization of people who are homeless, the policy of taking children away from their mothers because the mom has psychiatric problems, and the insensitivity that is exhibited by some caregivers who recommend treatment that is impossible for a homeless person to carry out. Hepburn (1993, p. 28) reminds us that "we live in a society characterized by inequality and in which we must act responsibly and care for those who are dependent on us."

When grappling with ethical dilemmas that require decisions about treatment choices and about the disposition of a homeless child whose parent may require hospitalization, Hepburn (p. 33) recommends an approach that involves a "sensitive moral analysis" of the dilemma after "obtaining as much of the contextual detail as possible [to] provide insights as to how principles should be ordered" in making a moral decision about the dilemma. By **searching for** additional **information**, the nurse tries to obtain the contextual detail to which Hepburn refers. The nurse wants to know more about the history regarding past placement of the daughter. She also wants to know how bad the ulcer is, whether the client will need to be on antibiotics, and whether she will need to be hospitalized. If so, the nurse wants to know where the daughter will go while her mother is in the hospital.

◣ SCENE THREE

When you ask Molly where her daughter is, she indicates that she has her sitting in the hospital cafeteria. She shares that Marie has been expelled from her school due to tardiness and absenteeism. Molly begins to cry and says, "Marie wants to stay with me and doesn't want to be in school or in another foster home. If you try to take Marie away, I'll kill myself." You suspect that Molly will require admission for treatment of her ulcer.

The Nurse's Response

Upon discharge from the hospital, I will work with Molly to get her clustered and to connect her with a therapist whom she feels comfortable seeing. And it's not enough to just get them an appointment and then have them go to see the therapist; you want to make sure that there's hope for some kind of a relationship to form between the client and the therapist. I would take Molly to the therapists myself, sit with her during a couple of meetings, and help her to connect with the other therapist.

I don't know what causes somebody to be schizophrenic or what causes one schizophrenic to do better than another. I don't know if it's a biochemical difference, the genetic makeup of a person, if it's the environment they come from, or the support they get. I do believe that environmental support makes a big difference. Each person has a different history, so it's hard to say. That's schizophrenia. I think it is probably the worst psychiatric disease there is. If we can find a medication that works and we can keep it at the lowest dose, I think that helps. We try to keep people from having exacerbations, so they don't get worse. But there are a lot of schizophrenics out there that are homeless, and if you put me on the streets, then I'm going to get suicidal. And I'm probably going to be doing drugs after awhile. I work with a lot of people like that, who basically are not really chronically mentally ill, but because of their circumstances, such as being homeless, they have a psychotic break.

◣ *Thinking Activities*

1. How does **recognizing a lack of fit** with a **pattern** help the nurse when initially reasoning about this case?

2. Describe a situation in your practice when **recognizing a lack of fit** with a **pattern** helped you to reason about a case.

3. Provide an example from your practice that supports Hepburn's (1993, p. 28) statement that "we live in a society characterized by inequality and in which we must act responsibly for those who are dependent on us."

4. Provide an example from your practice that demonstrates the usefulness of **searching for** additional **information** when making a moral decision about a dilemma.

Clinical Dilemma Three

SCENE ONE

It is 7:00 A.M. Your shift has just started with report, where you learned that PES has been busy all night with high-acuity patients. Your patient Joy was brought in at 3:00 A.M. and is currently sitting on a couch bed in the corner of the dayroom, chatting loudly to herself.

Joy is a 37-year-old, black, single woman who was brought into PES by the police at 3:00 A.M., following a disturbance at her Tenderloin hotel, the Lone Star. The hotel manager reports that Joy was in her hotel room when he heard screaming and banging from her room. He looked up to see Joy, naked, chasing a man down the stairs. She was screaming, "You play, you pay, you SOB!" The man had a laceration on his forehead, was dripping blood, and said, "That woman tried to kill me."

The Nurse's Response

I'm sure that her chatting is going over big with the other patients because the dayroom is rather small and everyone is lined up next to each other. Oh, the other patients are not going to be happy. Well, I don't blame her for wanting to be paid. Okay, she's out there prostituting. She's making some money. I would suspect that she's also been doing some drugs. She came into PES naked. It always amazes me that these patients are brought naked in the cop cars to the PES. I mean, they have to get to PES before anyone gives them a blanket to cover up with. It always amazes me that they're not covered up in the police cars. I mean, many times the police have brought women into PES while they're still naked. The nursing staff then run for a blanket or something to cover the patient with.

SCENE TWO

When you see Joy at 7:00 A.M., she is wearing a hospital gown and has a yellow turban on her head. As you enter the dayroom to interview her, you notice that she has her gown pulled up over her head. The RN in the dayroom indicates that Joy has been exposing herself off and on all night. Joy jumps up and runs to greet you saying, "Honey, have you got a cigarette? These people won't let me smoke."

The Nurse's Response

I don't remember hearing that she was wearing a turban when she came in. Maybe she washed her hair. That could be it. I would tell her, "You can't smoke because this is a nonsmoking facility, but I can get you some Nicorette gum." We don't have a diagnosis on this person yet, but she sounds like she's a manic depressive. You see a lot of nakedness and hypersexuality with manic disease. Sometimes prostituting might go with it. But then again, it could be drugs; we have to rule that out. So I would want to know if a toxicology screen had been done on this woman.

At least she knows who I am this time. This is good. I'm pleased with that. I'd want to know what's going on that causes her to run around without any clothes on.

Having lived through the period of controversy when the psychiatric units at our hospital switched from a smoking to a nonsmoking facility, having smoked for years a long time ago, I understand where the patient is coming from. Being allergic to cigarette smoke myself, I also understand what it's like for the staff to be on a unit that's filled with smoke, and I realize the dangers of secondary smoke for those who don't smoke. On most of the inpatient units, after a patient has been there 24 hours, they are allowed to go outside for cigarette breaks a couple of times a day. PES doesn't allow cigarette breaks for their patients; they just went nonsmoking 3 months ago. But a lot of patients really do want to have a cigarette. We know that research has demonstrated that patients who don't smoke need much lower doses of psychotherapeutic medications than those who do.

SCENE THREE

You calmly explain that you have no cigarette and that you want Joy to come with you to an interview room so you can sort things out with her. She shouts, "I won't go! I'm out of here!" She rips her gown off and runs for the exit.

The Nurse's Response

In which case, several staff members would drop on her and carry her off to a seclusion room. Now I really want to know what her toxicology screen showed because it does sound like her behavior is caused by amphetamines or cocaine, or else she is in a manic episode. Again, she probably needs to be medicated. She obviously needs to be secluded because she's quite overwhelmed at this point.

The world is rather twisted, but I can't change that. I can only try to offer comfort and to hope that the client wants it and that I can help them to move along in the right direction. One of the primary things I learned a long time ago was that I have my problems and the clients have theirs. Their problems are their own. I can only offer what I have to offer. I'm very open with my clients about that.

If they need housing, then I can offer them a hotel. But it often is one that may have roaches, and perhaps there will be drug deals going on outside the front door. That's what I can offer them, or they can go to a shelter. I really put every-thing out on the table for my clients so that they know what I can and cannot give them.

It took me a long time to get to the point where I could say to my clients, "Hey, that's your problem, not mine." I can sit there and cry over the fact that some-body's homeless, but that's not going to do them any good, or me. I do think the world's in a terrible state. I think there's a lot going on that's not right, and I know that most of the community mental health money has dried up. Every year that I remain in practice and try to help these types of clients, there are less and less resources. So, I put it all out there, and then I find that my clients are pretty amazing what they can come up with to help themselves. I've found that they have their own strength.

Commentary

Early on, when thinking about this case, the nurse **generates** two working **hypo-theses** to explain her client's extravagant behavior: *We don't have a diagnosis on this* *person yet, but she sounds like she's a manic depressive. You see a lot of nakedness and hypersexuality with manic disease. Sometimes prostituting might go with it. But then again, it could be drugs; we have to rule that out.* Barrows and Pickell (1991, p. 58) explain that a hypothesis is "a fixed constellation of facts or ideas from the clinician's memory; when a hypothesis proves to be incorrect, unlikely, or too vague, it is replaced by another hypothesis. It is the clinician's internal representation or synthesis of the patient's problem under investigation that develops, grows, and changes during the clinical-reasoning process. The clinician attempts to put together an enlarging concept of the patient's problem from the data he has obtained following the initial concept, data obtained from inquiry guided by the hypothesis."

Even after obtaining the information provided in the last scene of this dilemma, the nurse does not seem to have confirmed either hypothesis (drugs or manic disease) to explain the client's behavior. Nonetheless, the nurse is clear about what she can and cannot do to help the client: *I can only try to offer comfort and to hope that the client wants it and that I can help them to move along in the right direction. . . . If they need housing, then I can offer them a hotel. But it often is one that may have roaches, and perhaps there will be drug deals going on outside the front door. That's what I can offer them, or they can go to a shelter. I really put everything out on the table for my clients so that they know what I can and cannot give them.*

The nurse also seems very clear about who is responsible for the clients' problems: *One of the primary things I learned a long time ago was that I have my problems and the clients have theirs. Their problems are their own. . . . It took me a long time to get to the point where I could say to my clients, "Hey, that's your problem, not mine." I can sit there and cry over the fact that somebody's homeless, but that's not going to do them any good, or me.* The nurse's attitude demonstrates the distinction between empathy and sympathy. Barry (1996, p. 15) explains, "In empathy the helper borrows the patient's feelings in order to understand them fully, but is always aware of his or her own separateness. Sympathetic understanding, on the other hand, involves a process in which the helper loses his or her separate identity and takes on the patient's feelings and circumstances, as if the helper were in the patient's place."

The nurse explains that when she is honest with her clients about what she can and cannot do and when she insists that her clients assume the responsibility for their own problems, *then I find that my clients are pretty amazing what they can come up with to help themselves. I've found that they have their own strength.* Caregivers must realize that the people whom they help are responsible for their own lives and that they have forces within themselves that will allow them to achieve their optimal potential. The caregiver may facilitate this process, but it is the clients themselves who must ultimately resolve their own problems (Gertis, Edgman-Levitan, Daley, & Delbanco, 1993).

Thinking Activities

1. Comment on the nurse's frank disclosure regarding what she can and cannot do for the client. Do you think that her approach is helpful or unhelpful to the client? Justify your response.

2. Do you have any difficulty distinguishing between empathic and sympathetic behavior in your practice? Explain your response.

3. Describe a situation in your practice where you discovered that your clients had their own strength and were able to come up with a way to help themselves.

4. What strategies have you found that assisted your clients in finding their own inner strength?

Clinical Dilemma Four

◣ SCENE ONE

Everyone else on the crisis resolution team is working a full caseload of 10 patients, and you currently have a caseload of 9 patients. It is Monday, 8:30 A.M. Jane is a 25-year-old brought into PES by her boyfriend. The charge nurse, Mary, has already spoken with Jane, who says she would like some help with her situation.

Mary gives you a report. Jane is having suicidal ideations. She cannot form a no-harm contract. She's crying and between sobs is talking about how close she was to killing herself. Her plan was to cut her wrists with a straight razor. She is extremely upset because her mother died recently. Jane has no previous psychiatric history. Mary has placed her in a seclusion room so that she will not harm herself. Mary removed Jane's earrings and took her matches. She has been checking on her every 15 minutes.

The Nurse's Response

As is appropriate, the nurse in PES is letting me know that I have a new patient. Jane is asking to speak to me. After getting the report from Mary, I would go into the seclusion room to find out what's been going on in Jane's life that would cause her to feel suicidal.

◣ SCENE TWO

You go in to see Jane, who is sitting on the floor in the corner with her knees drawn up. She is sobbing, so you cannot understand what she is saying. After you give her some time to compose herself, Jane tells how close she was to her mom. She considered her mother to be her "soul mate." Jane lived at home with her mother and was financially dependent on her. Jane has no other living family.

The Nurse's Response

I'd probably go sit on the floor with Jane if it's not too cruddy. Or else I might just sit on the bed and have her come sit next to me. There's a bed in the room. I'd just sit there with her. If she's crying that hard, I would just sit there, let her pull herself together. What I do a lot with patients who are crying and not able to stop is to get them to talk about what they're thinking rather than about why they're crying. That's part of my approach to switch back and forth between feelings and thinking. Most of time, you hear nurses in psychiatry say, "How do you feel?" I very rarely ask that, unless I'm working with a client who always talks about what they're thinking, rather than what they're feeling. Then I might say, "Gee, you really should look at your feelings a little bit."

So I would ask this client what kinds of thoughts were going through her mind, to` catch a thought and to talk about it, to let me know what it was. That way, I could get a sense of what the tears were about. Because let's face it, if she is crying, then she has much stuff rattling around in her mind. So, it gives me a sense of what's on her mind that she might not be able to verbalize any other way. So, I'll bring in many Kleenex, sit there, and try to get her to verbalize. I'll just sit there with her to see what's going on.

Often, just being someone with whom the client has made a connection, someone whom the patient knows is there to help them, can make a major difference in their affect. I've had patients come in who were rip-roaring mad or who were crying and really despondent. After I had spent some time with them, they would walk out feeling pretty good about themselves. And much of it is just being there to listen, just reassuring them with my presence, letting them know that they're not alone. After a half hour or an hour, most people feel a big difference.

Commentary

It's interesting to hear this nurse **making a choice** for an action that is almost identical to that described by the psychiatric nurse in Chapter 24 when responding to a dilemma involving an agitated client on the inpatient HIV psychiatric unit. This approach of just being with a client in a centered and caring therapeutic manner seems to be common to psychiatric nursing practice. The concept of presence has been identified as an important component of healing in nursing practice (Mc-Kivergin & Daubenmire, 1994).

Another approach that this nurse has found helpful when a client is upset and crying, as is the case with this client, is *to get them to talk about what they're thinking rather than about why they're crying. . . . So I would ask this client what kinds of thoughts were going through her mind, to catch a thought and to talk about it, to let me know what it was. That way, I could get a sense of what the tears were about. . . . It gives me a sense of what's on her mind that she might not be able to verbalize any other way.*

The nurse indicates that she gets positive results from just spending some time listening to her clients: *And much of it is just being there to listen, just reassuring them with my presence, letting them know that they're not alone. After a half hour or an hour, most people feel a big difference.* According to Jackson (1992, p. 1623), "A healer is a person to whom a sufferer tells things; out of his or her listening, the healer develops the basis for therapeutic interventions."

Thinking Activities

1. Speculate as to why just spending time in the presence of a client would be a common action that nurses in psychiatry would choose in their practice.

2. Describe a situation in your practice when you have taken this action. What impact did this have on your client's outcome?

3. Do you ever ask clients what thoughts are on their mind in a given moment? How has this assisted with your care?

4. In your practice, how often do you get to spend a concentrated amount of time listening to a client? How does this assist your care?

SCENE THREE

After you have spent a half hour talking with Jane, she seems to have a slightly brighter affect. She is now sitting on the bed, and her crying has stopped for the moment. You need to get your calendar from your office to set up a weekly time to meet with her. You tell Jane that you will be back shortly, but she is begging you to stay with her. She says she doesn't want to be left alone. You ask Mary to keep an eye on her.

When you return with your calendar, you discover that Jane has taken a straight razor to her wrist, and there is a pool of blood on the floor. Mary is nowhere in sight.

The Nurse's Response

The PES staff didn't do a good job of searching Jane, and I'm going to find out why. It's really hard to blame anybody for these incidences because the client is responsible for what she does. But I do question what happened with the search. Where did this razor come from? Patients are supposed to be searched before they are put into seclusion. I'm not sure what happened, where she had this hidden. I would probably try to find out where it was hidden. If the staff just did a pocket search, which many times is all that is done, then the client may have had empty pockets. Bras are great places to hide things. So, it's hard to say where she had this razor. Patients do hide things in very interesting places, however. Clients are checked every 15 minutes when they are in seclusion, but a lot can happen in 15 minutes.

I tend to be pretty cool in these kinds of situations. I would grab a towel and throw it on top of whatever she's cut. And I would ask her, "What is this all about?" I would see this very much as manipulation on the patient's part. I walked away, so she tried to get back at me. Well, I'm not going to be gotten back at. I would deal with it in a very matter of fact way. I'd say, "Okay, what is this all about?" and see what she says.

I'm a great actress. I might not be calm inside. I would not want to respond with a lot of emotion. The most important thing is to appear calm and collected: "Okay, so you've cut yourself. Let me see how we deal with that. What's this all about? You tell me. I'm not going to play guessing games. I'm not going to get angry with you." Why should I victimize someone who's already victimizing herself? And why should I be fearful and angry and upset? This is her problem, and she needs to deal with it. I'm not going to act it out.

The kind of response I'm describing comes with experience. I am now at the point where I don't feel that I have to take responsibility for the other person's behavior. And that took a lot of self-work, which as a psychiatric nurse, I think is very important.

If it was a serious cut, then I would take her over to the medical emergency room, where the surgeons would check her out. It would depend on how bad it is. When she returns from the medical emergency department, she'll probably be strip-searched. Once we know that a client is a danger to herself, we will strip-search her. Most of the time the staff will just pat down the pockets and take away the client's sharps and matches and things like that.

I will also do a suicide assessment when she returns. Is she willing to agree to a no-harm contract? I've sent a lot of patients out of the hospital who still had suicidal ideations. I work a lot with clients as outpatients who are suicidal, and I see them very frequently, sometimes daily. Depending on where this client lives and depending on how much support she has out in the community, I might let her go. I would tell her something like, "Okay, you're feeling really suicidal. You're not sure if you're going to do anything. Okay, fine. If you feel like you will hurt yourself, you call suicide prevention. You come to PES. You call me and you come in." This becomes a contract. I really place the responsibility on the patient. They do have a choice. If they want help, they can come and talk to me. They don't have to cut themselves. They don't have to do any of the other things that people do. They can call me and talk, or they can talk to a counselor if I place them in a residential program and things like that.

Commentary

The nurse's first reaction to discovering that her client has cut herself with a razor is to **draw the conclusion** that the PES staff didn't do a very good job searching the client. She admits, however, that *patients do hide things in very interesting places*. She wonders, *Where did this razor come from?* But ultimately, she concludes, the client is responsible for what she does.

The nurse describes how through experience she has learned to hide her emotions in these situations and to appear calm and collected. She reiterates that this suicidal attempt is the client's responsibility, not hers. *I am now at the point where I don't feel that I have to take responsibility for the other person's behavior. And that took a lot of self-work, which as a psychiatric nurse, I think is very important.* Barry (1996, p. 18) suggests that "one of the most important characteristics of helpers is the attainment of healthy levels of personal growth. . . . Nurses must be able to analyze honestly their normal way of relating to patients if they plan to be effective in a counseling situation."

Thinking Activities

1. Where would you place the responsibility for this client's cutting herself with the razor blade? Justify your response.

2. Describe a situation in your practice where you felt that it was important that you act calm and collected, even if you didn't really feel that way.

3. Was this difficult for you to do? Why or why not?

4. Have you found that your ability to act calm and collected in a stressful situation in practice has improved with experience? Justify your response.

Clinical Dilemma Five

SCENE ONE

It is 9:30 A.M. on a Tuesday when you get a call from PES to come to see a client who is being referred to the crisis resolution team. The clinician tells you that the client is a 19-year-old black woman who lost her mother 1 year ago to suicide. She was raised in the Potrero Hill projects by her mother, never knew her father, and has no other siblings or known family. She has been displaced the past year, staying with boyfriends, in shelters, and on the streets. The clinician asks if it's possible to meet with Sonia today and start her on the 30-day plan.

The Nurse's Response

Of course I can see her today, because if somebody's going to be discharged from PES, I will go ahead and meet with them and do an intake and offer my services. My services are totally voluntary; if the patient is not interested, then that's their choice.

SCENE TWO

It's 11:30 A.M., and you meet with Sonia and the clinician who referred her. After an introduction, the clinician leaves. It is obvious that Sonia is uncomfortable and anxious. Her answers to your questions are curt, simply responding with a yes or no. You tell Sonia that the crisis team is here to help her in any way possible and that she can talk freely. You let Sonia know that your primary goal is to get her housing and to help her with food and to provide therapy. She gets tears in her eyes and begins to cry. As you comfort her, Sonia says that she is to blame for her mother's suicide and hopes that God can forgive her.

The Nurse's Response

Sonia's uncomfortable and anxious. If I felt that I was to blame for my mother's suicide, then that would make me pretty anxious, too. I'd ask her what she has been told about my services and then go from there. I'd say, "I'm here to work with you, so what do you want?"

If she starts talking about the fact that her mother is dead and she's to blame, then I'd be concerned that she might be thinking about what she can do to punish herself further. I would try to find out why she feels she killed her mother, why she's to blame. A lot of people feel that what has happened in their past, be it the death of a parent, the suicide of a parent, or the fights between their parents, was all their fault. If they got beat up, then it was their fault. If their father got drunk or their mother got drunk, then it was their fault. They see themselves as the center of the world, and everything revolves around them. A lot of times people feel like they've done something that caused another person to go over the edge. Let's face it, nobody can really cause another person to go over the edge.

Commentary

Here again, the nurse is trying to sort out who is responsible for what. The client is responsible for her own behavior, but not that of her parents. The nurse indicates that she will try to get her client to recognize this.

SCENE THREE

It is now 3:00 P.M., and you just got word of a group home placement for Sonia. You drive her to the placement, and on the way, Sonia tells you that her mother was involved with drugs for as long as she can remember, which led to neglect, physical abuse, going hungry, and men coming and going throughout her childhood.

By the time Sonia was a junior in high school, she began to follow her mother's footsteps by drinking and using drugs. Her grades dropped; she stopped going to class and eventually dropped out of high school just 2 months short of graduation. It was Sonia who found her mother dead 2 weeks after she should have graduated. Sonia claims to be dry now and wants to start a new life.

The Nurse's Response

It sounds like this client had several strikes against her from the start. Heaven only knows what her dad was doing or what genetics are involved there. Her mom obviously wasn't into motherhood. Who knows how she got pregnant! Sonia was one of those people, and it seems like there are millions of them, who just wasn't wanted and therefore was neglected or beaten. Why does this woman have a drug habit? Why does she prostitute? She grew up with it; this is how she learned to cope, and this is how her life is; it looks pretty bleak.

If you're doing drugs and whatever else, then you're going to drop out of school because your grades are going to fall. Because mom decided to kill herself 2 weeks after the client's graduation should have taken place, then the client blames herself, which is not realistic. Obviously, the mom had her own problems.

When clients tell me that they want to start a new life, I am optimistic, despite their circumstances. That's the one thing I don't get too jaded about. So, if a patient tells me that they want to start a new life (and many of them at that instant really do mean it), then I reply, "Okay, it's your life. You're the one who's got to do it. I'll be here for whatever you need, but you've got to do it. I can't do it for you." And then it's up to them. And all I can do is support them in that effort. With this kind of a patient, I'd do a lot of therapy centered around trying to discover what the drugs really mean to her, what she uses them for. A lot of patients use drugs basically to medicate themselves because they are depressed, and some of them do have major organic depressions. Is it any wonder that Sonia is depressed? This client's life has been pretty awful.

I would work with her on how she deals with stress. What can she do better? What kinds of things does she want to change? I would try to help her to look at where she can make some changes in her life. I'd get her hooked up with some kind of drug treatment program if that's what she wants. Again, it's whatever she wants. I'll meet with her once or twice a week, or daily, depending on what she wants.

Commentary

The nurse expresses empathetic understanding of this client's situation: *It looks pretty bleak. . . . Is it any wonder that Sonia is depressed? This client's life has been pretty awful*. The nurse **makes** several **choices** for intervention: *I would work with her on how she deals with stress. What can she do better? What kinds of things does she want to change? I would try to help her to look at where she can make some changes in her life. I'd get her hooked up with some kind of drug treatment program if that's what she wants.*

SCENE FOUR

The next morning there is a message when you return to work at 7:30 A.M. Apparently, Sonia slipped out with no one knowing. At 5:30 A.M., she returned, pounding on the front door, shouting to let her in, and appeared to be under the influence of alcohol.

It is 10:00 A.M. when you meet Sonia at her group home. Sonia begins to sob and tells you she is totally confused and doesn't know what she wants. She also tells you she's 6 weeks pregnant.

The Nurse's Response

Gee whiz, does that surprise me? No. Like I said, at the moment people do want to change their lives, but stopping drugs and alcohol abuse is really hard. Coming out of the detox stage is just so difficult; your body just craves that stuff. And people do leave their placements. Sometimes they don't even make it through the interview and they're gone, so she at least lasted a little while, which is pretty good. And many times they do come back to pound on the door of the residential placement, begging, "Let me back in!" The residential staff would reply, "Well, you're kind of drunk and loaded. I think you need to go to a detox center." So that's probably what happened. She was probably sent off to a detox center. The residential staff will call transportation to have the client picked up.

Like I said before, this is the patient's problem; it's not mine. It is not mine. And all I can do is to be there to help her look at what happened, what made her go out and get drunk. I see clinicians that get very angry over this type of behavior, but why? Her leaving doesn't hurt me as a person. Yes, it bothers me that she's hurting herself, but that's her choice. And I really do throw everything back onto the patient; it's their responsibility. It's their life. They've got to do it, not me.

Community placement is voluntary, so the patient has the right to walk out at any point. If the staff knows that somebody wants to leave, then they'll try to encourage them to stay, or they'll try to figure out what's going on. Patients want to leave for multiple reasons. Sometimes they're very paranoid, and the staff will talk to them to help them feel more comfortable; they'll make some adjustments in rooms, etc., and then the patient may stay. But patients sneak out all the time. The doors are not locked. They may be locked on the outside, to keep people from coming in, but patients can walk out at any point in time. It's a voluntary placement; it's up to the patient to decide what they want.

She starts to sob and tells me that she is totally confused and doesn't know what she wants. She's probably confused because she's still detoxing. One of the biggest things that I've learned about working with people who do drugs is that it takes a long, long time for their brains to become unconfused. Until then, they have a lot of trouble thinking clearly. I tell them, "It'll get better."

She tells me that she's 6 weeks pregnant. Oh dear! What drugs was she doing? Well, again, what does she want to do with this pregnancy? I know what I'd do with that pregnancy, but it's her pregnancy, not mine. I might mention to her some of the problems associated with fetal alcohol syndrome or cocaine babies and things like that, but it is her child, it's her body. She doesn't know what she wants. I hear that a lot, because most people don't really know what they want. They have an idea. And that's when I'll usually say, "Well, what's your idea? Let's work with that." If their idea is a three-bedroom house by the ocean or in the Marina district, which I have had requests for, then I'll tell her, "I can get you into a residential hotel."

She may say, "I really would like to be able to stop using drugs. I would really like to stop drinking. I really want to do something about the anger that I feel towards my mother or the rage I feel, or I want to do something so that when I have this child I don't abuse it like my mother abused me." So, we'll start with that. "In the ideal world, what would be the best-case scenario? What would you like? How can I help you?" And then we work with what is available and with what we can and what we can't do.

Commentary

The nurse reiterates that these are the client's problems, not hers. She states that not all clinicians can maintain this perspective: *I see clinicians that get very angry over this type of behavior, but why? Her leaving doesn't hurt me as a person. Yes, it bothers me that she's hurting herself, but that's her choice. And I really do throw everything back onto the patient; it's their responsibility. It's their life. They've got to do it, not me.*

Barry (1996, p. 19) cautions that "too much warmth from the caregiver is threatening. It is especially so for those with whom a close relationship with another is difficult. . . . Too much support by a helper also risks a sympathetic rather than empathetic relationship."

The client doesn't really know what she wants to do about her problems. The nurse says this is common, that *most people don't really know what they want.* But they have an idea, so she works with that: *We'll start with that. "In the ideal world, what would be the best-case scenario?"* The nurse can then evaluate this ideal with the client, helping her to distinguish between *what we can and what we can't do.*

Thinking Activities

1. Describe a situation in your practice where you found that too much warmth from you, the caregiver, was threatening to a client.

2. What did you learn from this experience that will help you in future practice situations?

3. Do you think that the nurse's generalization that "most people don't really know what they want" is more likely to be true for clients in psychiatry or in general for clients in all areas or practice? Justify your response.

4. What are the advantages and disadvantages of **making generalizations** such as this?

Clinical Dilemma Six

It is 8:00 A.M., and Barbara is asking for help. Barbara, a 45-year-old white woman, has three children—Resa, 8; Susan, 5; and John, 10—who are suspected of stealing clothes at Kiddie Land Clothing. The PES nurse has called you for further evaluation of Barbara.

You see that she is agitated and anxious. Barbara says she is scared about her children because they are not with her; they are in juvenile hall. "I want my children back. We are the Messiah's messengers. My children are the angels." She starts crying, "When can I see the children? I have no money, and we have been living in our car for the last 2 years. I've been doing some housekeeping for a friend. Where are my children? I want to see them now! The children are my only family. Please help me. I don't want to lose the children."

The Nurse's Response

The truth is I can't do too much if the children are removed. I really have no power. Basically, I think I'd just deal with the client in terms of the moment, when she's here in the hospital.

She probably has not been taking her meds. I don't know. I'm assuming she hasn't. Or she's been under so much stress that, even with the meds, she's having breakthrough symptoms. If she thinks she's the "Messiah's messenger," then she's really having some breakthrough symptoms.

I would talk to her about the children, tell her that they are safe. I might try to find out if they are in juvenile hall, which probably they are because of the shoplifting.

I'd see if she could possibly talk to them. And I would probably put her back in the hospital, just to be restabilized or to find out what's going on and try to put the clinical data together.

Most likely her kids would probably not be returned to her. It's really pathetic because a lot of schizophrenic patients, a lot of personality disorder patients, and a lot of drug-using patients lose their children very fast. And what I see is a constant series of pregnancies as these patients try to keep replacing the children that keep being taken away. So, it's really very sad. And there is no treatment center in the city that will take a woman with her children. There is no treatment program anywhere that a woman can go to with a child, including new mothers with infants. There's a plan to open one hopefully within the year. I'm not sure. It's still going through a lot of litigation.

But, many of these patients really do lose their children, especially if they're letting them steal and things like that. They're seen as inadequate parents and not good role models, and they're in the hospital all the time. It is very, very sad, and it's very difficult. What can I say to somebody whose child is being taken away? I don't have any power to do anything, and the reality of it is that the patient just has to deal with their loss.

Commentary

The nurse recognizes her limitations in this situation. She doubts that she will be able to help the client maintain custody of her children. She recognizes that this is *very, very sad, and it's very difficult.* But it is nonetheless an honest appraisal of the situation. Moreover, the nurse admits that there is not much that she can say to comfort the client about the loss of her children: *What can I say to somebody whose child is being taken away? I don't have any power to do anything, and the reality of it is that the patient just has to deal with their loss.*

References

Barrows, H., & Pickell, G. (1991). *Developing clinical problem-solving skills. A guide to more effective diagnosis and treatment.* New York: Norton Medical Books.

Barry, P. (1996). *Psychosocial nursing: Care of physically ill patients and their families.* Philadelphia: Lippincott.

Gertis, M., Edgman-Levitan, S., Daley, J., & Delbanco, T. (1993). *Through the patient's eyes: Understanding and promoting patient-centered care.* San Francisco: Jossey-Bass.

Hepburn, E. (1993). Women and ethics: A "seeing" justice? *Journal of Moral Education, 23*(1), 27–38.

Jackson, S. (1992). The listening healer in the history of psychological healing. *Journal of Psychiatry, 149*(12), 1623–1632.

McKivergin, M., & Daubenmire, M. (1994). The healing process of presence. *Journal of Holistic Nursing, 12*(1), 65–81.

Walters, A. (1995). A heideggerian hermeneutic study of the practice of critical care nurses. *Journal of Advanced Nursing, 21,* 492–497.

26 *Clinical Dilemmas Related to Interpreting Laboratory Data*

The nurse responding to the clinical dilemmas in this chapter has 35 years of nursing practice experience, primarily in medical-surgical nursing. She is recognized for her expertise in reasoning about laboratory data and diagnostic procedures, has conducted research, and has published extensively on this subject.

Clinical Dilemma One

Mr. Jones is admitted to your unit because of a clotted shunt. You are asked to oversee and manage his care during hospitalization. He is 72 years old and has been on dialysis for 3 years. In 1992, he had a stroke due to a blood clot thrown during dialysis and has residual left-sided weakness.

He has been on warfarin (Coumadin), 5 mg/day, since that time and comes to the outpatient department for a weekly international normalized ratio (INR).

His admitting laboratory values are as follows: INR, 1.6; red blood cell count (RBC), 3.6 million/mm³; hemoglobin, 10 gm/dL; hematocrit, 25%; blood urea nitrogen (BUN), 57 mg/dL; creatinine, 5.9 mg/dL; and potassium, 6.0 mEq/L.

The Nurse's Response

He definitely has a clotting problem; I would think about that. He's got a clotted shunt. He had a stroke because of a blood clot thrown during dialysis. So what if he had some sort of dysrhythmia? Is that from the dialysis?

Because he is on dialysis, that degree of anemia is expected and for him would be sort of normal. I wouldn't be so concerned about his anemia. In fact, that's a very good value for somebody who has chronic renal failure.

The BUN is pretty high to have been on dialysis. I wonder when he was last dialyzed. His creatinine is sky-high for somebody who is on dialysis. And his potassium is high. Now what I need to find out is what his normal lab values are because I've got to use the norms for somebody who is on dialysis. That's too high a potassium, but he might be able to tolerate that better than somebody who hasn't been in renal failure.

I assume that he probably doesn't have a therapeutic dose of warfarin. The INR is too low. So he's not adequately anticoagulated. The INR should be 2 to 3. I have several concerns. One of my major concerns is that he is not adequately anticoagulated. I need to find out if he has been taking his warfarin regularly. Does he understand about it? There's a possibility of noncompliance here. I would consult with the physician to find out how long he has been on the warfarin. What's happened?

I assume he's going to need dialysis because that's a very high BUN and creatinine. The problem is he's got a clotted shunt, so there's going to have to be some other access, like a catheter or something. In the meantime, he has a history of having thrown a clot. So that would be a real problem.

Commentary

This dilemma concerns an elderly client on dialysis who is being anticoagulated to prevent the recurrence of a blood clot, which had been a problem in the past and resulted in a stroke. The possibility of another clot's forming is heightened by the fact that he currently has a clotted shunt. The nurse is given data about the client's recent laboratory values, in addition to a little bit of data about the client's history. Her interpretation of the meaning of these values is based on the information that she has been given about this client as well as her previous experience with dialysis clients.

The thinking strategies **judging the value** and **drawing conclusions** predominate in the nurse's thoughts about this case. She uses **judging the value** to determine that *the INR is too low, his BUN is pretty high, his creatinine is sky-high, and his potassium is high*. She uses **drawing conclusions** to determine that *he definitely has a clotting problem* and *that degree of anemia is expected and for him would be sort of normal*. The thinking strategy called **judging the value** is narrow and specific, while the thinking strategy **drawing conclusions** is broad and general. **Judging the value** of discrete pieces of data, such as individual laboratory values, assists the nurse to **draw** more general **conclusions** about the client's overall status and to determine the probability that a blood clot will reoccur.

Thinking Activities

1. Give examples of the laboratory data about which you are the most comfortable in **judging the value**?

2. Give examples of the laboratory data about which you are the least comfortable in **judging the value**?

3. Describe the factors that contribute to your comfort in **judging the value** of certain laboratory data.

4. Describe the factors that contribute to your discomfort in **judging the value** of certain laboratory data.

5. Provide examples of how you use the thinking strategy **drawing conclusions** when interpreting laboratory data.

6. What relationship do you see between the thinking strategy **judging the value** and the thinking strategy **drawing conclusions**?

Clinical Dilemma Two

It is 10:00 A.M. Wednesday, and you've just admitted a new client to the medical-surgical unit where you work. Mrs. Smith is a 74-year-old woman with diverticulitis. She has a history of ventricular tachycardia with occasional premature ventricular contractions. Over the last 3 days she has become increasingly short of breath, requiring three pillows at night in order to sleep. On admission, her laboratory values are as follows: white blood cell count (leukocytes, WBC), 15,000/mm³; neutrophils, 80%; eosinophils, 3%; basophils, 1%; lymphocytes, 14%; monocytes 2%; RBC, 3.0 million/mm³; hemoglobin, 10 gm/dL; hematocrit, 32%; albumin, 2.8 gm/dL; globulin, 2.0 gm/dL; sodium, 130 mEq/L; chloride, 95 mEq/L; potassium, 2.9 mEq/L; and total CO_2 content, 28 mEq/L. Her usual medications at home are digoxin, 0.25 qd, and a multivitamin.

The Nurse's Response

When I see that someone has to have three pillows at night in order to sleep, I know that's somebody who is probably in congestive [heart] failure. I don't see anything else in her history that right now I would pinpoint as being very worrisome.

The WBC is a little high, but the neutrophils are quite high too. I'm looking for what's not here that would help me to see if she possibly has an infection. She's anemic with an RBC at 3 million[/mm³], hemoglobin 10 [gm/dL], hematocrit 32%. But she's elderly, 74. She's got diverticulitis. I've sort of tucked that in the back of my mind: Is that something she's had for a period of time? Is that nutritional? It could be from blood loss. I don't know what it means, but I'd think about it. Her albumin is not low. Her globulin is 2 [gm/dL]. But when I look at her electrolytes, right away I think this is dilutional, with a sodium of 130 [mEq/L]. That is supported by the fact that she's increasingly short of breath, indicating that she's probably got a fluid volume overload. I wonder if she's on digitalis for her congestive heart failure. Her potassium is low, which could partly be due to her fluid overload. It's also likely that she's on a diuretic and has probably lost potassium in her urine. Being on the digitalis, a low potassium would be something to think about. Her bicarbonate is okay, as reflected in her total CO_2 content.

So, looking back at her history (that she's got some congestive failure), her low sodium is the number one concern I see with her. That would be my primary worry. In fact, I'd put on hold until later my plan to find out more about her WBC, whether or not that's a concern, and the same with regards to her anemia. That's not an immediate concern. I'd do an assessment, listen for breath sounds, see if she's got fluid in her lungs, and see if she has a dysrhythmia. My intuitive feeling would be here's somebody that hasn't been taking their digoxin. What sometimes happens is that people get to feeling good and they don't think they need the digitalis, and then they are admitted in heart failure.

Commentary

In this clinical dilemma, the nurse is given a limited amount of data to reason about the case and to establish an initial hypothesis regarding the primary concerns for this client. Her first reaction to the information that she has been given about this client is to **recognize a pattern**: *When I see that someone has to have three pillows in order to sleep, I know that's somebody who is probably in congestive [heart] failure*. Thus, the nurse's initial working hypothesis is that the client is in congestive heart failure (CHF). She uses this hypothesis to support her interpretation of each of the client's laboratory values: *Right away I think this is dilutional, with a sodium of 130 [mEq/L]. . . . Her potassium is low, which could partly be due to her fluid overload. It's also likely that she's on a diuretic and has probably lost potassium in her urine*.

After reviewing all of this client's laboratory values, the nurse **draws the conclusion** that the main concern is the low sodium (which would indicate fluid volume overload, presumably from CHF). She has a hunch (hypothesis) about what may have caused the heart failure: *What sometimes happens is that people get to feeling good and they don't think they need the digitalis, and then they are admitted in heart failure*.

The thinking strategy **generating a hypothesis** assists in framing client problems and provides a context for further reasoning about and exploration of these problems (Kassirer & Kopelman, 1991). In this case, the hypothesis that CHF is the client's primary problem provides a context and framework for interpreting and explaining the client's various laboratory values and for further exploration of the CHF: *I'd do an assessment, listen for breath sounds, see if she's got fluid in her lungs, and see if she has a dysrhythmia*. **Generating a hypothesis** about the possible cause of the client's CHF (*My intuitive feeling would be here's somebody that hasn't been taking their digoxin*) provides a framework for the approach to take to help resolve the dilemma (e.g., determine if the client is on digoxin and if she's been taking it as prescribed; determine if her digoxin level is within therapeutic range; see if the client is also taking a diuretic and determine if that is contributing to potassium loss; teach the client about how to achieve optimum therapeutic benefit and minimum harm from her medications).

Thinking Activities

1. Describe your understanding of what it means to "frame a problem."

2. How does framing a problem assist one's reasoning about the problem?

3. Think about your practice. Describe instances where using the thinking strategy **generating a hypothesis** has assisted you in framing a problem.

Clinical Dilemma Three

You are caring for a 70-year-old man who was admitted to the medical-surgical unit 2 days ago with abdominal pain. He's been scheduled for exploratory laparotomy surgery tomorrow at 7:00 A.M. The surgical consent has been signed, and his orders are for nothing by mouth after midnight.

You received his preoperative laboratory results at 8:00 P.M., and they are as follows: WBC, 7000/mm³; RBC, 2.9 million/mm³; hemoglobin, 9.6 gm/dL; and hematocrit, 27%. Although you're a little concerned about these results, your charge nurse says there is nothing to worry about because the surgeon will be up to look at them early tomorrow morning, long before surgery is to begin.

The Nurse's Response

The WBC is okay. His RBC is not okay. That's too low for somebody that's going to surgery. His hemoglobin is not okay. So he's definitely quite anemic; that's a concern for somebody going to surgery. He looked pretty standard until I saw what his hemoglobin and hematocrit were.

The charge nurse's response is problematic because in the days before we were so concerned about blood transfusions, anybody whose hematocrit was lower than 30[%] or hemoglobin less than 10 [gm/dL] would have automatically been transfused. But that's no longer true because of all the concerns about blood transfusions. So it's a gray area; it really is. It's the surgeon's decision whether or not to transfuse with a hemoglobin that's borderline, and I would still want the surgeon to know that tonight. I think it's really important not to leave this until the morning. That decision needs to be made by the surgeon. The client's being scheduled for an exploratory lap[arotomy]. I would feel very differently if this was somebody that just came in for something else entirely but their hemoglobin was low. But I see that as most likely a part of his pathology, leading to his need for surgery. So my concern is if he goes to surgery with his hemoglobin being pretty low, although I know that these days they sometimes do. He's an ill man. He probably has something going on with his GI [gastrointestinal] system; that's a very common reason to be anemic. That's the most common thing with a malignancy; anemia is going to be what brings them in. But no matter what, the surgeon needs to know that his hemoglobin and hematocrit are low. That's a procedural thing; you don't wait till the morning of surgery.

Then, I would do a little detective work by going and assessing the client to see if he was having black stools from the bleeding. It may be that these lab values are a lot lower than the surgeon expected them to be. It used to be pretty standard that no one would go to surgery with a hematocrit lower than 30[%]. But clients with a low hematocrit and hemoglobin seem to do very well with surgery. A long time ago, we used to routinely type and crossmatch all clients who were scheduled for surgery, but it became very costly. What is done now is a type and screening, and I think the surgeon would type and screen and not type and crossmatch. But I can't imagine the surgeon would take somebody like this to surgery without first doing a type and screen.

Commentary

When thinking about this dilemma, the nurse again uses the thinking strategy **judging the value** to determine the significance of the laboratory data. She quantifies each laboratory value using descriptive terms indicating intensity or degree of desirability: *The WBC is okay. His RBC is not okay. That's too low. . . . He's definitely quite anemic.* Interpreting the meaning of numerical values in more descriptive terms is a reflection of this nurse's expertise in interpretation of laboratory data. She does not just accept particular numerical values but rather transforms them into language that is more contextually relevant to this particular client's case. For example, an RBC of 2.9 million/mm³, hemoglobin of 9.6, and hematocrit of 27%, although always indicative of anemia, are *not okay* and are *a concern for somebody going to surgery.* Understanding the significance of these values in the context of a client who is scheduled for an exploratory laparotomy at 7:00 A.M. the next day provides a rationale for why the nurse wants the surgeon to know these values tonight and *not to leave this until the morning.*

The endeavor to judge information in a context-specific manner has been identified in the literature as a characteristic associated with expertise within a specific domain, reflecting a well-organized and extensive knowledge base (Chi, Glaser, & Farr, 1988; Ericsson & Straszewski, 1989).

Thinking Activities

1. Think about ways that context influences your language in practice. Give some examples of the type of context-specific language that you use to evaluate clinical data in your practice.

2. How does the use of context-specific language influence your thinking in practice?

Clinical Dilemma Four

It is 8:00 A.M., and you are just beginning to make rounds on the clients admitted in the last 24 hours. Your first new client is known as John Doe and appears to be in his 50s and transient. He was brought in by the police at 2:00 A.M. after being found unarousable behind an abandoned gas station in the middle of town. He has been unable to give any history since admission. His diagnosis is uncertain, but he is suspected to have encephalopathy with associated jaundice. You examine his initial laboratory values to gain further insight and find the following: sodium, 150 mEq/L; chloride, 115 mEq/L; total CO_2 content, 26 mEq/L; serum osmolality, 315 mOsm/kg H_2O; total bilirubin, 2.4 mg/dL; indirect bilirubin, 1.7 mg/dL; alanine aminotransferase (SGPT), 800 U/L; and aspartate aminotransferase (SGOT), 400 U/L.

The Nurse's Response

He was found unarousable . . . I'm running through some possible causes, like drug overdose or being in insulin shock. Those would be the things I would think of. The suspected encephalopathy with jaundice makes me think that he probably has cirrhosis. The most common reason for an elevated sodium is dehydration, fluid volume deficit. So probably he's dehydrated.

His chloride is not too bad; potassium is okay; bicarbonate is okay. His serum osmolality is high, and that supports that he's dehydrated, so maybe he's been unconscious for a day or so. His total bilirubin is high, and the indirect bilirubin is quite high. That points to liver failure. His SGPT is high, and his SGOT is elevated, so he definitely has liver involvement.

This is a complicated client. Anybody who's unarousable is complicated, and then looking at his dehydration, his osmolality . . . whether or not part of that could be a dehydration due to alcohol abuse. He's jaundiced. Looks like probably that he has cirrhoses. He may be unconscious from his encephalopathy. I'd look for other lab values that aren't given here, like ammonia level. I always think about somebody unresponsive possibly being hypoglycemic. I assume that they would have given him glucose in the emergency department to see if he were hypoglycemic. And maybe they did a drug screen on him. He's suspected of having encephalopathy, and he is jaundiced, and it's mostly the indirect bilirubin, rather than direct, so that really means liver failure or liver involvement. To determine whether or not he's in a hepatic coma, I would want to see if his ammonia level was high. I don't know what's going on. He's jaundiced. He's got elevated liver enzymes. I'm thinking that it's hepatic encephalopathy. I'm looking for his serum ammonia levels. And I want to rule out those other things like drug overdose. What evidence is there for some of it? And if his ammonia turns out to be high and his blood sugar is all right, then I would worry about him still not being arousable. Clients can have encephalopathy that may not be because of liver failure. We have some evidence that he's jaundiced. He's going to need extra fluids to get him hydrated, and he's going to need fluids just for maintenance. And then we need to know what's causing this. If he has a high ammonia level, and I would suspect he does, then there are medications that can be given to get the ammonia level down, things like lactulose.

I'm wondering if a drug screen was done on this client. If somebody's unarousable, the possibility of an overdose is very, very, very high. But I assume that they would probably have given him naloxone in the emergency department. I assume they probably would have given him glucose also. If he were in insulin shock, neither one of those drugs would have hurt him. So, I assume this has been ruled out.

If he has a liver problem, his prothrombin time is going to be elevated. There's a whole thing that looking at a client would give me, a sense that this is a client with advanced cirrhosis and possibly that he has encephalopathy. I would look for the possibility that he's bleeding from esophageal varices. That would put somebody into a coma. It's a complex client. It might be a terminal condition if it's somebody who has severe liver failure with hepatic encephalopathy and is unarousable.

Commentary

When reasoning about this dilemma, the nurse's analysis of the facts that she is given moves from uncertainty (an unexplained set of facts) to greater certainty (a set of facts explained by a probable clinical hypothesis). This form of reasoning has been described in cognitive science literature as forward reasoning and is defined as explaining each piece of information within the framework of the predominant working hypothesis (Patel, Evans, & Groen, 1989). In this case, the predominant hypothesis that explains what is wrong with the client and why he is unarousable is that he has hepatic encephalopathy. The nurse indicates that this is the most likely explanation because of a **pattern** that she **recognizes** characterized by the following features: unarousable, dehydrated, jaundiced, elevated indirect and direct bilirubin, and a suspected diagnosis of encephalopathy. Experienced clinicians' reasoning is often characterized by **pattern recognition**, seeing the strong resemblance in the features of a current case to cases previously encountered in practice that were characterized by similar features.

Elstein (1995) proposes that the ability to **recognize a pattern** is strongly influenced by the context of a situation. In this case, the client is a John Doe, a transient found unarousable behind an abandoned gas station. This context might easily lead one to think the client got drunk and passed out. Additionally, he is suspected to have encephalopathy and jaundice and has elevated liver enzymes and total and indirect bilirubin, all of which are findings often associated with liver damage due to alcohol abuse. Kassirer and Kopelman (1991, p. 8) describe this manner of **recognizing a pattern** as "relying on the resemblance of a set of findings to some well-defined clinical entity." This then evokes a hypothesis to describe what is going on with a client. This type of **pattern recognition** can easily lead to errors in judgment, however, if it causes clinicians to ignore or discount other less characteristic data or if it causes clinicians to prematurely choose an approach to care based on a hypothesis that was arrived at by using incomplete and somewhat ambiguous data.

To guard against such errors in judgment, clinicians should continue to investigate and question all available data and should purposefully look for further evidence to support or refute their initial hunches. When reasoning about this dilemma, the nurse identifies other competing hypotheses that could account for the clinical findings, including hypoglycemia and drug overdose (a possibility that she describes as being *very, very, very high*). To assist in confirming her predominant hypothesis, the nurse indicates that she would like to be able to look at (rather than just read about) the client: *There's a whole thing that looking at a client would give me, a sense that this is a client with advanced cirrhosis and possibly that he has encephalopathy.*

The nurse also stresses the need to give the client extra fluids initially *to get him hydrated* and then continue to give him fluids *just for maintenance*. This can be initiated before the client's diagnosis is clearly established because the benefit of treating the dehydration can just as easily be achieved without proof of diagnosis.

Thinking Activities

1. Think about your practice. When you are first confronted with a new client problem, do you tend to have one predominant hypothesis in mind regarding the cause of the problem or multiple hypotheses?

2. What are the advantages of having one versus multiple hypotheses regarding the cause of a problem?

3. What are the disadvantages of having one versus multiple hypotheses regarding the cause of a problem?

Clinical Dilemma Five

For the past 2 weeks, you have been following a 75-year-old female patient after discharge from the hospital. She is recovering from a five-vessel coronary artery bypass and graft and also has non–insulin-dependent diabetes.

You last visited Mrs. Nelson in her home on Friday, and it is now Monday morning. In reviewing the weekend records, you note that the nurse covering received two calls from Mrs. Nelson. Both times she complained that she felt feverish and her right leg incision was red and sore. Prior to your follow-up visit scheduled for this afternoon, you review the laboratory results from blood drawn this morning by the visiting laboratory technician. The laboratory data reveal RBC, 3.87 million/mm³; WBC, 13,500/mm³; hemoglobin, 10.8 gm/dL; hematocrit, 31.8%; and glucose, 400 mg/dL.

The Nurse's Response

Okay, right then that's a big red flag: somebody who's diabetic and is getting an infection. I would always be concerned when anyone post-op got a wound infection; I'd be doubly so with someone who is a diabetic.

Her RBC, hemoglobin, and hematocrit are low, but she's 75 and she had bypass surgery 2 weeks ago, major surgery. She probably had some blood loss with that, so these low values are probably not a big deal.

Her WBC is not that high yet. She's had some infection, and she's hyperglycemic. She's not insulin dependent. She may need some insulin during the time that she has the infection. She's going to need treatment for the infection as well as treatment for her hyperglycemia. Everybody who has diabetes and gets an infection is going to be out of control for as long as they have an infection. They're going to have to have better control of their blood sugar. I'm going to have a consultation with her physician because she's probably going to need to receive some insulin to stay controlled until the infection is resolved. Also, many elderly people tend to have a little bit lower WBC to begin with, and certainly, a person that's 75 cannot respond as quickly to an infection. So, given that, a WBC of 13,000 [/mm³] may be the best this client can do at 75. When I went out to visit her, I'd want to see that she's doing all right with the bypass graft. But since she's already 2 weeks post-op, I'm assuming she's probably doing fine. She's probably going to have some edema, so I wouldn't be surprised if her right ankle might be a little bit swollen. That's not uncommon after a vein has been removed. If she had atherosclerosis bad enough that she needed a bypass graft on the coronary arteries, she probably has that pathology in all of her arteries to some extent, and she probably doesn't have very good arterial circulation. But the arterial circulation in her legs wouldn't have been made any worse because she had a vein removed. And I wouldn't be surprised if she didn't haven't such good pulses in her feet. But if her feet felt warm, and so forth, I would figure that's pretty good for someone who is 75 years old and probably has pretty extensive atherosclerosis. The immediate problem is this infection.

Commentary

The nurse's initial response to this clinical dilemma demonstrates another type of **pattern recognition**, identifying *a big red flag* that in this instance is characterized by the combined clinical features of *somebody who's diabetic and is getting an infection.* In her study of expert critical care nurses' clinical reasoning, Fonteyn (1991) described identifying critical indicators, or what subjects referred to as "red flags," as a reasoning strategy that nurses use to mentally tag significant data so that it will be remembered and focused on to direct a line of inquiry. One subject in this study stated that red flags "put up an alert that I need to watch [the client] very closely" (p. 110), and another described using red flags to "consider things that could progress to something worse" (p. 108). In this clinical dilemma, recognizing a red flag assists the nurse to focus on essential interventions: *She's going to need treatment for the infection as well as treatment for her hyperglycemia. . . . I'm going to have a consultation with her physician.*

Another approach that the nurse uses to think about this dilemma is **making predictions**. In their study of critical care nurses' reasoning about patient care immediately after surgery, Fisher and Fonteyn (1995) describe how subjects use **making predictions** to anticipate patient responses and outcomes. Evans and Gadd's (1989) study of expert physicians describe how subjects use **making predictions** to confirm previously generated hypotheses. In response to this dilemma, the nurse uses **making predictions** to anticipate assessment findings: *She's probably going to have some edema, so I wouldn't be surprised if her right ankle might be a little bit swollen. . . . And I wouldn't be surprised if she didn't have such good pulses in her feet.*

Thinking Activities

1. Reflect on your practice. What critical indicators are red flags for you?

2. How does identifying red flags assist you in your practice?

3. Describe ways that you have used **making predictions** to anticipate patient responses and outcomes.

4. Give several examples of how **making predictions** has helped your thinking in practice.

References

Chi, M., Glaser, R., & Farr, M. (Eds.). (1988). *The nature of expertise*. Hillsdale, NJ: Lawrence Erlbaum Associates.

Elstein, A. (1995). Clinical reasoning in medicine. In J. Higgs and M. Jones (Eds.), *Clinical reasoning in the health professions* (pp. 49–59). Oxford, England: Butterworth-Heinemann.

Ericsson, K. A., & Straszewski, J. J. (1989). Skilled memory and expertise: Mechanisms of exceptional performance. In D. Kalhr & K. Kotovsky (Eds.), *Complex information processing: The impact of Herbert A. Simon* (pp. 235–268). Hillsdale, NJ: Lawrence Erlbaum Associates.

Evans, D., and Gadd, C. (1989). Managing coherence and context in medical problem-solving discourse. In D. Evans and V. Patel (Eds.), *Cognitive science in medicine* (pp. 211–256). Cambridge, MA: MIT Press.

Fisher, A., & Fonteyn, M. (1995). An innovative methodological approach for examining nurses' heuristic use in clinical practice. *Journal of Scholarly Inquiry, 9*(3), 263–276.

Fonteyn, M. (1991). *A descriptive analysis of expert critical care nurses' clinical reasoning*. Unpublished doctoral dissertation, University of Texas, Austin.

Kassirer, J., & Kopelman, R. (1991). *Learning clinical reasoning*. Baltimore: Williams & Wilkins.

Patel, V., Evans, D., & Groen G. (1989). Biomedical knowledge and clinical reasoning. In D. Evans & V. Patel (Eds.), *Cognitive science in medicine: Biomedical modeling* (pp. 53–112). Cambridge, MA: MIT Press.

27 Final Thoughts: Implications for Research, Education, and Practice

As was explained in Unit One, this book is based on research examining how nurses with extensive knowledge and experience in a specific area of practice (domain) think when reasoning about dilemmas within that domain. Identifying and describing the thinking strategies that nurses use in practice has implications for nursing research, education, and practice.

Implications for Research

Despite the fairly extensive body of research describing nurses' thinking in practice, our understanding of this phenomenon remains incomplete. Additional research is needed to provide a fuller understanding of how nurses think in practice. Until we have a full description of nurses' thinking, our practice, much of which is an exercise in clinical judgment, will be less precise and scientific. As Pless and Clayton (1993, p. 428) remind us, "The important first step of establishing a clear concept that defines critical thinking has not been accomplished." Recently, a Delphi study has been initiated to obtain a consensus definition of critical thinking in nursing from a panel of expert researchers and theoreticians (Scheffer, personal communication, July 16, 1996).

The thinking strategies that nurses use in practice that were identified and described in this text assist in building the body of knowledge about nurses' thinking in practice.

Implications for Education

In nursing education, an intense interest in teaching and assessing critical thinking has emerged, due in part to National League for Nursing (NLN) requirements for accreditation, but also due to an increasing number of educators who are realizing the profound need to improve students' skill in critical thinking and clinical judgment so that they will be better prepared for the demands of practice. As Fonteyn (1995, p. 67) explains, "Educators are realizing that the amount of clinical knowledge and information is increasing too rapidly to expect that students can possibly remember all of the information that they will need for practice. Moreover, possessing an encyclopedic memory of facts and concepts will not ensure effective clinical reasoning."

In response to the NLN's requirement for outcomes' assessment, and as a natural consequence of nurse educators' increased focus on developing and improving students' critical thinking strategies, nursing programs have begun to include some type of critical thinking assessment tool in their program assessment plan. Among the commercially available instruments for assessment of critical thinking skills, the Watson-Glaser Critical Thinking Appraisal has been, by far, the most widely used (Scriven & Fisher, 1997). Recently, however, the California Critical Thinking Skills Test (CCTST) has begun to gain national recognition and increasing popularity among schools of nursing. CCTST assesses the critical thinking skills that were derived from the Delphi Report's (Facione, 1993) expert consensus definition of critical thinking. The CCTST assesses five critical thinking skills: interpretation, analysis, evaluation, inference, and explanation. Psychometric studies of the instrument have demonstrated fairly high scores on a range of validity and reliability measures.

Close analysis of CCTST by the author of this text revealed its unique comprehensiveness in assessing all 12 of the dominant thinking strategies identified by the Thinking in Practice (TIP) Study and emphasized throughout this book. The fit of the findings of the TIP Study with the CCTST is as follows:

1. The critical thinking skill of interpretation is defined as comprehending and expressing the meaning or significance of a wide variety of experiences, situations, data, and so on by categorization, decoding significance, and clarifying meaning. The thinking strategies that represent a component of the skill of interpretation include **recognizing a pattern**, **forming relationships**, and **stating a proposition**.

2. The critical thinking skill of analysis is defined as identifying the intended and actual inferential relationships among statements, questions, concepts, descriptions, or other forms of representation intended to express beliefs, judg-

ments, and reasons by examining ideas, detecting arguments, and analyzing arguments. The thinking strategies that represent a component of the skill of analysis include **forming relationships**, **stating a proposition**, and **asserting a practice rule**.

3.   The critical thinking skill of evaluation is defined as assessing the credibility of statements and assessing the logical strength of actual or intended inferential relationships by assessing claims and assessing arguments. The thinking strategies that represent a component of the skill of evaluation include **judging the value** and **drawing conclusions**.

4.   The critical thinking skill of inference is defined as identifying and securing elements needed to draw reasonable conclusions, forming conjectures and hypotheses, considering relevant information, and educing the consequences flowing from data, evidence, or judgments by querying evidence and conjecturing alternatives. The thinking strategies that represent a component of the skill of inference include **generating hypotheses**, **setting priorities**, **searching for information**, **making predictions**, and **drawing conclusions**.

5.   The critical thinking skill of explanation is defined as stating the results of one's reasoning, justifying that reasoning in terms of the evidential, conceptual, methodologic, criteriologic, and contextual considerations on which one's results were based, and presenting one's reasoning in the form of cogent arguments by stating results, justifying procedures, and presenting arguments. The thinking strategies that represent a component of the skill of explanation include **stating a proposition**, **asserting a practice rule**, **making choices**, and **providing explanations**.

Thus, the thinking strategies identified and described in this text provide a conceptualization of the critical thinking cognitive skills identified in the Delphi study and measured by the CCTST as they uniquely pertain to nursing practice. Conversely, the CCTST provides an excellent measure of all 12 of the dominant thinking strategies identified and described in this text.

Implications for Practice

By identifying and describing nurses' thinking strategies, this text has implications for nursing practice. The ultimate goal of this text is to improve nurses' thinking in their practice. By providing an understanding of the thinking strategies that nurses use in practice, by suggesting methods for developing and improving each strategy, by depicting excellence in nurses' thinking in a variety of areas of practice, and by offering numerous thinking activities, this text will improve nurses' metacognition, knowledge of one's own thinking. When resolving problems or dilemmas encountered in clinical practice, metacognition assists nurses to identify the problem(s), frame the problem within the context in which it is encountered, devise a plan for solving the problem, and evaluating the solutions. This approach is not dissimilar to the nursing process that has traditionally guided our practice.

Metacognition maintains our awareness of how we are conceptualizing our care and of our thinking as we carry out the nursing process.

References

Facione, P. (1993). *Critical thinking: A statement of expert consensus for purposes of educational assessment and instruction.* Milbrae, CA: The California Academic Press.

Fonteyn, M. (1995). Clinical reasoning in nursing. In J. Higgs & M. Jones (Eds.), *Clinical reasoning in the health professions.* Oxford, England: Butterworth-Heinemann.

Pless, B., & Clayton, G. (1993). Clarifying the concept of critical thinking in nursing. *Journal of Nursing Education, 32*(9), 425–428.

Scriven, M., & Fisher, A. (forthcoming). *Critical thinking: Defining and assessing it.*

INDEX